Oxford Handbook of Clinical Haematology

Second edition

Drew Provan
Senior Lecturer in Haematology,
Barts and The London, Queen Mary's School of Medicine and Dentistry,
University of London

Charles R. J. Singer
Consultant Haematologist, Royal United Hospital, Bath, UK

Trevor Baglin
Consultant Haematologist, Addenbrookes NHS Trust, Cambridge, UK

John Lilleyman
Professor of Paediatric Oncology & Consultant Paediatric Haematologist,
Barts and The London, Queen Mary's School of Medicine and Dentistry,
University of London

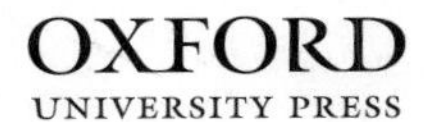
OXFORD
UNIVERSITY PRESS

OXFORD
UNIVERSITY PRESS

Great Clarendon Street, Oxford OX2 6DP

Oxford University Press is a department of the University of Oxford.
It furthers the University's objective of excellence in research, scholarship,
and education by publishing worldwide in

Oxford New York

Auckland Cape Town Dar es Salaam Hong Kong Karachi
Kuala Lumpur Madrid Melbourne Mexico City Nairobi
New Delhi Shanghai Taipei Toronto

With offices in

Argentina Austria Brazil Chile Czech Republic France Greece
Guatemala Hungary Italy Japan Poland Portugal Singapore
South Korea Switzerland Thailand Turkey Ukraine Vietnam

Published in the United States
by Oxford University Press, Inc., New York

First edition published 1998
Reprinted 1999, 2000, 2003
Second edition published 2004
Reprinted 2005 (with correction), 2006, 2007, 2008 (with correction)

British Library Cataloguing in Publication Data
Data available

Typeset by Drew Provan and EXPO, Malaysia
Printed by Asia Pacific Offset, China

ISBN 978-0-19-852652-0

5 7 9 10 8 6

Foreword to the first edition

The Concise Oxford Dictionary defines a handbook as 'a short manual or guide'. Modern haematology is a vast field which involves almost every other medical speciality and which, more than most, straddles the worlds of the basic biomedical sciences and clinical practice. Since the rapidly proliferating numbers of textbooks on this topic are becoming denser and heavier with each new edition, the medical student and young doctor in training are presented with a daunting problem, particularly as they try to put these fields into perspective. And those who try to teach them are not much better placed; on the one hand they are being told to decongest the curriculum, while on the other they are expected to introduce large slices of molecular biology, social science, ethics and communication skills, not to mention a liberal sprinkling of poetry, music and art.

In this over-heated educational scene the much maligned 'handbook' could well stage a come-back and gain new respectability, particularly in the role of a friendly guide. In the past this genre has often been viewed as having little intellectual standing, of no use to anybody except the panic-stricken student who wishes to try to make up for months of mis-spent time in a vain, one-night sitting before their final examination. But given the plethora of rapidly changing information that has to be assimilated, the carefully prepared précis is likely to play an increasingly important role in medical education. Perhaps even that ruination of the decent paragraph and linchpin of the pronouncements of medical bureaucrats, the 'bullet-point', may become acceptable, albeit in small doses, as attempts are made to highlight what is really important in a scientific or clinical field of enormous complexity and not a little uncertainty.

In this short account of blood diseases the editors have done an excellent service to medical students, as well as doctors who are not specialists in blood diseases, by summarising in simple terms the major features and approaches to diagnosis and management of most of the blood diseases that they will meet in routine clinical practice or in the tedious examinations that face them. And in condensing this rapidly expanding field they have, remarkably, managed to avoid one of the great difficulties and pitfalls of this type of teaching; in trying to reduce complex issues down to their bare bones, it is all too easy to introduce inaccuracies.

One word of warning from a battle-scarred clinician however. A précis of this type suffers from the same problem as a set of multiple-choice questions. Human beings are enormously complex organisms, and sick ones are even more complicated; during a clinical lifetime the self-critical doctor will probably never encounter a 'typical case' of anything. Thus the outlines of the diseases that are presented in this book must be used as approximate guides, and no more. But provided they bear this in mind, students will find that it is a very valuable summary of modern haematology; the addition of the Internet sources is a genuine and timely bonus.

D. J. Weatherall
April 1998

Preface to the second edition

Haematology has seen many changes since 1998 when the first edition of this small book was written. Most notably, there are major advances in the treatments of malignant blood disorders with the discovery of tyrosine kinase inhibitors which have transformed the outlook for patients with CML, the rediscovery of arsenic for AML and many other new therapies. Progress has been slower in the non-malignant arena since there is still limited evidence on which to base decisions. We have attempted to update each section in the book in order to ensure that it reflects current practice. Although molecular diagnostics have seen huge changes through the Human Genome Project and other methodological developments, we have not included these in great detail here because of lack of space. We have attempted to focus more on clinical aspects of patient care.

This edition welcomes two new authors: Professor Sir John Lilleyman, immediate Past-President of the Royal College of Pathologists, is a Paediatric Oncologist at Barts and The London, Queen Mary's School of Medicine and Dentistry, University of London. John is a leading figure in the world of paediatric haematology with an interest in both malignant and non-malignant disease affecting children. He has extensively revised the Paediatric section of the book, in addition to Immunodeficiency. Dr Trevor Baglin, Consultant Haematologist at Addenbrookes Hospital, Cambridge is Secretary of the British Committee for Standards in Haematology Haemostasis and Thrombosis Task Force. Trevor is the author of many evidence-based guidelines and peer-reviewed scientific papers. He has rewritten the Haemostasis section of the book and brought this in line with modern management.

Other features of this edition include the greater use of illustrations such as blood films, marrows and radiological images which we hope will enhance the text and improve readers' understanding of the subject. We have increased the number of references and provided URLs for key websites providing easy access to organisations and publications.

There will doubtless be omissions and errors and we take full responsibility for these. We are very keen to receive feedback (good or otherwise!) since this helps shape future editions. If there is something you feel we have left out please complete the Readers comment card.

DP
CRJS
TB
JL

January 2004

Preface to the first edition

This small volume is intended to provide the essential core knowledge required to assess patients with possible disorders of the blood, organise relevant investigations and initiate therapy where necessary. By reducing extraneous information as much as possible, and presenting key information for each topic, a basic understanding of the pathophysiology is provided and this, we hope, will stimulate readers to follow this up by consulting the larger haematology textbooks.

We have provided both a patient-centred and disease-centred approach to haematological disease, in an attempt to provide a form of 'surgical sieve', hopefully enabling doctors in training to formulate a differential diagnosis before consulting the relevant disease-orientated section.

We have provided a full review of haematological investigations and their interpretation, handling emergency situations, and included the commonly used protocols in current use on Haematology Units, hopefully providing a unified approach to patient management.

There are additional sections relating to patient support organisations and Internet resources for further exploration by those wishing to delve deeper into the subject of blood and its diseases.

Obviously with a subject as large as clinical haematology we have been selective about the information we chose to include in the handbook. We would be interested to hear of diseases or situations not covered in this handbook. If there are inaccuracies within the text we accept full responsibility and welcome comments relating to this.

DP
MC
ASD
CRJS
AGS

1998

Acknowledgements

We are indebted to many of our colleagues for providing helpful suggestions and for proofreading the text. In particular we wish to thank Dr Helen McCarthy, Specialist Registrar in Haematology; Dr Jo Piercy, Specialist Registrar in Haematology; Dr Tanay Sheth, SHO in Haematology, Southampton; Sisters Clare Heather and Ann Jackson, Haematology Day Unit, Southampton General Hospital; Dr Mike Williams, Specialist Registrar in Anaesthetics; Dr Frank Boulton, Wessex Blood Transfusion Service, Southampton; Dr Paul Spargo, Consultant Anaesthetist, Southampton University Hospitals; Dr Sheila Bevin, Staff Grade Paediatrician; Dr Mike Hall, Consultant Neonatologist; Dr Judith Marsh, Consultant Haematologist, St George's Hospital, London; Joan Newman, Haematology Transplant Coordinator, Southampton; Professor Sally Davies, Consultant Haematologist, Imperial College School of Medicine, Central Middlesex Hospital, London; Dr Denise O'Shaughnessy, Consultant Haematologist, Southampton University Hospitals NHS Trust; Dr Kornelia Cinkotai, Consultant Haematologist, Barts and The London NHS Trust; Dr Mansel Haeney, Consultant Immunologist, Hope Hospital, Salford; Dr Simon Rule, Derriford Hospital, Plymouth; Dr Adam Mead, Specialist Registrar Barts and The London; Dr Chris Knechtli, Consultant Haematologist, Royal United Hospital, Bath. And finally, we would like to thank Alastair Smith, Morag Chisholm and Andrew Duncombe for their contributions to the first edition of the handbook.

Warm thanks are also extended to Oxford University Press, and in particular Catherine Barnes, commissioning editor for medicine. She has been a calming influence throughout the reworking of the handbook. Kate Martin, production manager, has helped immensely with artwork and matters of book design. Our thanks also go to Georgia Pinteau, PA to Catherine, who has facilitated throughout, chasing up electronic artwork and other materials required for the book.

Typographical notes—the entire book was typeset using Quark Express™ 4.11 on a Mac G4 minitower. Body text is a modified Gill Sans (designed and very kindly supplied by Jonathan Coleclough) with headings/subheadings in Frutiger and Gill Sans. Symbols comprise Universal Greek w. Math Pi, Zapf Dingbats, Universal News w. Commercial Pi, and a modified version of Murray Longmore's OUP font (modified by Jonathan Coleclough).

Symbols and abbreviations

🕮	cross-reference
►	important
►►	very important
↓	decreased
↑	increased
↔	normal
♂:♀	male: female ratio
1°	primary
2°	secondary
2,3 DPG	2,3 diphosphoglycerate
2-CDA	2-chlorodeoxyadenosine
α2-M	alpha$_2$ microglobulin
6-MP	6-mercaptopurine
^{99m}Tc-MIBI	^{99m}Tc methoxyisobutyl-isonitride *or* ^{99m}Tc-MIBI scintigraphy
AA	aplastic anaemia *or* reactive amyloidosis
Ab	antibody
ABVD	adriamycin (doxorubicin), bleomycin, vinblastine, dacarbazine
ACD	acid-citrate-dextrose *or* anaemia of chronic disease
ACE	angiotensin converting enzyme
ACL	anticardiolipin antibody
ACML	atypical chronic myeloid leukaemia
ADA	adenosine deaminase
ADE	cytosine arabinoside (Ara-C) daunorubicin etoposide
ADP	adenosine 5-diphosphate
AFB	acid fast bacilli
Ag	antigen
AIDS	acquired immunodeficiency syndrome
AIHA	autoimmune haemolytic anaemia
AIN	autoimmune neutropenia
AL	(primary) amyloidosis
ALB	serum albumin
ALG	anti-lymphocyte globulin
ALIPs	abnormal localisation of immature myeloid precursors
ALL	acute lymphoblastic leukaemia
ALS	advanced life support
ALT	alanine aminotransferase

AML	acute myeloid leukaemia
AMP	adenosine monophosphate
ANA	antinuclear antibodies
ANCA	anti-neutrophilic cytoplasmic antibody
ANAE	alpha naphthyl acetate esterase
APC	activated protein C
APCR	activated protein C resistance
APL	antiphospholipid antibody
APML	acute promyelocytic leukaemia
APS	antiphospholipid syndrome
APTR	activated partial thromboplastin ratio
APTT	activated partial thromboplastin time
APTT ratio	activated partial thromboplastin time ratio
ARDS	adult respiratory distress syndrome
ARF	acute renal failure
ARMS	amplification refractory mutation system
AST	aspartate aminotranferase
ASCT	autologous stem cell transplantation
AT (ATIII)	antithrombin III
ATCML	Adult-type chronic myeloid (granulocytic) leukaemia
ATG	anti-thymocyte globulin
ATLL	adult T-cell leukaemia/lymphoma
ATP	adenosine triphosphate
ATRA	all-*trans* retinoic acid
A-V	arteriovenous
BAL	broncho-alveolar lavage
B-CLL	B-cell chronic lymphocytic leukaemia
bd	*bis die* (twice daily)
BEAC	BCNU, etoposide, cytosine & cyclophosphamide
BEAM	BCNU, etoposide, cytarabine (ara-C), melphalan
β_2-M	β_2-microglobuline
BFU-E	burst-forming unit-erythroid
BJP	Bence Jones protein
BL	Burkitt lymphoma
BM	bone marrow
BMJ	*British Medical Journal*
BMT	bone marrow transplant(ation)
BNF	British National Formulary
BP	blood pressure
BPL	BioProducts Laboratory
BSS	Bernard–Soulier syndrome

Symbols and abbreviations

BU	Bethesda Units
Ca	carcinoma
Ca^{2+}	calcium
CABG	coronary artery by pass graft
cALL	common acute lymphoblastic leukaemia
CBA	collagen binding activity
CBV	cyclophosphamide, carmustine (BCNU), etoposide (VP16)
CCF	congestive cardiac failure
CCR	complete cytogenetic response
CD	cluster designation
CDA	congenital dyserythropoietic anaemia
cDNA	complementary DNA
CEL	chronic eosinophilic leukaemia
CGL	chronic granulocytic leukaemia
CHAD	cold haemagglutinin disease
CHOP	cyclophosphamide, adriamycin, vincristine, prednisolone
C/I	consolidation/intensification
CJD	Creutzfeldt–Jakob disease (v = variant)
Cl^-	chloride
CLD	chronic liver disease
CLL	chronic lymphocytic ('lymphatic') leukaemia
CMC	chronic mucocutaneous candidiasis
CML	chronic myeloid leukaemia
CMML	chronic myelomonocytic leukaemia
CMV	cytomegalovirus
CNS	central nervous system
COAD	chronic obstructive airways disease
COC	combined oral contraceptive
COMP	cyclophosphamide, vincristine, methotrexate, prednisolone
CR	complete remission
CRF	chronic renal failure
CRP	C-reactive protein
CRVT	central retinal renous thrombosis
CSF	cerebrospinal fluid
CT	computed tomography
CTZ	chemoreceptor trigger zone

CVA	cerebrovascular accident
CVP	cyclophosphamide, vincristine, prednisolone; central venous pressure
CVS	cardiovascular system
CXR	chest x-ray
CyA	cyclosporin A
CytaBOM	cytarabine, bleomycin, vincristine, methotrexate
d	day
DAGT	direct antiglobulin test
DAT	direct antiglobulin test; daunorubicin, cytosine (Ara-C), thioguanine
dATP	deoxy ATP
DBA	Diamond–Blackfan anaemia
DC	dyskeratosis congenita
DCS	dendritic cell system
DCT	direct Coombs' test
DDAVP	desamino D-arginyl vasopressin
DEAFF	detection of early antigen fluorescent foci
DEB	diepoxy butane
DFS	disease-free survival
DHAP	dexamethasone, cytarabine, cisplatin
DI	delayed intensification
DIC	disseminated intravascular coagulation
dL	decilitre
DLBCL	diffuse large B-cell lymphoma
DLI	donor leucocyte/lymphocyte infusion
DMSO	dimethyl sulphoxide
DNA	deoxyribonucleic acid
DOB	date of birth
DPG	diphosphoglycerate
DRVVT	dilute Russell's viper venom test
DTT	dilute thromboplastin time
DVT	deep vein thrombosis
DXT	radiotherapy
EACA	epsilon aminocaproic acid
EBV	Epstein–Barr virus
EBVP	etoposide bleomycin vinblastine prednisolone
ECG	electrocardiograph
ECOG	European Co-operative Oncology Group
EDTA	ethylenediamine tetraacetic acid
EFS	event-free survival
EGF	epidermal growth factor

ELISA	enzyme-linked immunosorbent assay
EMU	early morning urine
Epo	erythropoietin
EPOCH	doxorubicin/epirubicin, vincristine, etoposide over 96h IVI with bolus cyclophosphamide and oral prednisolone
EPS	electrophoresis
ESHAP	etoposide, methylprednisolone, cytarabine, platinum
ESR	erythrocyte sedimentation rate
ET	essential thrombocythaemia *or* exchange transfusion
FAB	French–American–British
FACS	fluorescence-activated cell sorter
FBC	full blood count (complete blood count, CBC)
FCM	fludarabine, cyclophosphamide, melphalan
FDP	fibrin degradation products
FDG-PET	2^{18} fluoro–D–2–deoxyglucose positron emission tomography
Fe	iron
FEIBA	factor eight inhibitor bypassing activity
FEL	familial erythrophagocytic lymphohistiocytosis
$FeSO_4$	ferrous sulphate
FFP	fresh frozen plasma
FFS	failure-free survival
FH	family history
FISH	fluorescence *in situ* hybridisation
FITC	fluorescein isothiocyanate
FIX	factor IX
fL	femtolitre
FL	follicular lymphoma
FNA	fine needle aspirate
FOB	faecal occult blood
α-FP	alpha-fetoprotein
FVIII	factor VIII
FVL	factor V Leiden
g	gram
G6PD	glucose-6-phosphate dehydrogenase
GA	general anaesthetic
G-CSF	granulocyte colony stimulating factor
GIT	gastrointestinal tract

GM-CSF	granulocyte macrophage colony stimulating factor
GP	glycoprotein
GPI	glycosylphosphatidylinositol
G&S	group, screen and save
GvHD	graft versus host disease
GvL	graft versus leukaemia
h	hour
HAV	hepatitis A virus
Hb	haemoglobin
HbA	haemoglobin A
HbA_2	haemoglobin A_2
HbF	haemoglobin F (fetal Hb)
HbH	haemoglobin H
HBsAg	hepatitis B surface antigen
HBV	hepatitis B virus
HCII	heparin cofactor II
HCD	heavy chain disease
HCG	human chorionic gonadotrophin
HCL	hairy cell leukaemia
HCO_3^-	bicarbonate
Hct	haematocrit
HCV	hepatitis C virus
HDM	high dose melphalan
HDN	haemolytic disease of the newborn
HDT	high dose therapy
HE	hereditary elliptocytosis
HELLP	haemolysis, elevated liver enzymes and low platelets
HES	hypereosinophilic syndrome
HHT	hereditary haemorrhagic telangiectasia
HIT(T)	heparin-induced thrombocytopenia (with thrombosis)
HIV	human immunodeficiency virus
HL	Hodgkin's lymphoma (Hodgkin's disease)
HLA	human leucocyte antigen
HLH	haemophagocytic lymphohistiocytosis
H/LMW	high/low molecular weight
HMP	hexose monophosphate shunt
HMWK	high molecular weight kininogen
HPA	human platelet antigen
HPFH	hereditary persistence of fetal haemoglobin
HPLC	high performance liquid chromatography
HPP	hereditary pyropoikilocytosis

HRT	hormone replacement therapy
HS	hereditary spherocytosis
HTLV-1	human T-lymphotropic virus type 1
HUS	haemolytic uraemic syndrome
IAGT	indirect antiglobulin test
IAHS	Infection-associated haemophagocytic syndrome
ICE	ifosfamide, carboplatin, etoposide
ICH	intracranial haemorrhage
IDA	iron deficiency anaemia
IF	involved field [radiotherapy]
IFA	intrinsic factor antibody
IFN-α	interferon alpha
Ig	immunoglobulin
IgA	immunoglobulin A
IgD	immunoglobulin D
IgE	immunoglobulin E
IgG	immunoglobulin G
IgM	immunoglobulin M
IL-1	interleukin-1
IM	intramuscular
IMF	idiopathic myelofibrosis
INR	International normalised ratio
inv	chromosomal inversion
IPI	International Prognostic Index
IPSS	International Prognostic Scoring System
IT	intrathecal
ITP	idiopathic thrombocytopenic purpura
ITU	Intensive Therapy Unit
iu/IU	international units
IUT	intrauterine transfusion
IV	intravenous
IVI	intravenous infusion
IVIg	intravenous immunoglobulin
JCMML	juvenile chronic myelomonocytic leukaemia
JML	juvenile myelomonocytic leukaemia
JVP	jugular venous pressure
kg	kilogram
L	litre

LA	lupus anticoagulant
LAP	leucocyte alkaline phosphatase (score)
LC	light chain
LCH	Langerhans cell histiocytosis
LDH	lactate dehydrogenase
LFTs	liver function tests
LFS	leukaemia free survival
LGL	large granular lymphocyte
LLN	lower limit of normal
LMWH	low molecular weight heparin
LN	lymph node(s)
LP	lumbar puncture
LPD	lymphoproliferative disorder
LSCS	lower segment Caesarian section
M&P	melphalan and prednisolone
MACOP-B	methotrexate, doxorubicin, cyclophosphamide, vincristine, bleomycin, prednisolone
MAHA	microangiopathic haemolytic anaemia
MALT	mucosa-associated lymphoid tissue
m-BACOD	methotrexate, bleomycin, adriamycin (doxorubicin), cyclophosphamide, vincristine, dexamethasone
MC	mast cell(s)
MCH	mean cell haemoglobin
MCHC	mean corpuscular haemoglobin concentration
MCL	mantle cell lymphoma
MCP	mitoxantrone, chlorambucil, prednisolone
MCR	major cytogenetic response
M-CSF	macrophage colony stimulating factor
MCV	mean cell volume
MDS	myelodysplastic syndrome
MetHb	methaemoglobin
MF	myelofibrosis
mg	milligram
MGUS	monoclonal gammopathy of undetermined significance
MHC	major histocompatibility complex
MI	myocardial infarction
min(s)	minute(s)
MM	multiple myeloma
MMC	mitomycin C
MNC	mononuclear cell(s)
MO	month(s)
MoAb	monoclonal antibody

MPD	myeloproliferative disease
MPO	myeloperoxidase
MPS	mononuclear phagocytic system
MPV	mean platelet volume
MRD	minimal residual disease
MRI	magnetic resonance imaging
mRNA	messenger ribonucleic acid
MRSA	methicillin-resistant *Staphylococcus aureus*
MSBOS	maximum surgical blood ordering schedule
Mst II	a restriction enzyme
MSU	midstream urine
MT	mass: thoracic
MTX	methotrexate
MUD	matched unrelated donor (transplant)
Na^+	sodium
NADP	nicotinamide adenine diphosphate
NADPH	nicotinamide adenine diphosphate (reduced)
NAIT	neonatal alloimmune thrombocytopenia
NAP	neutrophil alkaline phosphatase
NBT	nitro blue tetrazolium
NEJM	*New England Journal of Medicine*
NHL	non-Hodgkin's lymphoma
NRBC	nucleated red blood cells
NS	non-secretory [myeloma]
NSAIDs	non-steroidal antiinflammatory drugs
NSE	non-specific esterase
OCP	oral contraceptive pill
od	*omni die* (once daily)
OPG	orthopantomogram
OR	overall response
OS	overall survival
PA	pernicious anaemia
PAI	plasminogen activator inhibitor
PaO_2	partial pressure of O_2 in arterial blood
PAS	periodic acid–Schiff
PB	peripheral blood
PBSC	peripheral blood stem cell
PC	protein C
PCC	prothrombin complex concentrate

PCH	paroxysmal cold haemoglobinuria
PCL	plasma cell leukaemia
PCP	*Pneumocystis carinii* pneumonia
PCR	polymerase chain reaction
PCV	packed cell volume
PDGF	platelet-derived growth factor
PDW	platelet distribution width
PE	pulmonary embolism
PEP	post-expoure prophylaxis
PET	pre-eclamptic toxaemia *or* position emission tomography
PF	platelet factor
PFA	platelet function analysis
PFK	phosphofructokinase
PFS	progression-free survival
PGD2	prostaglandin D2
PGE1	prostaglandin E1
PGK	phosphoglycerate kinase
Ph	Philadelphia chromosome
PIG	phosphatidylinositol glycoproteins
PIVKA	protein induced by vitamin K absence
PK	pyruvate kinase
PLL	prolymphocytic leukaemia
PML	promyelocytic leukaemia
PNET	primitive neuroectodermal tumour
PNH	paroxysmal nocturnal haemoglobinuria
PO	*per os* (by mouth)
PPH	post-partum haomorrhage
PPI	proton pump inhibitor
PPP	primary proliferative polycythaemia
PRCA	pure red cell aplasia
PRN	as required
ProMACE	prednisolone, doxorubicin, cyclophosphamide, etoposide
PRV	polycythaemia rubra vera
PS	protein S
PSA	prostate-specific antigen
PT	prothrombin time
PTP	post-transfusion purpura
PUVA	phototherapy with psoralen plus UV-A
PVO	pyrexia of unknown origin
PV	polycythaemia vera
QoL	quality of life

qds	*quater die sumendus* (to be taken 4 times a day)
℞	treatment
RA	refractory anaemia
RAEB	refractory anaemia with excess blasts
RAEB-t	refractory anaemia with excess blasts in transformation
RAR	retinoic acid receptor
RARα	retinoic acid receptor α
RARS	refractory anaemia with ring sideroblasts
RBC	red blood cell *or* red blood count
RCC	red blood cell count
RCM	red cell mass
RCMD	refractory cytopenia with multilineage dysplasia
RDS	respiratory distress syndrome
RDW	red cell distribution width
RE	relative erythrocytosis; reticuloendothelial
RES	reticuloendothelial system
RFLP	restriction fragment length polymorphism
Rh	Rhesus
rhG-CSF	recombinant human granulocyte colony stimulating factor
rHuEPO	recombinant human erythropoietin
RI	remission induction
RIA	radioimmunoassay
RiCoF	ristocetin cofactor
RIPA	ristocetin-induced platelet aggregation
RS	Reed–Sternberg *or* ringed sideroblasts
RT-PCR	reverse transcriptase polymerase chain reaction
s	seconds
SAA	serum amyloid A protein
SAGM	saline adenine glucose mannitol
SaO_2	arterial oxygen saturation
SAP	serum amyloid P protein
SBP	solitary plasmacytoma of bone
SC	subcutaneous
SCA	sickle cell anaemia
SCBU	special care baby unit
SCD	sickle cell disease
SCID	severe combined immunodeficiency
SCT	stem cell transplant(ation)

SD	standard deviation
SE	secondary erythrocytosis
SEP	extramedullary plasmacytoma
SLE	systemic lupus erythematosus
SLL	small lymphocytic lymphoma
SLVL	splenic lymphoma with villous lymphocytes
SM	systemic mastocytosis
SmIg	surface membrane immunoglobulin
SOB	short of breath
SPB	solitary plasmacytoma of bone
SPD	storage pool deficiency
stat	statim (immediate; as initial dose)
sTfR	soluble transferrin receptor
SVC	superior vena cava
SVCO	superior vena caval obstruction
T° (↑T°)	temperature (fever)
$t_{1/2}$	half-life
T4	thyroxine
TAM	transient abnormal myelopoiesis
TAR	thrombocytopenia with absent radius
TB	tuberculosis
TBI	total body irradiation
TCR	T-cell receptor
tds	*ter die sumendum* (to be taken 3 times a day)
TdT	terminal deoxynucleotidyl transferase
TEC	transient erythroblastopenia of childhood
TENS	transcutaneous nerve stimulation
TF	tissue factor
TFT	thyroid function test(s)
TGF-β	transforming growth factor-β
TIAs	transient ischaemic attacks
TIBC	total iron binding capacity
tiw	three times in a week
TNF	tumour necrosis factor
topo II	topoisomerase II
TORCH	toxoplasmosis, rubella, cytomegalovirus, herpes simplex
TPA	tissue plasminogen activator
TPI	triphosphate isomerase
TPN	total parenteral nutrition
TPO	thrombopoietin
TPR	temperature, pulse, respiration

TRAP	tartrate-resistant acid phosphatase
TRM	treatment related mortality
TSH	thyroid-stimulating hormone
TT	thrombin time
TTP	thrombotic thrombocytopenic purpura
TXA	tranexamic acid
TXA2	thromboxane A2
U&E	urea and electrolytes
u/U	units
UC	ulcerative colitis
UFH	unfractionated heparin
URTI	upper respiratory tract infection
USS	ultrasound scan
UTI	urinary tract infection
VAD	vincristine adriamycin dexamethasone regimen
VBAP	vincristine, carmustine (BCNU), doxorubicin (adriamycin), prednisolone
VBMCP	vincristine, carmustine, melphalan, cyclophosphamide, prednisolone
VIII:C	Factor VIII clotting activity
VDRL	screening test for syphilis (Venereal Disease Research Laboratory
VF	ventricular fibrillation
Vit K	vitamin K
VMCP	vincristine, melphalan, cyclophosphamide, prednisolone
VOD	veno-occlusive disease
VTE	venous thromboembolism
vWD	von Willebrand's disease
vWF	von Willebrand factor
vWFAg	von Willebrand factor antigen
WBC	white blood count *or* white blood cell
WCC	White cell count
WM	Waldenström's macroglobulinaemia
XDPs	cross-linked fibrin degradation products
X match	cross-match
μg	microgram

Clinical approach

1

History taking in patients with haematological disease

Approach to patient with suspected haematological disease

An accurate history combined with a careful physical examination are fundamental parts of clinical assessment. Although the likely haematological diagnosis may be apparent from tests carried out before the patient has been referred, it is nevertheless essential to assess the clinical background fully—this may influence the eventual plan of management, especially in older patients.

It is important to find out early on in the consultation what the patient may already have been told prior to referral, or what he/she thinks the diagnosis may be. There is often fear and anxiety about diagnoses such as leukaemia, haemophilia or HIV infection.

Presenting symptoms and their duration

A full medical history needs to be taken to which is added direct questioning on relevant features associated with presenting symptoms:

- Non-specific symptoms such as fatigue, fevers, weight loss.
- Symptoms relating to anaemia e.g. reduced exercise capacity, recent onset of breathlessness and nature of its onset, or worsening of angina, presence of ankle oedema.
- Symptoms relating to neutropenia e.g. recurrent oral ulceration, skin infections, oral sepsis.
- Evidence of compromised immunity e.g. recurrent oropharyngeal infection.
- Details of potential haemostatic problems e.g. easy bruising, bleeding episodes, rashes.
- Anatomical symptoms, e.g. abdominal discomfort (splenic enlargement or pressure from enlarged lymph nodes), CNS symptoms (from spinal compression).
- Past medical history, i.e. detail on past illnesses, information on previous surgical procedures which may suggest previous haematological problems (e.g. may suggest an underlying bleeding diathesis) or be associated with haematological or other sequelae e.g. splenectomy.
- Drug history: ask about prescribed and non-prescribed medications.
- Allergies: since some haematological disorders may relate to chemicals or other environmental hazards specific questions should be asked about occupational factors and hobbies.
- Transfusion history: ask about whether the patient has been a blood donor and how much he/she has donated. May occasionally be a factor in iron deficiency anaemia. History of previous transfusion(s) and their timing is also critical in some cases e.g. post-transfusion purpura.
- Tobacco and alcohol consumption is essential; both may produce significant haematological morbidity.
- Travel: clearly important in the case of suspected malaria but also relevant in considering other causes of haematological abnormality, including HIV infection.

- Family history also important, especially in the context of inherited haematological disorders.

A complete history for a patient with a haematological disorder should provide all the relevant medical information to aid diagnosis and clinical assessment, as well as helping the haematologist to have a working assessment of the patient's social situation. A well taken history also provides a basis for good communication which will often prove very important once it comes to discussion of the diagnosis.

Physical examination

This forms part of the clinical assessment of the haematology patient. Pay specific attention to:

General examination—e.g. evidence of weight loss, pyrexia, pallor (*not* a reliable clinical measure of anaemia), jaundice, cyanosis or abnormal pigmentation or skin rashes.

The mouth—ulceration, purpura, gum bleeding or infiltration, and the state of the patient's teeth. Hands and nails may show features associated with haematological abnormalities e.g. koilonychia in chronic iron deficiency (rarely seen today).

Record—weight, height, T°, pulse and blood pressure; height and weight give important baseline data against which sequential measurements can subsequently be compared. In myelofibrosis, for example, evidence of significant weight loss in the absence of symptoms may be an indication of clinical progression.

Examination—of chest and abdomen should focus on detecting the presence of lymphadenopathy, hepatic and/or splenic enlargement. Node sizes and the extent of organ enlargement should be carefully recorded.

Lymph node enlargement—often recorded in centimetres e.g. 3cm × 3cm × 4cm; sometimes more helpful to compare the degree of enlargement with familiar objects e.g. pea. Record extent of liver or spleen enlargement as maximum distance palpable from the lower costal margin.

Erythematous margins of infected skin lesions—mark these to monitor treatment effects.

Bones and joints—recording of joint swelling and ranges of movement are standard aspects of haemophilia care. In myeloma, areas of bony tenderness and deformity are commonly present.

Optic fundi—examination is a key clinical assessment in the haematology patient. May yield the only objective evidence of hyperviscosity in paraproteinaemias (📖*Emergencies p510*) or hyperleucocytosis (📖*Emergencies p510*) such as in e.g. CML. Regular examination for haemorrhages should form part of routine observations in the severely myelosuppressed patient; rarely changes of opportunistic infection such as candidiasis can be seen in the optic fundi.

Neurological examination—fluctuations of conscious level and confusion are clinical presentations of hyperviscosity. Isolated nerve palsies in a patient with acute leukaemia are highly suspicious of neurological involvement or disease relapse. Peripheral neuropathy and long tract signs are well recognised complications of B_{12} deficiency.

Clinical approach

Splenomegaly

Many causes. Clinical approach depends on whether splenic enlargement is present as an isolated finding or with other clinical abnormalities e.g. jaundice or lymphadenopathy. Mild to moderate splenomegaly have a much greater number of causes than massive splenomegaly.

Causes of splenomegaly

Infection	Viral	EBV, CMV, hepatitis
	Bacterial	SBE, miliary tuberculosis, *Salmonella, Brucella*
	Protozoal	Malaria, toxoplasmosis, leishmaniasis
Haemolytic	Congenital	Hereditary spherocytosis, hereditary elliptocytosis Sickle cell disease (infants), thalassaemia Pyruvate kinase deficiency, G6PD deficiency
	Acquired	AIHA (idiopathic or 2°)
Myeloproliferative & leukaemic		Myelofibrosis, CML, polycythaemia rubra vera Essential thrombocythaemia, acute leukaemias
Lymphoproliferative		CLL, hairy cell leukaemia, Waldenström's, SLVL, other NHL, Hodgkin's disease, ALL & lymphoblastic NHL
Autoimmune disorders & Storage disorders		Rheumatoid arthritis, SLE, hepatic cirrhosis Gaucher's disease, histiocytosis X Niemann–Pick disease
Miscellaneous		Metastatic cancer, cysts, amyloid, portal hypertension, portal vein thrombosis, tropical splenomegaly

Clinical approach essentially involves a working knowledge of the possible causes of splenic enlargement and determining the more likely causes in the given clinical circumstances by appropriate further investigation. There are fewer causes of massive splenic enlargement, i.e. the spleen tip palpable below the level of the umbilicus.

Massive splenomegaly

- Myelofibrosis.
- Chronic myeloid leukaemia.
- Lymphoproliferative disease—CLL and variants including SLVL, HCL and marginal zone lymphoma.
- Tropical splenomegaly.
- Leishmaniasis.
- Gaucher's disease.
- Thalassaemia major.

Clinical approach

Lymphadenopathy

Occurs in a range of infective or neoplastic conditions; less frequently enlargement occurs in active collagen disorders. May be isolated, affecting a single node, localised, involving several nodes in an anatomical lymph node grouping, or generalised, where nodes are enlarged at different sites. As well as enlargement in the easily palpable areas (cervical, axillary and iliac) node enlargement may be hilar or retroperitoneal and identifiable only by imaging. Isolated/localised lymphadenopathy usually results from local infection or neoplasm. Generalised lymphadenopathy may result from systemic causes, especially when symmetrical, as well as infection or neoplasm. Rarely drug-associated (e.g. phenytoin).

Causes of lymphadenopathy		
Infective	Bacterial	Tonsillitis, cellulitis, tuberculous infections & primary syphilis usually produce isolated or localised node enlargement
	Viral	EBV, CMV, rubella, HIV, HBV, HCV
	Other	Toxoplasma, histoplasmosis, chlamydia, cat-scratch
Neoplastic		Hodgkin's disease (typically isolated or localised lymphadenopathy), NHL isolated, generalised or localised, CLL, metastatic carcinoma, acute leukaemia (ALL especially, but occasionally AML)
Collagen and other systemic disorders		E.g. rheumatoid arthritis, SLE, sarcoidosis

History and examination—points to elicit

- Age.
- Onset of symptoms, whether progressing or not.
- Systemic symptoms, weight loss (>10% body weight loss in <6 months).
- Night sweats.
- Risk factors for HIV infection.
- Local or systemic evidence of infection.
- Evidence of systemic disorder such as rheumatoid arthritis.
- Evidence of malignancy; if splenic enlargement present then lymphoreticular neoplasm is more likely.
- Specific disease-related features e.g. pruritus and alcohol induced lymph node pain associated with Hodgkin's disease.
- Determine the duration of enlargement ± associated symptoms, whether nodes are continuing to enlarge and whether tender or not. Distribution of node enlargement should be recorded as well as size of node.

Investigations

1. FBC and peripheral blood film examination.
2. ESR or plasma viscosity.
3. Screening test for infectious mononucleosis and serological testing for other viruses.

4. Imaging—e.g. chest radiography and abdominal ± pelvic USS to define hilar, retroperitoneal and para-aortic nodes. CT scanning may also be helpful.
5. Microbiology—e.g. blood cultures, indirect testing for TB and culture of biopsied or aspirated lymph node material.
6. Lymph node biopsy for definitive diagnosis especially if a neoplastic cause suspected. Aspiration of enlarged lymph nodes is generally unsatisfactory in providing effective diagnostic material.
7. Bone marrow examination should be reserved for staging in confirmed lymphoma or leukaemia cases—it is not commonly a useful primary investigation of lymphadenopathy.

Unexplained anaemia

Evaluate with the combined information from clinical history, physical examination and results of investigations.

History—focus on

- Duration of symptoms of anaemia—short duration of dyspnoea and fatigue etc. suggests recent bleeding or haemolysis.
- Specific questioning on blood loss—include system-related questions e.g. GIT and gynaecological sources, ask about blood donation.
- Family history—e.g. in relation to hereditary problems such as HS or ethnic Hb disorders such as thalassaemia or HbSS.
- Past history—e.g. association of gastrectomy with later occurrence of Fe and/or B_{12} deficiency.
- Drug history—including prescribed and non-prescribed medication.
- Dietary factors—mainly relates to folate and Fe deficiency, rarely B_{12} in vegans. Fe deficiency always occurs because Fe losses exceed intake (it is extremely rare in developed countries for diet to be the sole cause of Fe deficiency).

Examination

- May identify indirectly helpful signs e.g. koilonychia in chronic Fe deficiency (rare), jaundice in haemolytic disorders.
- Lymphadenopathy suggesting lymphoreticular disease or viral infection.
- Hepatosplenomegaly in lymphoproliferative or myeloproliferative disorders, or metabolic diseases.

Full blood count

Laboratory investigation of anaemia is discussed fully in section 2. Anaemia in adult ♂ if Hb <13.0g/dL and in adult ♀ if Hb <11.5g/dL.

MCV useful for initial anaemia evaluation	
↓ MCV (<76fL)	Fe deficiency α & β thalassaemia, HbE, HbC Anaemia of chronic disorders
Normal MCV (78–98fL)	Recent bleeding Anaemia of chronic disorders Most non-haematinic deficiency causes Combined Fe + B_{12}/folate deficiency
↑ MCV (>100fL)	Folate or B_{12} deficiency Haemolytic anaemia Liver disease Marrow dysplasia & failure syndromes including aplastic anaemia 2° to antimetabolite drug therapy e.g. hydroxyurea

The need for film examination, reticulocyte counting and additional tests on the FBC sample such as checking for Heinz bodies is based on the initial clinical and FBC findings. The findings from the initial FBC examination have a major influence in determining the nature and urgency of further clinical investigation.

Serum ferritin level will identify iron deficiency and focus on the need for detailed investigation for blood loss which, for adult males and postmenopausal females, will frequently require large bowel examination with colonoscopy or barium enema, and gastroscopy. BM examination may occasionally be required.

Anaemia is not a diagnosis—it is an abnormal clinical finding requiring an explanation for its cause. There is no place for empirical use of Fe therapy for management and treatment of 'anaemia' in modern medical practice.

Patient with elevated haemoglobin

Finding a raised Hb concentration requires a systematic clinical approach for differential diagnosis and further investigation. Initially it is essential to check whether the result ties in with the known clinical findings—if unexpected the FBC should be re-checked to exclude a mix-up over samples or a sampling artefact. Dehydration and diuretic therapy may ↑ the Hct and these should be excluded in the initial phase of assessment.

Having determined that the ↑ Hb concentration is genuine the issue is whether there is a genuine increase in red cell mass or not, and the explanation for the elevated Hb.

Anoxia is a major stimulus to RBC production and will result in an increase in erythropoietin with consequent erythrocytosis.

History and examination should assess

- Recent travel and residence at high altitude (>3000m).
- COAD, other hypoxic respiratory conditions, cyanotic congenital heart disease, other cardiac problems causing hypoxia.
- Smoking—heavy cigarette smoking causes ↑ carboxyHb levels leading to ↑ RBC mass to compensate for loss of O_2 carrying capacity.
- Ventilatory impairment 2° to gross obesity, alveolar hypoventilation (Pickwickian syndrome).
- Possibility of high-affinity Hb abnormalities arises if there is a FH of polycythaemia, otherwise requires assessment through Hb analysis.
- If obvious secondary causes excluded possibilities include:

Spurious polycythaemia—pseudopolycythaemia or Gaisbock's syndrome, associated features can include cigarette smoking, obesity, hypertension and excess alcohol consumption; sometimes described as 'stress polycythaemia'.

Primary proliferative polycythaemia (polycythaemia rubra vera)—plethoric facies, history of pruritus after bathing or on change of environmental temperature and presence of splenomegaly are helpful clinical findings to suggest this diagnosis.

Inappropriate erythropoietin excess—occurs in a variety of benign and malignant renal disorders. Rare complication of some tumours including hepatoma, uterine fibroids and cerebellar haemangioblastoma.

Part of clinical assessment must also include an evaluation of thrombotic risk; previous thrombosis or a family history of such problems increase the urgency of investigation and appropriate treatment

📖 *p240–249.*

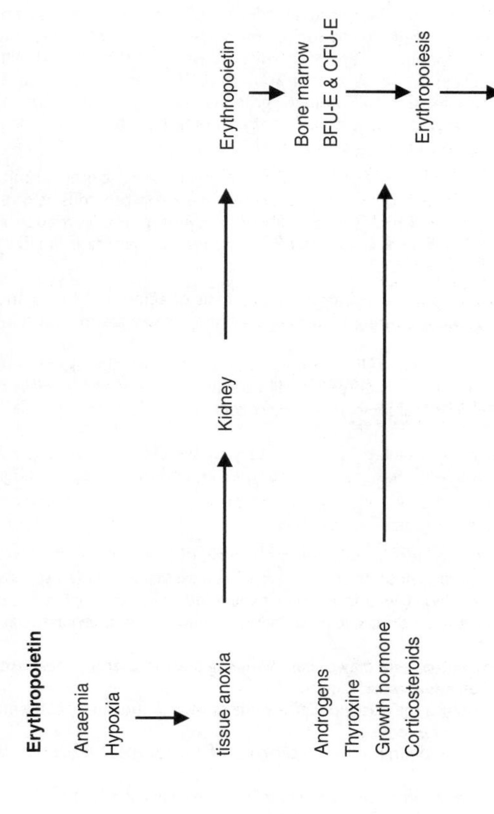
Erythropoietin
Anaemia
Hypoxia
tissue anoxia
Kidney
Erythropoietin
Bone marrow
BFU-E & CFU-E
Erythropoiesis
Increased RBC mass
Androgens
Thyroxine
Growth hormone
Corticosteroids

Elevated WBC

Leucocytosis is defined as elevation of the white cell count >2 SD above the mean. The detection of leucocytosis should prompt immediate scrutiny of the automated WBC differential (generally accurate except in leukaemia) and the other FBC parameters. Blood film should be examined and a manual differential count performed. Important to evaluate leucocytosis in terms of the age-related absolute normal ranges for neutrophils, lymphocytes, monocytes, eosinophils and basophils (📖 p688, 690) and the presence of abnormal cells: immature granulocytes, blasts, nucleated red cells and 'atypical cells'.

Leukaemoid reaction—leucocytosis >50 × 10^9/L defines a neutrophilia with marked 'left shift' (band forms, metamyelocytes, myelocytes and occasionally promyelocytes and myeloblasts in the blood film). Differential diagnosis is chronic granulocytic leukaemia (CGL) and in children, juvenile CML. Primitive granulocyte precursors are also frequently seen in the blood film of the infected or stressed neonate, and any seriously ill patient e.g. on ITU.

Leucoerythroblastic blood film—contains myelocytes, other primitive granulocytes, nucleated red cells and often tear drop red cells, is due to bone marrow invasion by tumour, fibrosis or granuloma formation and is an indication for a bone marrow biopsy. Other causes include anorexia and haemolysis.

Leucocytosis due to blasts—suggests diagnosis of acute leukaemia and is an indication for cell typing studies and bone marrow examination.

FBC, blood film, white cell differential count and the clinical context in which the leucocytosis is detected will usually indicate whether this is due to a 1° haematological abnormality or reflects a 2° response.

▶ It is clearly important to seek a history of symptoms of infection and examine the patient for signs of infection or an underlying haematological disorder.

Neutrophilia

- 2° to acute infection is most common cause of leucocytosis.
- Usually modest (uncommonly >30 × 10^9/L), associated with a left shift and occasionally toxic granulation or vacuolation of neutrophils.
- Chronic inflammation causes less marked neutrophilia often associated with monocytosis.
- Moderate neutrophilia may occur following steroid therapy, heatstroke and in patients with solid tumours.
- Mild neutrophilia may be induced by stress (e.g. immediate postoperative period) and exercise.
- May be seen in the immediate aftermath of a myocardial infarction or major seizure.
- Frequently found in states of chronic bone marrow stimulation (e.g. chronic haemolysis, ITP) and asplenia.
- Primary haematological causes of neutrophilia are less common. CML is often the cause of extremely high leucocyte counts (>200 × 10^9/L), predominantly neutrophils with marked left shift, basophilia and occa-

sional myeloblasts. A low LAP score and the presence of the Ph chromosome on karyotype analysis are usually helpful to differentiate CGL from a leukaemoid reaction.
- Less common are juvenile CML, transient leukaemoid reaction in Down syndrome, hereditary neutrophilia and chronic idiopathic neutrophilia.

Bone marrow examination is rarely necessary in the investigation of a patient with isolated neutrophilia. Investigation of a leukaemoid reaction, leucoerythroblastic blood film and possible CGL or juvenile CML are firm indications for a bone marrow aspirate and trephine biopsy. Bone marrow culture, including culture for atypical mycobacteria and fungi, may be useful in patients with persistent pyrexia or leucocytosis.

Lymphocytosis

- Lymphocytosis $>4.0 \times 10^9/L$.
- Normal infants and young children <5 have a higher proportion and concentration of lymphocytes than adults.
- Rare in acute bacterial infection except in pertussis (may be $>50 \times 10^9/L$).
- Acute infectious lymphocytosis also seen in children, usually associated with transient lymphocytosis and a mild constitutional reaction.
- Characteristic of infectious mononucleosis but these lymphocytes are often large and atypical and the diagnosis may be confirmed with a heterophil agglutination test.
- Similar atypical cells may be seen in patients with CMV and hepatitis A infection.
- Chronic infection with brucellosis, tuberculosis, secondary syphilis and congenital syphilis may cause lymphocytosis.
- Lymphocytosis is characteristic of CLL, ALL and occasionally NHL.

Where primary haematological cause suspected, immunophenotypic analysis of the peripheral blood lymphocytes will often confirm or exclude a neoplastic diagnosis. BM examination is indicated if neoplasia is strongly suspected and in any patient with concomitant neutropenia, anaemia or thrombocytopenia.

Reduced WBC

Although not entirely synonymous, it is uncommon for absolute leucopenia (WBC <4.0 × 10^9/L) to be due to isolated deficiency of any cell other than the neutrophil though in marked leucopenia several cell lines are often affected.

▶ Neutropenia

Defined as a neutrophil count <2.0 × 10^9/L. The risk of infective complications is closely related to the absolute neutrophil count. More severe when neutropenia is due to impaired production from chemotherapy or marrow failure rather than to peripheral destruction or maturation arrest where there is often a cellular marrow with early neutrophil precursors and normal monocyte counts. Type of infection determined by the degree and duration of neutropenia. Ongoing chemotherapy further increases the risk of serious bacterial and fungal opportunistic infection and the presence of an indwelling intravenous catheter increases the incidence of infection with coagulase-negative staphylococci and other skin commensals. Patients with chronic immune neutropenia may develop recurrent stomatitis, gingivitis, oral ulceration, sinusitis and peri-anal infection.

Neutrophil count	Risk of infection
1.0–1.5 × 10^9/L	No significant increased risk of infection.
0.5–1.0 × 10^9/L	Some increase in risk; some fevers can be treated as an outpatient.
<0.5 × 10^9/L	Major increase in risk; treat all fevers with broad spectrum IV antibiotics as an inpatient.

The history and physical examination provide a guide to the subsequent management of a patient with neutropenia. Simple observation is appropriate initially for an asymptomatic patient with isolated mild neutropenia who has an unremarkable history and examination. If there has been a recent viral illness or the patient can discontinue a drug which may be the cause, follow-up over a few weeks may see resolution of the abnormality.

Investigations

BM examination—if there is concomitant anaemia or thrombocytopenia, if there is a history of significant infection or if lymphadenopathy or organomegaly are detected on examination. Usually unhelpful in patients with an isolated neutropenia >0.5 × 10^9/L. However, if neutropenia persists, bone marrow aspiration, biopsy, cytogenetics and serology for collagen diseases, anti-neutrophil antibodies, HIV and immunoglobulins should be performed.

Differential diagnoses

Isolated neutropenia may be the presenting feature of myelodysplasia, aplastic anaemia, Fanconi's anaemia or acute leukaemia but these conditions will usually be associated with other haematological abnormalities.

Post-infectious (most usually post-viral) neutropenia may last several weeks and may be followed by prolonged immune neutropenia.

Severe sepsis particularly at the extremes of life.

Drugs—cytotoxic agents, and many others, notably phenothiazines, many antibiotics, NSAIDs, anti-thyroid agents and psychotropic agents. Recovery of neutrophils usually starts within a few days of stopping the offending drug.

Autoimmune neutropenia due to anti-neutrophil antibodies may occur in isolation or in association with haemolytic anaemia, immune thrombocytopenia or SLE.

Felty's syndrome neutropenia is accompanied by seropositive rheumatoid arthritis, and splenomegaly.

Chronic benign neutropenia of infancy and childhood is associated with fever and infection but resolves by age 4, probably also has an immune basis.

Benign familial neutropenia is a feature of rare families and of certain racial groups, notably negroes, is associated with mild neutropenia but no propensity to infection.

Chronic idiopathic neutropenia is a diagnosis of exclusion, associated with severe neutropenia but often a benign course.

Cyclical neutropenia is a condition of childhood onset and dominant inheritance characterised by severe neutropenia, fever, stomatitis and other infections occurring with a periodicity of ~4 weeks.

Hereditary causes (less common) include Kostmann syndrome (📖 *p459*), Shwachman–Diamond–Oski syndrome (📖 *p459*), Chediak–Higashi syndrome (📖 *p465*), reticular dysgenesis and dyskeratosis congenita, and Gaucher's disease.

Management

Febrile episodes should be managed according to the severity of the neutropenia (see table) and the underlying cause (bone marrow failure is associated with more life-threatening infections). Broad spectrum IV antibiotics may be required and empirical systemic antifungal therapy may be required in those who fail to respond to antibiotics. Prophylactic antibiotic and antifungal therapy may be helpful in some patients with chronic neutropenia as may G-CSF. Antiseptic mouthwash is of value and regular dental care is important.

▶ Lymphopenia

Lymphopenia ($<1.5 \times 10^9$/L) may be seen in acute infections, cardiac failure, pancreatitis, tuberculosis, uraemia, lymphoma, carcinoma, SLE and other collagen disease, corticosteroid therapy, radiation, chemotherapy and anti-lymphocyte globulin. Most common cause of chronic severe lymphopenia in recent years has been HIV infection (📖 *p414*).

Chronic severe lymphopenia ($<0.5 \times 10^9$/L) is associated both with opportunistic infections notably *Candida* species, *Pneumocystis carinii*, CMV, Herpes zoster, *Mycoplasma* spp., *Cryptosporidium* and toxoplasmosis and with an increased incidence of neoplasia particularly NHL, Kaposi's sarcoma and skin and gastric carcinoma.

Clinical approach

Elevated platelet count

Thrombocytosis is defined as a platelet count >450 × 10^9/L. May be due to a *primary* myeloproliferative disorder (MPD) or a *secondary* reactive feature. If the platelet count is markedly elevated a patient with a myeloproliferative disorder has a risk of haemorrhage (due to the production of dysfunctional platelets), or thrombosis, or both. The patient's history may reveal features of the condition to which the elevated platelet count is secondary. Clinical examination may provide similar clues or reveal the presence of palpable splenomegaly which suggests a myeloproliferative disorder. FBC may provide useful information: marked leucocytosis with left shift (in the absence of a history of infection), basophilia or an elevated haematocrit and red cell count are highly suggestive of a myeloproliferative disorder when associated with thrombocytosis. Unusual for reactive thrombocytosis to cause a platelet count >1000 × 10^9/L. *Note:* platelet counts below this may occur in myeloproliferative disorders.

Differential diagnosis

Myeloproliferative disorders	Disorders associated with ↑ platelets
Primary thrombocythaemia	Haemorrhage
Polycythaemia rubra vera	Trauma
Chronic granulocytic leukaemia	Surgery
Idiopathic myelofibrosis	Iron deficiency anaemia
	Malignancy (ca lung, ca breast, Hodgkin's disease)
	Acute & chronic infection
	Inflammatory disease e.g. rheumatoid arthritis, UC
	Post-splenectomy

Investigation

- BM aspirate may show megakaryocyte abnormalities in MPD.
- BM trephine biopsy may show clusters of abnormal megakaryocytes and increased reticulin or fibrosis in MPD.

Management

- In reactive thrombocytosis treat the underlying condition.
- Unusual for treatment to ↓ the platelet count to be necessary in a patient with reactive thrombocytosis.
- Consider low dose aspirin (or if contraindicated, dipyridamole).
- Reactive thrombocytosis is generally transient.
- If secondary to iron deficiency—review FBC after iron therapy: the platelet count normalises if thrombocytosis was due to iron deficiency.
- Iron deficiency may have masked PRV—this will be revealed by iron therapy.
- If impossible to define the cause of thrombocytosis then a watch-and-wait policy should be followed in an asymptomatic patient.
- If MPD is suspected—📖 *Essential thrombocythaemia, p250.*

Clinical approach

Reduced platelet count

Thrombocytopenia is defined as platelet count $<150 \times 10^9$/L. Although there is no precise platelet count at which a patient will or will not bleed, most patients with a count $>50 \times 10^9$/L are asymptomatic. The risk of spontaneous haemorrhage increases significantly $<20 \times 10^9$/L. Purpura is the most common presenting symptom and is usually found on the lower limbs and areas subject to pressure. May be followed by bleeding gums, epistaxis or more serious life-threatening haemorrhage. A patient with newly diagnosed severe thrombocytopenia with or without purpura is a medical emergency and should be admitted for further investigation and treatment.

Confirm low platelet count by examination of the blood sample for clots and the blood film for platelet aggregates (causing pseudothrombocytopenia). History and examination will determine the clinical severity of the thrombocytopenia and should also reveal the duration of symptoms, presence of any prodromal illness, causative medication or underlying disease.

Determine whether the cause of thrombocytopenia is failure of production or increased consumption. FBC may be helpful as the mean platelet volume (MPV) is often elevated in the latter group (large platelets may also be seen on the blood film). May also reveal additional haematological abnormalities (normocytic anaemia or neutropenia) suggestive of a bone marrow disorder. A coagulation screen should also be performed. Examination of the bone marrow is the definitive investigation in all patients with moderate or severe thrombocytopenia—may reveal normal megakaryocytes or compensatory hyperplasia in peripheral destruction syndromes or marrow hypoplasia or infiltration. Tests for platelet antibodies are unreliable but an autoimmune screen may be helpful to exclude lupus.

Management

Treat underlying condition. Most patients with a platelet count $>30 \times 10^9$/L require no specific therapy. Avoid aspirin. In the event of life-threatening haemorrhage platelet transfusion should be administered to thrombocytopenic patients *with the exception of those with heparin-induced thrombocytopenia and TTP*.

Failure of production	Increased consumption
Drugs & chemicals (p392)	ITP (p388)
Viral infection	Drugs (p392)
Radiation	DIC (p512)
Aplastic anaemia (p122)	Infection
Leukaemia	Massive haemorrhage & transfusion (p524)
Marrow infiltration (p120, 634)	SLE
Megaloblastic anaemia (p60–64)	CLL & lymphoma (p168, 194)
HIV (p414)	Heparin (p588) TTP (p530) Hypersplenism (p392) Post-transfusion purpura (p392) HIV (p414)

Easy bruising

Evaluation of a patient who complains of easy bruising involves a detailed history, physical examination with particular attention to any current haemorrhagic lesions and the performance of basic haemostatic investigations. More common in ♀ and often difficult to evaluate. Also a frequent complaint in the elderly.

History

Careful attention to the history is essential to the diagnosis of all the haemorrhagic disorders and one must attempt to define the nature of the bruising in a patient with this complaint. *Note*: many normal healthy people believe that they have excessive bleeding or bruising. Conversely some people with haemorrhagic disorders and abnormal bleeding histories will not volunteer the information unless asked directly or indeed may consider their bleeding to be normal. Remember that excessive bruising may be a manifestation of a blood vessel disorder rather than a coagulopathy or platelet disorder.

Ask about

Presenting complaint—How long and how frequently has easy bruising occurred? Is it ecchymoses or purpura? How extensive are bruises? Are they located in areas subject to trauma (e.g. limbs) or pressure (e.g. waist band)? Do petechiae occur? Are bruises painful? Is there a palpable knot or cord? How long to resolution? How many currently?

Associated symptoms

Has there been gum bleeding? Has the patient experienced prolonged bleeding after skin trauma, dental extraction, childbirth or surgery? Has there been any other form of haemorrhage e.g. epistaxis, menorrhagia, joint or soft tissue haematoma, haematemesis, melaena, haemoptysis or haematuria? Is there a history of poor wound healing?

Family history

Has any other family member a history of excessive bleeding or bruising?

Drug history

Is the patient on any medication (remember self-medication of vitamins and food supplements), most notably aspirin, anticoagulant therapy?

Systematic enquiry

Is there evidence of a disorder associated with a haemorrhagic tendency e.g. hepatic or renal failure, malabsorption, leukaemia, connective tissue disorder or amyloid?

Physical examination

Haemorrhagic skin lesions are likely to be present in a patient with a serious problem and their distribution will often indicate the extent to which they are likely to be related to trauma. Senile purpura is almost invariably on the hands and forearms. True purpura is easily differentiated from erythema and telangiectasis by pressure. Petechiae are highly suggestive of a platelet or vascular disorder whilst palpable purpura is associated with anaphylactoid purpura. In addition there may be other physical findings which may indicate an underlying disorder e.g. splenomegaly or lymphadenopathy in leukaemia, signs of hepatic failure, telangiectasia in Osler–Rendu–Weber syndrome or hyperextensible joints and paper-thin scars in Ehlers–Danlos syndrome.

Basic haemostatic investigations

All patients should be investigated except those in whom history and examination has given strong grounds for believing that they are normal and in whom there is a history of a normal response to a haemostatic challenge e.g. surgery or dental extraction.

Screening tests

- FBC and blood film.
- APTT.
- PT.
- Thrombin clotting time and/or fibrinogen.
- Bleeding time (a largely obsolete investigation, of dubious utility).

If these investigations are normal there is no indication for further haemostatic investigations unless the history provides strong grounds for believing that there is indeed a haemostatic disorder. The appropriate further investigation of the haemostatic mechanism is discussed in Section 10.

Differential diagnoses

- Common diagnoses
  - Simple easy bruising (purpura simplex).
  - Trauma (including non-accidental injury in children).
  - Senile purpura.
- Haemostatic defects
  - Thrombocytopenia.
  - Platelet function defects.
  - Coagulation abnormalities (rarely).
- Vascular defects
  - Corticosteroid excess.
  - Collagen diseases.
  - Uraemia.
  - Dysproteinaemias.
  - Anaphylactoid purpura.
  - Ehlers–Danlos syndrome.
  - Scurvy.
  - Vasculitis.

Recurrent thromboembolism

A hypercoagulable state should be suspected in all patients with recurrent thromboembolic disease, family history of thrombosis, thrombosis at a young age or at an unusual site (in addition to recurrent thromboembolism) associated with inherited thrombophilia. Further important aspects of the history are precipitating factors at the time of thrombosis and lifestyle considerations e.g. smoking, exercise and obesity. Clinical examination may reveal signs suggestive of an associated underlying condition.

Hypercoagulable states	
Inherited	Activated protein C resistance (factor V Leiden) Protein C deficiency Protein S deficiency Prothrombin gene mutation Hyperhomocysteinaemia Sickle cell disease Antithrombin deficiency and some very rare abnormalities of fibrinogen, plasminogen and plasminogen activator
Acquired	Immobilisation Oral contraceptive or oestrogen therapy Postpartum Old age Postoperative Malignancy (notably Ca pancreas) Nephrotic syndrome Myeloproliferative disorders Hyperhomocysteinaemia Antiphospholipid syndrome (lupus anticoagulant) Hyperviscosity Paroxysmal nocturnal haemoglobinuria Thrombotic thrombocytopenic purpura Heparin-induced thrombocytopenia

Laboratory Investigation

📖 *Thrombophilia p394.*

Clinical approach

Pathological fracture

Fracture in a bone compromised by the presence of a pathological process resulting in fracture occurring following relatively minor trauma. Most commonly due to local neoplastic involvement or osteoporosis.

Haematological causes

- Local bony damage.
- Myelomatous deposits.
- Lymphoma.
- Metastatic carcinoma (± marrow infiltration); breast, prostate and lung are commoner primary sites.
- Gaucher's disease.
- Sickle cell anaemia.
- Homozygous thalassaemia.
- Osteoporosis from prolonged corticosteroid therapy e.g. for autoimmune disease.

Clinically

Presentation as local pain, discomfort and restriction of mobility.

Diagnosis

Confirmed by x-ray or other imaging.

Management

- Awareness of risk/possibility and early diagnosis.
- Analgesia.
- Orthopaedic—immobilisation and support as appropriate for nature and site of injury, surgical intervention including pinning or other fixation.
- Radiotherapy—local management of fracture 2° to local malignancy.
- Mobilisation—physiotherapy.
- Treatment of underlying condition predisposing to fracture.

Clinical approach

Raised ESR

The ESR remains an established, empirical test clinically useful as a method for identifying and monitoring the acute phase response. It is influenced by changes in fibrinogen, α-macroglobulins and immunoglobulins which enhance red cell aggregation *in vitro*.

Plasma viscosity is also an effective measure of acute phase reactants and can be used as an alternative to the ESR in clinical practice; increases in ESR and plasma viscosity generally parallel each other.

Normal ranges

- 0–10mm/h for ♂ 18–65 years.
- 1–20mm/h for ♀ 18–65 years.
- Upper limits of normal increase by 5–10mm/h for patients >65 years.
- Other factors e.g. Hct influence the ESR.
- Should be regarded as semiquantitative.
- Marked elevations are clinically significant.
- Modest elevations can be more problematic to interpret.

The main advantages to the ESR are its low cost and technical simplicity allied to the absence of a more accurate, inexpensive and technically simple alternative.

Causes of raised ESR	
Pregnancy	Increases in pregnancy; maximal in 3rd trimester
Infections	Acute and chronic infections, including TB *Note*: ↑ ESR also occurs in HIV infection
Collagen disorders	Rheumatoid, SLE, polymyalgia rheumatica, vasculitides etc. (including temporal arteritis); ESR useful as non-specific monitor of disease activity
Other inflammatory processes	Inflammatory bowel disease, sarcoidosis, post-MI
Neoplastic conditions	Carcinomatosis, NHL, Hodgkin's disease and paraproteinaemias (benign & malignant)

Investigations

Given the wide range of situations in which a raised ESR can arise, further investigation depends on a carefully conducted history and examination. In the absence of likely causes from these, simple initial laboratory and radiology assessments to include urinalysis, full blood count and film examination, urea, electrolytes, plasma protein electrophoresis, an autoimmune profile and CXR should represent a practical and pragmatic primary diagnostic screen.

📖 *p632.*

Clinical approach

Serum or urine paraprotein

Differential diagnosis

Common

- Monoclonal gammopathy of undetermined significance (MGUS).
- Myeloma.
- Solitary plasmacytoma.
- Lymphoproliferative disorders e.g. CLL, NHL, Waldenström's.

Less common

- Autoimmune disorders e.g. rheumatoid arthritis, SLE.
- Polymyalgia rheumatica.

Rare

- AL amyloid (primary amyloid).
- Plasma cell leukaemia.
- Heavy chain disease.
- Gaucher's disease.

Discriminating clinical features

MGUS—no symptoms or signs, normal FBC and biochemical profile, paraprotein level <30g/L and stable, no immuneparesis (rarely present), BM plasma cells <10%, no lytic lesions.

Plasmacytoma—localised bone pain, low paraprotein level, isolated bony lesion.

Myeloma—symptoms and signs of anaemia or hyperviscosity (📖 *p510*); bone pain or tenderness, raised Ca^{2+}, creatinine, urate; high β-2 microglobulin and low albumin; immuneparesis; ***paraprotein >30g/L of IgG or >20g/L of IgA or heavy BenceJones proteinuria; BM >10% plasma cells; lytic bone lesions on x-ray***. Minimum diagnostic criteria are at least 2 of emboldened items.

Plasma cell leukaemia—as myeloma but fulminant history. Plasma cells seen on blood film.

Heavy chain disease—rare, characterised by a single heavy chain only in serum or urine electrophoresis. Presence of any light chain excludes.

Amyloid—myriad clinical features. Diagnosis on biopsy of affected site or, if inaccessible, by BM or rectal biopsy—characteristic fibrils stain with Congo Red and show green birefringence in polarised light.

CLL and NHL—systemic symptoms e.g. fever, night sweats, weight loss. Lymphadenopathy or hepatosplenomegaly likely. Confirm on BM or node biopsy.

Waldenström's—as for CLL but with symptoms or signs of hyperviscosity (📖 *p284*).

Autoimmune disorders—suggested by joint pain, skin rashes, multisystem disease. Confirm on autoimmune profile including rheumatoid factor, ANA, ANCA.

📖 *p272*.

Clinical approach

Anaemia in pregnancy

Physiological changes in red cell and plasma volume occur during pregnancy.

- Red cell mass ↑ by ≤30%.
- Plasma volume ↑ ≤60%.
- Net effect to ↑ blood volume by ≤50% with lowering of the normal Hb concentration to 10.0–11.0g/dL during pregnancy. MCV increases during pregnancy.
- Iron deficiency is a common problem and cause of anaemia in pregnancy.

Cause of ↑ requirements	Amount of additional Fe
↑ Red cell mass	~500mg
Fetal requirements	~300mg
Placental requirements	~5mg
Basal losses over pregnancy (1.0–1.5mg/d)	~250mg

These result in a total requirement of ≤1000mg Fe requiring an average daily intake of 3.5–4.0mg/d. Average Western diet provides <4.0mg Fe/d so that balance is marginal during pregnancy. Diets with Fe mainly in non-haem form (e.g. vegetables) provide less Fe available for absorption. Thus a high risk of developing Fe deficiency anaemia which is exacerbated if pre-conception Fe stores are reduced.

Folate requirements are increased during pregnancy because of increased cellular demands; folate levels tend to drop during pregnancy.

Prophylaxis recommendation to give 40–60mg elemental Fe/d which will increase availability of dietary absorbable Fe and protect against chronic Fe deficiency; debated whether supplements required by all pregnant women or only for those in at-risk socio-economic and nutritionally deficient groups. Folate supplementation is recommended for all and also appears to reduce incidence of neural tube defects.

- Dilutional anaemia—Hb seldom <10.0g/dL (requires no therapy).
- Fe deficiency—may occur with normal MCV because of ↑ MCV associated with pregnancy; check serum ferritin and give Fe replacement; assess and treat the underlying cause.
- Blood loss—sudden ↓ in Hb may signify fetomaternal bleeding or other forms of concealed obstetric bleeding.
- Folate deficiency—macrocytic anaemia in pregnancy almost invariably will be due to folate deficiency (B_{12} deficiency is extremely rare during pregnancy).
- Microangiopathic haemolysis/DIC may be seen in eclampsia or following placental abruption or intrauterine death. HELLP syndrome (*p34*) is rare but serious cause of anaemia.
- Anaemia may also arise during pregnancy from other unrelated causes and should be investigated.

Clinical approach

Thrombocytopenia in pregnancy

A normal uncomplicated pregnancy is associated with a platelet count in the normal range though up to 10% of normal deliveries may be associated with mild thrombocytopenia (>100 × 10^9/L). Detection of thrombocytopenia in a pregnant patient requires consideration not only of the diagnoses listed in the previous section but also the conditions associated with pregnancy which cause thrombocytopenia. An additional important consideration is the possible effect on the fetus and its delivery.

If thrombocytopenia is detected late in pregnancy, most women will have a platelet count result from the booking visit (at 10–12 weeks) for comparison. Mild thrombocytopenia (100–150 × 10^9/L) detected for the first time during an uncomplicated pregnancy is not associated with any risk to the fetus nor does it require special obstetric intervention other than hospital delivery.

Non-immune thrombocytopenia

- Thrombocytopenia may develop in association with pregnancy-induced hypertension, pre-eclampsia or eclampsia. Successful treatment of hypertension may be associated with improvement in thrombocytopenia which is believed to be due to consumption. Treatment of hypertension, pre-eclampsia or eclampsia may necessitate delivery of the fetus who is not at risk of thrombocytopenia.
  HELLP syndrome (haemolysis, elevated liver enzymes and low platelets) may occur in pregnancy.
- A number of obstetric complications, notably retention of a dead fetus, abruptio placentae and amniotic fluid embolism, are associated with DIC (📖 *p512*).

Immune thrombocytopenia may occur in pregnancy and women with chronic ITP may become pregnant. Therapeutic considerations must include an assessment of the risk to the fetus of transplacental passage of antiplatelet antibody causing fetal thrombocytopenia and a risk of haemorrhage before or during delivery. There is no reliable parameter for the assessment of fetal risk which, although relatively low, is most significant in women with pre-existing chronic ITP. Note: the severity of the mother's ITP has no bearing on the fetal platelet count.

Women with a platelet count <20 × 10^9/L due to ITP should receive standard prednisolone therapy or IVIg (📖 *p388*). If prednisolone fails or is contraindicated, IVIg should be administered and may need to be repeated at 3 week intervals. Splenectomy should be avoided (high rate of fetal loss). Enthusiasm has waned for assessing the fetal platelet count during pregnancy by cordocentesis followed by platelet transfusion. Fetal scalp sampling in early labour is unreliable and hazardous. Delivery should occur in an obstetric unit with paediatric support and the neonate's platelet count should be monitored for several days as delayed falls in the platelet count occur.

BCSH Guidelines (2003) Guidelines for the investigation and management of idiopathic thrombocytopenic purpura in adults, children and in pregnancy. *Br J Haematol*, **120**, 574–596.

Clinical approach

37

Prolonged bleeding after surgery

Prolonged bleeding following surgery often requires urgent haematological opinion and investigation. Usually the cause of the bleeding is surgical, i.e. due to local factors, and not a reflection of any underlying systemic bleeding disorder.

History and clinical assessment

- Past history in relation to previous haemostatic challenges e.g. previous surgery, dental extractions. Ask specific questions about whether blood transfusion was required.
- Presence of specific clinical problems e.g. impaired liver or renal function.
- Recent drug history—especially aspirin or NSAIDs which can affect platelet function. Also enquire about cytotoxic drugs and anticoagulants.
- Family history of bleeding problems especially after surgery.
- Nature of the surgery and intrinsic haemorrhagic risks of procedure.
- Whether surgery was elective or emergency (in emergency surgery known risk factors are less likely to have been corrected).
- Check case record or ask surgeon/anaesthetist for information on intraoperative bleeding, technical problems etc.
- Whether surgery involves a high risk of triggering DIC e.g. pancreatic or major hepatobiliary surgery.
- Detailed physical examination is not usually practical but bruising, ecchymoses or purpura should be assessed especially if remote from the site of surgery.
- What blood products have been used and over how long? Transfusion of several units of RBCs over a short period of time will dilute available clotting factors.
- Review preoperative investigation results and other information available in the record on past procedures and/or investigations.

Investigation

- Ensure samples not taken from heparinised line.
- FBC with platelet count and blood film examination.
- PT, APTT and fibrinogen.

  With normal platelets and coagulation screen bleeding is usually surgical and the patient should be supported with blood and urgent surgical re-exploration undertaken. Platelet function abnormalities may occur with aspirin/NSAIDs, uraemia or extracorporeal circuits. Prolongation of both PT and APTT suggests massive bleeding and inadequate replacement, DIC, underlying liver disease or oral anticoagulants. Disproportionate, isolated increases in either PT or APTR are more likely to indicate previously undiagnosed clotting factor deficiencies. A low platelet count may reflect dilution and consumption from bleeding or DIC if platelets were known to be normal preoperatively.

Treatment

- Low platelets or platelet function abnormalities:
  Give 1–2 adult doses of platelets stat.
- DIC—give 2 adult doses of platelets are 4 units FFP (10–20 units of cryoprecipitate if fibrinogen low) and recheck PT, APTT and FBC.
- Anticoagulant effect:
  heparin—reverse with protamine sulphate.

warfarin—reverse with FFP or PCC.
- Empirical tranexamic acid or aprotinin may be tried if bleeding continues despite the above.

Positive sickle test (HbS solubility test)

The decreased solubility of deoxyHbS forms the basis of this test. Blood is added to a buffered solution of a reducing agent e.g. sodium dithionate. HbS is precipitated by the solution and produces a turbid appearance. *Note*: does not discriminate between sickle cell *trait* and *homozygous disease*.

Use

This is a quick screening test (takes ~20 mins), often used preoperatively to detect HbS.

Action if sickle test +ve

- Delay elective operation until established whether *disease* or *trait*.
- Ask about family history of sickle cell anaemia or symptoms of SCA.
- FBC and film.

FBC and film features of sickle trait vs. disease	
Sickle cell trait	FBC— normal or ↓ MCV & MCH, no anaemia Film normal (may be microcytosis or target cells)
Sickle cell disease	FBC—Hb~7–8g/dL (range ~4–11g/dL) Film—sickled RBCs, target cells, polychromasia, basophilic stippling, NRBC (hyposplenic features in adults)

- Hb electrophoresis.
- Group and antibody screen serum.

False +ve results

- Low Hb.
- Severe leucocytosis.
- Hyperproteinaemia.
- Unstable Hb.

False –ve results

- Infants <6 months.
- HbS <20% (e.g. following exchange blood transfusion).

Sickle test not recommended as a screening test in pregnancy as it will not detect other Hb variants that interact with HbS e.g. β thalassaemia trait. Standard Hb electrophoresis of at-risk groups should be performed (and of all pregnant women if a high local ethnic population).

Clinical approa[illegible]

Red cell disorders

The peripheral blood film in anaemias

Morphological abnormalities and variants	
Microcytic RBCs	Fe deficiency, thalassaemia trait & syndromes, congenital sideroblastic anaemia, anaemia of chronic disorders
Macrocytic RBCs	Alcohol/liver disease (round macrocytes), MDS, pregnancy and newborn, haemolysis, B_{12} or folate deficiency, hydroxyurea and antimetabolites (oval macrocytes), acquired sideroblastic anaemia, hypothyroidism, chronic respiratory failure, aplastic anaemia
Dimorphic RBCs	Fe deficiency responding to iron, mixed Fe and B_{12}/folate deficiency, sideroblastic anaemia, post-transfusion
Polychromatic RBCs	Response to bleeding or haematinic Rx, haemolysis, BM infiltration
Spherocytes	HS, haemolysis e.g. warm AIHA, delayed transfusion reaction, ABO HDN, DIC and MAHA, post-splenectomy
Pencil/rod cells	Fe deficiency anaemia, thalassaemia trait & syndromes, PK deficiency
Elliptocytes	Hereditary elliptocytosis, MPD and MDS
Fragmented red cells	MAHA, DIC, renal failure, HUS, TTP
Teardrop RBCs	Myelofibrosis, metastatic marrow infiltration, MDS
Sickle cells	Sickle cell anaemia, other sickle syndromes (*not* sickle trait)
Target cells	Liver disease, Fe deficiency, thalassaemia, HbC syndromes.
Crenated red cells	Usually storage or EDTA artifact. Genuine RBC crenation may be seen post-splenectomy and in renal failure
Burr cells	Renal failure
Acanthocytes	Hereditary acanthocytosis, a-β-lipoproteinaemia, McLeod red cell phenotype, PK deficiency, chronic liver disease (esp. Zieve's)
Bite cells	G6PD deficiency, oxidative haemolysis
Basophilic stippling	Megaloblastic anaemia, lead poisoning, MDS, haemoglobinopathies
Rouleaux	Chronic inflammation, paraproteinaemia, myeloma
↑ Reticulocytes	Bleeding, haemolysis, marrow infiltration, severe hypoxia, response to haematinic therapy
Heinz bodies	Not seen in normals (removed by spleen), small numbers seen post-splenectomy, oxidant drugs, G6PD deficiency, sulphonamides, unstable Hb (Hb Zurich, Köln)
Howell-Jolly bodies	Made of DNA, generally removed by the spleen, dyserythropoietic states e.g. B_{12} deficiency, MDS, post-splenectomy, hyposplenism
H bodies	HbH inclusions, denatured HbH (β_4 tetramer), stain with methylene blue, seen in HbH disease ($--/-\alpha$), less prominent in α thalassaemia trait, not present in normals
Hyposplenic blood film	Howell–Jolly bodies, target cells, occasional nucleated RBCs, lymphocytosis, macrocytosis, acanthocytes

Red cell disorders

Anaemia in renal disease

Anaemia is consistently found in the presence of chronic renal failure. Severity generally relates to the degree of renal impairment. The dominant mechanism is inadequate production of erythropoietin. Other contributory factors include (i) suppressive effects of uraemia and (ii) ↓ in RBC survival. Uraemia impairs platelet function leading to blood loss and Fe deficiency. Small amounts of blood are inevitably left in the tubing following dialysis so that blood loss and Fe deficiency are further contributory factors in dialysis patients. Folate is lost in dialysis and supplementation is required to avoid deficiency. Aluminium toxicity (from trace amounts in dialysis fluids) and osteitis fibrosa from hyperparathyroidism are rare contributory factors.

Laboratory features

- Hb typically 5.0–10.0g/dL.
- MCV ↔.
- Blood film—mostly normochromic RBCs; schistocytes and acanthocytes present. No specific abnormalities in WBC or platelets.
- Microangiopathic haemolytic changes present in vasculitic collagen disorders with renal failure and classically in HUS and TTP.

Management

- Short term treatment with RBC transfusion, based on *symptoms* (not Hb).
- Correction of Fe and folic acid deficiencies.
- Erythropoietin (Epo) will correct anaemia in most patients.
  Start at 50–100units/kg SC × 3/week. Give IV iron at same time. Response apparent <10 weeks; reduced doses required as maintenance. Renal Association guidelines have been produced for application and monitoring of Epo therapy. Although expensive it improves quality of life and avoids transfusion dependency and iron overload.

Side effects of Epo

- ↑ BP.
- Pure red cell aplasia.
- Thrombotic tendency.

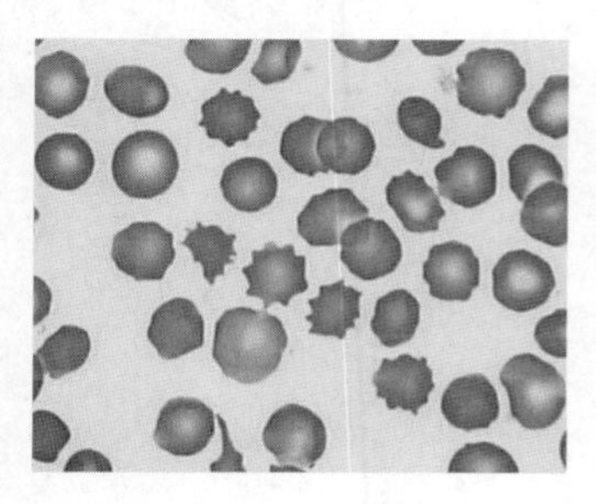

Blood film: chronic renal failure with burr (irregular shaped) cells.

www.nephronline.org/standards3/

Eschbach, J.W. *et al.* (1987) Correction of the anemia of end-stage renal disease with recombinant human erythropoietin. Results of a combined phase I and II clinical trial. *N Engl J Med*, **316**, 73–78; Levin, N., *et al.* (1997) National Kidney Foundation: Dialysis Outcome Quality Initiative--development of methodology for clinical practice guidelines. *Nephrol Dial Transplant*, **12**, 2060–2063.

Anaemia in endocrine disease

Anaemia and other haematological effects occur in various endocrine disorders. The abnormalities will usually correct as the endocrine abnormality is corrected.

Pituitary disorders

Deficiency/hypopituitarism is associated with normochromic, normocytic anaemia; associated leucopenia may also occur. Abnormalities correct as normal function is restored, by replacement therapy.

Thyroid disorders

Hypothyroidism may produce a mild degree of anaemia; MCV usually ↑ but may be normal. Corrects on restoration of normal thyroid function. Menorrhagia occurs in hypothyroidism and can result in associated Fe deficiency. B_{12} levels should be checked because of the association with other autoimmune disorders (e.g. pernicious anaemia).

Thyrotoxicosis may be associated with mild degrees of normochromic anaemia in 20% of cases which corrects as function is normalised. Erythroid activity is increased but a disproportionate increase in plasma volume means either no change in Hb concentration or mild anaemia. Haematinic deficiencies occur and should be excluded.

Adrenal disorders

Hypoadrenalism results in normochromic, normocytic anaemia; the plasma volume is ↓ which masks the true degree of associated anaemia. The abnormalities are corrected by replacement mineralocorticoids.

Hyperadrenalism (Cushing's) results in erythrocytosis with a typical net increase in Hb (by 1–2g/dL). Occurs whether Cushing's is primary or iatrogenic. Mechanism is unclear.

Parathyroid disorders—hyperparathyroidism may be associated with anaemia from impairment of erythropoietin production, or in some cases from secondary marrow sclerosis.

Sex hormones—androgens stimulate erythropoiesis and are occasionally used to stimulate red cell production in aplastic anaemia. The influence of androgens explains the higher Hb in adult ♂ *cf.* ♀.

Diabetes mellitus when poorly controlled may be associated with anaemia; however, the majority of haematological abnormalities in diabetes mellitus result from secondary disease related complications e.g. renal failure.

Red cell disorders

Anaemia in joint disease

Rheumatoid arthritis, psoriatic arthropathy and osteoarthritis may be complicated by anaemia. Various factors contribute to anaemia, commonly more than one is present, especially in rheumatoid arthritis. Some of the mechanisms that give rise to anaemia in rheumatoid also apply in other connective tissue disease, e.g. SLE, polyarteritis nodosa, etc.

Anaemia of chronic disorders (ACD)

ACD is a cytokine-driven suppression of red cell production. The clinical problem is to being able to recognise the presence of other contributory factors in pathogenesis of the anaemia. Bone marrow macrophages fail to pass their stored iron to developing RBCs and a lower than expected rise in erythropoietin suggesting some inhibition in its pathway. Marrow also appears less responsive to Epo. ↑ IL-1 has been identified. Detailed studies suggest a synergistic effect of IL-1 with T-cells to produce IFN-γ which can suppress erythroid activity. May also be ↑ levels of TNF-α which inhibits erythropoiesis through release of IFN-β from marrow stromal cells.

Typical features of ACD

- Hb range 7.0–11.0g/dL.
- MCV is usually ↔ but when longstanding the MCV is moderately ↓ (may look like iron deficiency).
- Ferritin usually ↔ but may be ↑.
- Serum iron ↔ or ↓, TIBC ↔ or ↓.
- Serum transferrin receptor levels normal.
- Bone marrow Fe stores plentiful.

Additional mechanisms of anaemia in rheumatoid disease	
Autoimmune phenomena	Warm antibody AIHA in association with rheumatoid and other collagen disorders; film will show reticulocytosis and +ve DAT Red cell aplasia
Drug related problems	Chronic blood loss (caused by medication) Drug side effects e.g. macrocytosis from antimetabolite immunosuppressives, e.g. azathioprine and methotrexate, oxidative haemolysis secondary to dapsone or sulfasalazine (occurs in normal individuals as well as those with G6PD deficiency) Anaemia secondary to gold therapy for rheumatoid arthritis Idiosyncratic reactions, unexplained or unforeseeable reactions such as marrow aplasia Rare autoimmune haemolysis due to mefenamic acid, diclofenac or ibuprofen
2° to other organ problems	Hypersplenism, Felty's syndrome in rheumatoid, renal failure in SLE or polyarteritis

Management

Supportive transfusion in symptomatic patients; coexistent Fe deficiency should be excluded and treated. Minority may be suitable for/responsive to erythropoietin therapy.

Bleeding and iron deficiency

Usually secondary to use of NSAIDs—consider and exclude other causes of blood loss which may occur in this patient group.

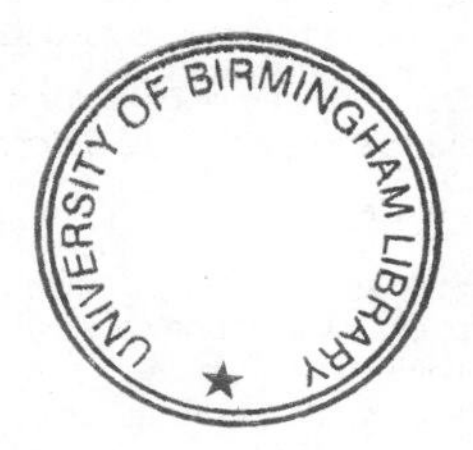

Bron, D., Meuleman, N. & Mascaux, C. (2001) Biological basis of anemia. *Semin Oncol*, **28**, 1–6.

Anaemia in gastrointestinal disease

Anaemia occurs in GIT disorders through mechanisms of blood loss, anaemia of chronic disease (ACD), specific disease-related complications or drug side effects/idiosyncrasy occurring singly or in various combinations.

Blood loss in gastrointestinal disease	
Acute	Immediately following acute haemorrhage—RBC indices usually normal Normochromic anaemia
Acute on chronic	RBC indices show low normal or marginally ↓, especially MCV Film shows mixture of normochromic & hypochromic RBCs ('dimorphic')
Chronic	RBC indices show established chronic Fe deficiency features ↓ MCV, MCH, platelets often ↑

Anaemia in GIT disorders can be simply considered against some of the commoner problems arising through the GIT:

Oesophageal—bleeding from peptic oesophagitis, association of oesophageal web and chronic Fe deficiency.

Gastric—pernicious anaemia and B_{12} deficiency, late effects of partial or total gastrectomy producing B_{12} and/or Fe deficiency. Microangiopathic haemolytic anaemia from metastatic adenocarcinoma.

Small bowel—malabsorption states e.g. Fe and/or folate deficiency 2° to coeliac disease, malabsorption from other problems including inflammatory bowel disease; hyposplenism secondary to coeliac with or without ↑ platelets.

Large bowel—blood loss anaemia from inflammatory bowel disorders. *Note*: these may also be associated with ACD. Rare occurrence of autoimmune haemolysis associated with ulcerative colitis.

Pancreas—anaemia of chronic disease associated with carcinoma or chronic pancreatitis, DIC associated with acute pancreatitis.

Liver—see *p54*.

Drug related anaemia arises through

- Upper GIT irritation causing blood loss—aspirin, NSAIDs, corticosteroids.
- Bleeding due to specific drugs e.g. warfarin and heparin.
- Drug-induced haemolysis e.g. oxidative (Heinz body) haemolysis due to sulphasalazine or dapsone.
- Production impairment e.g. aplasia secondary to mesalazine.

Red cell disorders

Anaemia in liver disease

Anaemia is common in chronic liver disorders. There are several possible causes including:

- Anaemia of chronic disease—part of marrow response to chronic inflammatory processes.
- Macrocytosis ± anaemia: specific effects on membrane lipids cause ↑ MCV.
- Alcohol—direct suppressive effect on erythropoiesis with ↑ MCV.
- Folate deficiency: seen in alcoholic liver disease⟶nutritional deficiency and/or direct effect of alcohol on folate metabolism.
- Blood loss from oesophageal varices⟶acute or chronic anaemia.
- Hypersplenism—portal hypertension can produce marked splenic enlargement leading to hypersplenism.
- Haemolytic anaemias e.g.
  - Autoimmune haemolytic anaemia in association with chronic active hepatitis.
  - Zieve's syndrome (hypertriglyceridaemia + self-limiting haemolysis due to acute alcohol excess).
  - Viral hepatitis may provoke oxidative haemolysis in those with G6PD deficiency.
  - Acute liver failure—DIC and MAHA may occur.
  - Acanthocytosis: acute haemolytic anaemia with acanthocytosis (spur cell anaemia). Rare. Usually late stage liver disease, with poor prognosis.

Red cell disorders

Iron deficiency anaemia

Microcytic anaemia is common and the commonest cause is chronic iron deficiency.

Iron physiology and metabolism

Normal (Western) diet provides ≅15mg of iron/d, of which 5–10% is absorbed in duodenum and upper jejunum. Ferrous (Fe^{2+}) iron is better absorbed than ferric (Fe^{3+}) iron. Total body iron store ≅ 4g. Around 1mg of iron/d lost in urine, faeces, sweat and cells shed from the skin and GIT. Iron deficiency is commoner in ♀ of reproductive age since menstrual losses account for ~20mg Fe/month and in pregnancy an additional 500–1000mg Fe may be lost (transferred from mother→fetus).

Causes of iron deficiency	
Reproductive system	Menorrhagia
GI tract	Oesophagitis, oesophageal varices, hiatus hernia (ulcerated), peptic ulcer, inflammatory bowel disease, haemorrhoids, carcinoma: stomach, colorectal, (rarely angiodysplasia, hereditary haemorrhagic telangiectasia)
Malabsorption	Coeliac disease, atrophic gastritis (*note*: may also result from Fe deficiency), gastrectomy
Physiological	Growth spurts, pregnancy
Dietary	Vegans, elderly
Genitourinary system	Haematuria (uncommon cause)
Others	PNH, frequent venesection e.g. blood donation, Gaucher's disease
Worldwide	Commonest cause is hookworm infestation

Assessment

Clinical history—review potential sources of blood loss, especially GIT loss.

Menstrual loss— quantitation may be difficult; ask about number of tampons used per day, how often these require changing, and duration.

Other sources of blood loss e.g. haematuria and haemoptysis (*these are not common causes of iron deficiency*). Ask patient if he/she has been a blood donor—regular blood donation over many years may cause chronic iron store depletion.

Drug therapy e.g. NSAIDs and corticosteroids may cause GI irritation and blood loss.

Past medical history e.g. previous gastric surgery (→malabsorption). Ask about previous episodes of anaemia and treatments with iron.

In patients with iron deficiency assume underlying cause is *blood loss* until proved otherwise. In developed countries pure dietary iron lack causing iron deficiency is almost unknown.

Examination

- General examination including assessment of mucous membranes (e.g. hereditary haemorrhagic telangiectasia).
- Seek possible sources of blood loss.
- Abdominal examination, rectal examination and sigmoidoscopy mandatory.
- Gynaecological examination also required.

Laboratory tests

- Hb ↓.
- ↓ MCV (<76FLz) and ↓ MCHC (*note:* ↓ MCV in thalassaemia and ACD).
- Red cell distribution width (RDW): ↑ in iron deficiency states with a greater frequency than in ACD or thalassaemia trait.
- Serum ferritin (measurement of iron/TIBC generally unhelpful). *Ferritin assay preferred—a low serum ferritin identifies the presence of iron deficiency but as an acute phase protein it can be ↑, masking iron deficiency. ↓ iron and ↑ TIBC indicates iron deficiency.*
- The soluble transferrin assay (sTfR) is useful in cases where ↑ ESR. sTfR is ↑ in iron deficiency but ↔ in anaemia in presence of ↑ ESR (e.g. rheumatoid, other inflammatory states). This assay is not universally available at present.
- % hypochromic RBCs—some modern analysers provide this parameter. 4% hypo RBCs are seen in iron deficiency but also thalassaemia, CRF on Epo where insufficient iron given.
- Zinc protoporphyrin (ZPP)—in the absence of iron, zinc is incorporated into protoporphyrin and can be measured.
- Examination of BM aspirate (iron stain) is occasionally useful.
- Theoretically FOB testing may be of value in iron deficiency but results can be misleading. False +ve results seen in high dietary meat intake.

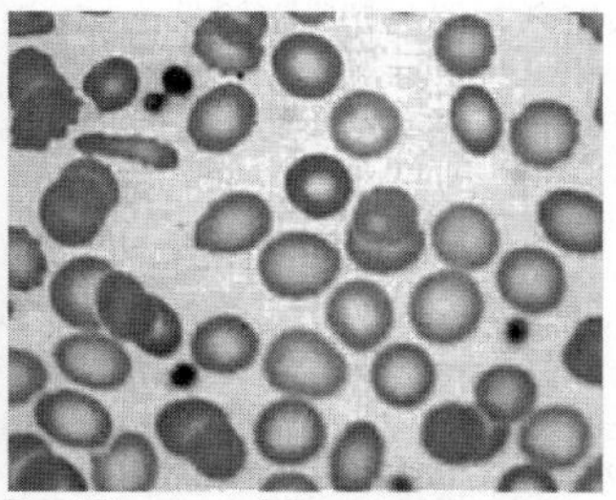

Blood film in iron deficiency anaemia: note pale red cells with pencil cell (top left).

Treatment of iron deficiency

Simplest, safest and cheapest treatment is oral ferrous salts, e.g. $FeSO_4$ (Fe gluconate and fumarate equally acceptable). Provide an oral dose of elemental iron of 150–200mg/d. Side effects in 10–20% patients (e.g. abdominal distension, constipation and/or diarrhoea)—try ↓ the daily dose to bd or od. Liquid iron occasionally necessary, e.g. children or adults with swallowing difficulties. Increasing dietary iron intake has no routine place in the management of iron deficiency except where intake is grossly deficient.

Response to replacement

A rise of Hb of 2.0g/dL over 3 weeks is expected. MCV will ↑ concomitantly with Hb. Reticulocytes may ↑ in response to iron therapy but is not a reliable indicator of response.

Duration of treatment

Generally ~6 months. After Hb and MCV are normal continue iron for at least 3 months to replenish iron stores.

Failure of response

- Is the diagnosis of iron deficiency correct?
  - *Consider anaemia of chronic disorders or thalassaemia trait.*
- Is there an additional complicating illness?
  - *Chronic infection, collagen disorder or neoplasm.*
- Is the patient complying with prescribed medication?
- Is the preparation of iron adequate in dosage and/or formulation?
- Is the patient continuing to bleed excessively?
- Is there malabsorption?
- Are there other haematinic deficiencies (e.g. B_{12} or folate) present?
- Reassess patient: ?evidence of continued blood loss or malabsorption.

Parenteral iron

Occasionally of value in genuine iron intolerance, if compliance is a problem, or if need to replace stores rapidly e.g. in pregnancy or prior to major surgery. *Note:* Hb will rise no faster than with oral iron.

Intravenous iron Iron may be administered IV as iron hydroxide sucrose complex.

Intramuscular iron e.g. iron sorbitol citrate. Usually ~10–20 IM injections over several week period *(note:* injections painful and lead to long-term skin discoloration at the injection site). Best avoided.

Andrews, N.C. (1999) Disorders of iron metabolism. *N Engl J Med*, **341**, 1986–1995; Kuhn, L.C. & Hentze, M.W. (1992) Coordination of cellular iron metabolism by post-transcriptional gene regulation. *J Inorg Biochem*, **47**, 183–195; Tapiero, H., Gate, L. & Tew, K.D. (2001) Iron: deficiencies and requirements. *Biomed Pharmacother*, **55**, 324–332.

Red cell disorders

Vitamin B_{12} deficiency

B_{12} deficiency presents with macrocytic, megaloblastic anaemia ranging from mild to severe (Hb <6.0g/dL). Symptoms are those of chronic anaemia, i.e. fatigue, dyspnoea on effort, etc. Neurological symptoms may also be present—classically peripheral paraesthesiae and disturbances of position and vibration sense. Occasionally neurological symptoms occur with no/minimal haematological upset. If uncorrected, the patient may develop subacute combined degeneration of the spinal cord→permanently ataxic.

Pathophysiology

B_{12} (along with folic acid) is required for DNA synthesis; B_{12} is also required for neurological functioning. B_{12} is absorbed in terminal ileum after binding to intrinsic factor produced by gastric parietal cells. Body stores of B_{12} are 2–3mg (sufficient for 3 years). B_{12} is found in meats, fish, eggs and dairy produce. Strictly vegetarian (vegan) diets are low in B_{12} although not all vegans develop clinical evidence of deficiency.

Presenting haematological abnormalities

- Macrocytic anaemia (MCV usually >110fL). In extreme cases RBC anisopoikilocytosis can result in MCV values lying just within normal range.
- RBC changes include oval macrocytosis, poikilocytosis, basophilic stippling, Howell–Jolly bodies, circulating megaloblasts.
- Hypersegmented neutrophils.
- Leucopenia and thrombocytopenia common.
- Bone marrow shows megaloblastic change; marked erythroid hyperplasia with predominance of early erythroid precursors, open atypical nuclear chromatin patterns, mitotic figures and 'giant' metamyelocytes.
- Iron stores usually ↑.
- Serum B_{12} ↓.
- Serum/red cell folate usually ↔ or ↑.
- LDH levels markedly ↑ reflecting ineffective erythropoiesis.
- Autoantibody screen in pernicious anaemia: 80–90% show circulating gastric parietal cell antibodies, 55% have circulating intrinsic factor antibodies. *Note*: parietal cell antibodies are not diagnostic since found in normals; IFA is only found in 50% of patients with PA but *is* diagnostic.

Causes of B_{12} deficiency

Pernicious anaemia	Commonest, due to autoimmune gastric atrophy resulting in loss of intrinsic factor production required for absorption of B_{12}. Incidence increases >40 years and often associated with other autoimmune problems, e.g. hypothyroidism.
Following total gastrectomy	May develop after major partial gastrectomy.
Ileal disease	Resection of ileum, Crohn's disease.

Blind loop syndromes	E.g. diverticulae or localised inflammatory bowel changes allowing bacterial overgrowth which then competes for available B_{12}.
Fish tapeworm	*Diphyllobothrium latum.*
Malabsorptive disorders	Tropical sprue, coeliac disease.
Dietary deficiency	E.g. vegans.
Other	Gaucher's disease

Management of B_{12} deficiency

1. Identify and correct cause if possible.
2. Above investigations are undertaken and a test of B_{12} absorption is carried out (e.g. Schilling test). Urinary excretion of a test dose of B_{12} labelled with trace amounts of radioactive cobalt is compared with excretion of B_{12} bound to intrinsic factor*; the test is done in two parts. B_{12} malabsorption corrected by intrinsic factor is diagnostic of pernicious anaemia (in absence of previous gastric surgery).
3. Management—hydroxocobalamin 1mg IM and folic acid PO should be given immediately.
4. Supportive measures—bed rest, O_2 and diuretics may be needed while awaiting response. Transfusion is best avoided but 2 units of concentrated RBCs may be used for patients *severely* compromised by anaemia (risk of precipitating cardiac failure); hypokalaemia is occasionally observed during the immediate response to B_{12} and serum $[K^+]$ should be monitored.
5. Response apparent in 3–5d with reticulocyte response of >10%; normoblastic conversion of marrow erythropoiesis in 12–24h. Patients frequently describe a subjective improvement within 24h.
6. B_{12} replacement therapy—initially hydroxocobalamin 5 × 1mg IM should be given during the first 2 weeks, thereafter maintenance injections are needed 3-monthly.
7. If dietary deficiency seems likely and B_{12} deficiency mild, worth trying oral B_{12} (cyanocobalamin 50–150μg or more, daily between meals)
8. Long term follow-up depends on the primary cause. Pernicious anaemia patients require lifelong treatment and should be checked annually with a full blood count and thyroid function; the incidence of gastric cancer is twice as high in these patients compared to the normal population.
9. Broad spectrum antibiotics should be given to suppress bacterial overgrowth in blind loop syndrome ± local surgery if appropriate. Long term IM B_{12} may be the pragmatic solution if blind loop cannot be corrected.

*Worldwide shortage of intrinsic factor at present, due to worries about human prion disease. This means that only part I Schilling test available in most centres.

Guidelines on the investigation and diagnosis of cobalamin and folate deficiencies. A publication of the British Committee for Standards in Haematology. BCSH General Haematology Test Force (1994). *Clin Lab Haematol*, **16**, 101–115; Toh, B.H., van Driel, I.R. & Gleeson, P.A. (1997) Pernicious anemia. *N Engl J Med*, **337**, 1441–1448.

Folate deficiency

Folate deficiency represents the other main deficiency cause of megaloblastic anaemia; haematological features indistinguishable from those of B_{12} deficiency. Distinction is on basis of demonstration of reduced red cell and serum folate.

▶▶ Megaloblastic anaemia patients should *never* receive empirical treatment with folic acid alone. ***If they lack B_{12}, folic acid is potentially capable of precipitating subacute combined degeneration of the cord.***

Pathophysiology

Adult body folate stores comprise 10–15mg; normal daily requirements are 0.1–0.2mg, i.e. sufficient for 3–4 months in absence of exogenous folate intake. Folate absorption from dietary sources is rapid; proximal jejunum is main site of absorption. Main dietary sources of folate are liver, green vegetables, nuts and yeast. Western diets contain ~0.5–0.7mg folate/d but availability may be lessened as folate is readily destroyed by cooking, especially in large volumes of water. Folate coenzymes are an essential part of DNA synthesis, hence the occurrence of megaloblastic change in deficiency.

Diagnosis

Haematological findings are identical to those seen in B_{12} deficiency—macrocytic, megaloblastic anaemia. Other findings also similar to B_{12} except parietal cell and intrinsic factor autoantibodies usually –ve. Reduced folate levels—*serum* folate levels reflect recent intake, *red cell folate* levels give a more reliable indication of folate status.

Causes of folate deficiency

↓ intake	Poor nutrition, e.g. poverty, old age, 'skid row' alcoholics.
↑ requirements/losses	Pregnancy, ↑ cell turnover, e.g. haemolysis, exfoliative dermatitis, renal dialysis.
Malabsorption	Coeliac disease, tropical sprue, Crohn's and other malabsorptive states.
Drugs	Phenytoin, barbiturates, valproate, oral contraceptives, nitrofurantoin may induce folate malabsorption.
Antifolate drugs	Methotrexate, trimethoprim, pentamidine *antagonise* folate *cf.* induce deficiency.
Alcohol	Poor nutrition *plus* a direct depressant effect on folate levels which can precipitate clinical folate deficiency.

Management

1. Treatment and support of severe anaemia as for B_{12} deficiency.

2. Folic acid 5mg/d PO (never on its own—*see above*), unless patient known to have normal B_{12} level.
3. Treatment of underlying cause e.g. in coeliac disease folate levels and absorption normalize once patient established on gluten-free diet. Long term supplementation advised in chronic haemolysis e.g. HbSS or HS.
4. Prophylactic folate supplements recommended in pregnancy and other states of increased demand e.g. prematurity.

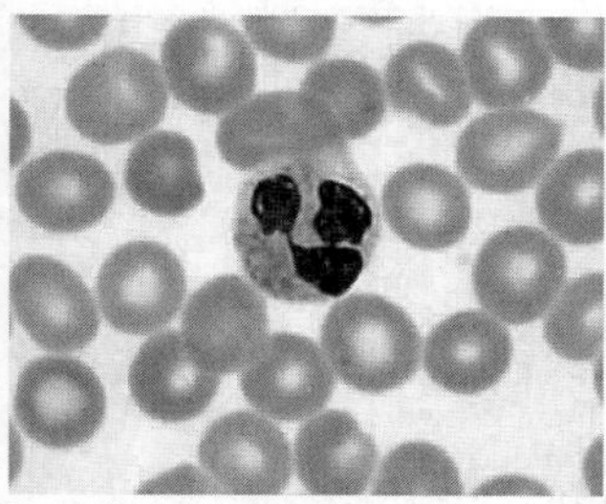

Blood film: normal neutrophil: usually has <5 lobes. This one has 3 lobes.

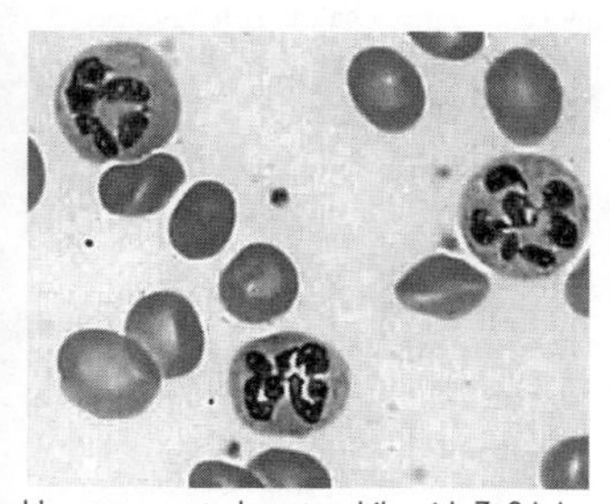

Hypersegmented neutrophils with 7–8 lobes: found in B_{12} *or* folate deficiency. *Note*: blood films and marrow appearances are identical in B_{12} and folate deficiencies.

Other causes of megaloblastic anaemia

Megaloblastic anaemia not due to actual deficiency of either B_{12} or folate is uncommon, but may occur in the following situations.

Congenital

- Transcobalamin II deficiency—absence of the key B_{12} transport protein results in severe megaloblastic anaemia (will correct with parenteral B_{12}).
- Congenital intrinsic factor deficiency—autosomal recessive, results in failure to produce intrinsic factor. Presents as megaloblastic anaemia up to age of 2 years and responds to parenteral B_{12}.
- Inborn errors of metabolism—errors in folate pathways, also occurs in orotic aciduria and Lesch–Nyhan syndrome.
- Megaloblastosis commonly present in the congenital dyserythropoietic anaemias (📖 p450).

Acquired

- MDS—often present in sideroblastic anaemia (RARS).
- Acute leukaemia—megaloblastic-like erythroid dysplasia in AML M6.
- Drug induced—secondary to antimetabolite drugs including 6-mercaptopurine, cytosine arabinoside, zidovudine and hydroxyurea.
- Anaesthetic agents—transient megaloblastic change after nitrous oxide.
- Alcohol excess—may result in megaloblastic change in absence of measurable folate deficiency.
- Vitamin C deficiency—occasionally results in megaloblastic change.

Red cell disorders

Anaemia in other deficiency states

Iron, folate or vitamin B_{12} deficiencies account for the majority of clinically significant deficiency syndromes resulting in anaemia. Anaemia is recognised as a complication in other vitamin deficiencies and in malnutrition.

Vitamin A deficiency

Produces chronic disorder like iron deficiency anaemia with ↓ MCV and MCH.

Vitamin B_6 (pyridoxine) deficiency

Can produce hypochromic microcytic anaemia; sideroblastic change may occur. Pyridoxine is given to patients on antituberculous therapy with isoniazid which is known to interfere with vitamin B_6 metabolism and cause sideroblastic anaemia.

Vitamin C deficiency

Occasionally associated with macrocytic anaemia (± megaloblastic change in 10%); since the main cause of vitamin C deficiency is inadequate diet or nutrition there may be evidence of other deficiencies.

Vitamin E deficiency

Occasionally seen in the neonatal period in low birth weight infants—results in haemolytic anaemia with abnormal RBC morphology.

Starvation

Normochromic anaemia ± leucopenia occurs in anorexia nervosa; features are not associated with any specific deficiency; bone marrow is typically hypocellular.

Red cell disorders

67

Haemolytic syndromes

Definition
Any situation in which there is a reduction in RBC life-span due to ↑ RBC destruction. Failure of compensatory marrow response results in anaemia. Predominant site of RBC destruction is red pulp of the spleen.

Classification—3 major types
1. Hereditary *vs.* acquired
2. Immune *vs.* non-immune
3. Extravascular *vs.* intravascular

Hereditary cause suggested if history of anaemia refractory to treatment in infancy ± FH e.g. other affected members, anaemia, gallstones, jaundice, splenectomy. ***Acquired*** haemolytic anaemia is suggested by sudden onset of symptoms/signs in adulthood. ***Intravascular*** haemolysis—takes place in peripheral circulation *cf.* ***extravascular*** haemolysis which occurs in RES.

Hereditary
- Red cell membrane disorders e.g. HS and hereditary elliptocytosis.
- Red cell enzymopathies e.g. G6PD and PK deficiencies.
- Abnormal Hb e.g. thalassaemias and sickle cell disease, unstable Hbs.

Acquired–immune
Alloimmune
- HDN
- RBC transfusion incompatibility

Autoimmune
- Warm AIHA–1° or 2° to SLE, CLL, drugs
- Cold–*Mycoplasma* or EBV infection,
- Cold haemagglutinin disease (CHAD)
- Lymphoproliferative disorders
- Paroxysmal cold haemoglobinuria (PCH)

Acquired–non-immune
- MAHA
- TTP/HUS
- Hypersplenism
- Prosthetic heart valves
- March haemoglobinuria
- Sepsis
- Malaria
- Paroxysmal nocturnal haemoglobinuria

Clinical features
Symptoms of anaemia e.g. breathlessness, fatigue. Urinary changes e.g. red or dark brown of haemoglobinuria. Symptoms of underlying disorder.

Confirm haemolysis is occurring
- Check FBC.
- Peripheral blood film—polychromasia, spherocytosis, fragmentation (schistocytes), helmet cells, echinocytes.
- ↑ reticulocytes.
- ↑ serum bilirubin (unconjugated).
- ↑ LDH.

- Low/absent serum haptoglobin (bind free Hb).
- Schumm's test (for intravascular haemolysis).
- Urinary haemosiderin (implies chronic intravascular haemolysis e.g. PNH).

Discriminant diagnostic features

Establish whether immune or non-immune—check DAT

?Immune if DAT +ve check IgG and C_3 specific reagents—suggest warm and cold antibody respectively. Screen serum for red cell alloantibodies.

?Cold antibody present—examine blood film for agglutination, check MCV on initial FBC sample and again after incubation at 37°C for 2h. High MCV at room temperature due to agglutinates falls to normal at 37°C. Check anti-I and anti-i titres for confirmation. Check *Mycoplasma* IgM and EBV serology, and for presence of Donath Landsteiner antibody (cold reacting IgG antibody with anti-P specificity).

?Warm antibody present—IgG +ve DAT only suggestive—examine film for spherocytes (usually prominent), lymphocytosis or abnormal lymphs to suggest LPD. Examine patient for nodes.

?Intravascular haemolysis—check for urinary haemosiderin, Schumm's test.

?Sepsis—check blood cultures.

?Malaria—examine thick and thin blood films for parasites.

?Renal/liver abnormality—examine for hepatomegaly, splenomegaly, LFTs and U&E.

?Low platelets—consider TTP/HUS.

?Haemoglobinopathy—check Hb electrophoresis.

?Red cell membrane abnormality—check family history and perform red cell fragility test.

?Red cell enzyme disorder—check family history and do G6PD and PK assay. *Note*: enzymes may be falsely normal if reticulocytosis.

?PNH—check immunophenotyping for CD55 + CD59 (Ham's acid lysis test now largely obsolete).

Treatment

Treat underlying disorder. Give folic acid and iron supplements if low.

Gehrs, B.C. & Friedberg, R.C. (2002) Autoimmune hemolytic anemia. *Am J Hematol*, **69**, 258–271.

Genetic control of haemoglobin production

Hb comprises 4 protein subunits (e.g. adult Hb = $2 \times \alpha + 2 \times \beta$ chains, $\alpha_2\beta_2$) each linked to a haem group. Production of different globin chains varies from embryo→adult to meet the particular environment at each stage. Globin genes are located on chromosomes 11 and 16. All globins related to α globin are located on chromosome 16; all those related to β globin are on chromosome 11. The sequence in which they are produced during development reflects their physical order on chromosomes such that ζ is the first α-like globin to be produced in life. After ζ expression stops, α production occurs ($\zeta \rightarrow \alpha$ switch). On chromosome 11 the arrangement of β-like globin genes follows the order (from left→right) $\varepsilon \rightarrow \gamma \rightarrow \delta \rightarrow \beta$ mirroring the β-like globin chains produced during development. As embryo develops into fetus, ζ production stops and α is produced. The α globin combines with γ chains and produces $\alpha_2\gamma_2$ (fetal Hb, HbF). After birth γ production ↓ and δ and β chains are produced. Adults have predominantly HbA ($\alpha_2\beta_2$) although small amounts of HbA$_2$ ($\alpha_2\delta_2$) and HbF are produced.

Hb switching is physiological but the mechanism is unclear. HbF ($\alpha_2\gamma_2$) binds O_2 more tightly than adult haemoglobin, ensuring adequate O_2 delivery to the fetus which must extract its O_2 from mother's circulation. After birth the lungs expand and the O_2 is derived from the air, with β production replacing that of γ, leading to an increase in adult haemoglobin ($\alpha_2\beta_2$).

Haemoglobin	Globin chains	Amount
Embryo		
Hb Gower 1	$\zeta_2\varepsilon_2$	42%*
Hb Gower 2	$\alpha_2\varepsilon_2$	24%*
Hb Portland	$\zeta_2\gamma_2$	
*by 5th week		
Fetus		
HbF	$\alpha_2\gamma_2$	85%
HbA	$\alpha_2\beta_2$	5–10%
Adult		
HbA	$\alpha_2\beta_2$	97%
HbA$_2$	$\alpha_2\delta_2$	2.5%
HbF	$\alpha_2\gamma_2$	0.5%

Haemoglobin abnormalities

Fall into 2 major groups: *structural abnormalities* of Hb due to alterations in DNA coding for the globin protein leading to an abnormal amino acid in the globin molecule, e.g. sickle haemoglobin (β^S). Second group of Hb disorders results from imbalanced globin chain production—globins produced are structurally normal but their relative amounts are incorrect and lead to *the thalassaemias*.

Haemoglobinopathies result in significant morbidity and mortality on a world-wide scale. Patients with these disorders are also seen in Northern Europe and the UK, especially in areas with significant Greek, Italian, Afro-Caribbean and Asian populations.

α-like genes on chromosome 16

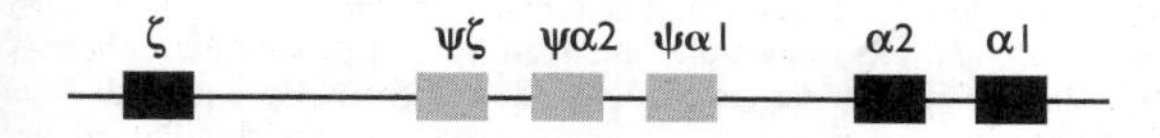

β-like genes on chromosome 11

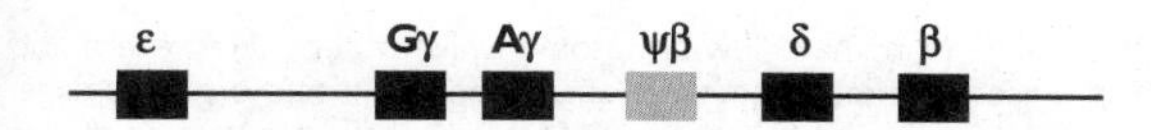

Arrangement of α-like and β-like globin genes (ψ indicates pseudogene)

α globin switching

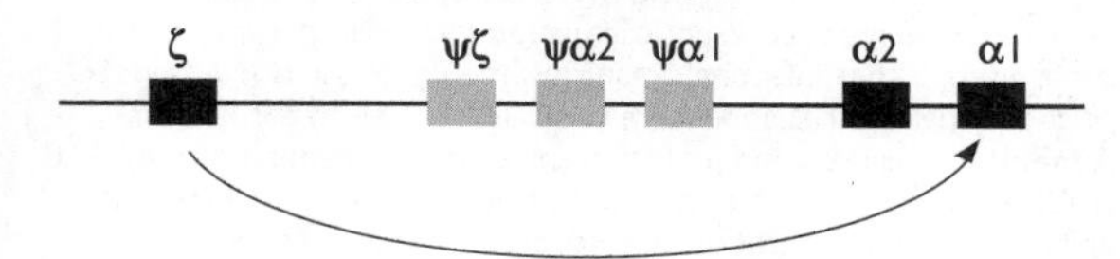

β globin switching

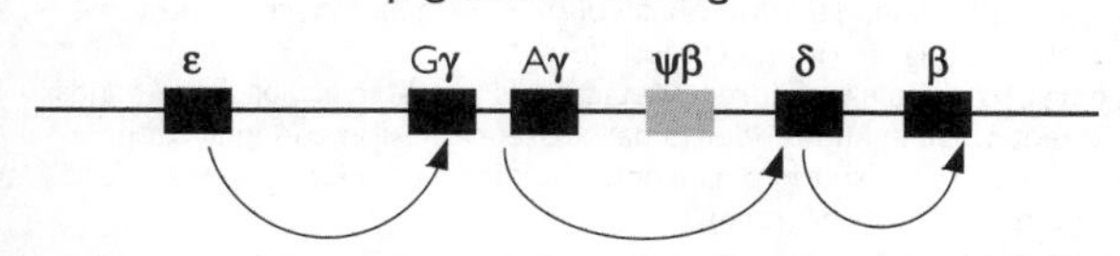

Globin gene switching during development

Sickling disorders

Sickle cell anaemia (homozygous SS, $\beta^S\beta^S$), HbSC ($\beta^S\beta^C$), HbS/β^+ or β° thalassaemia, and HbSD ($\beta^S\beta^D$) all produce significant symptoms but homozygous sickle cell anaemia is generally the most severe. The gene has remained at high frequency due to conferred resistance to malaria in heterozygotes. Inheritance is autosomal recessive.

Sickle cell anaemia (SCA, HbSS)

Pathogenesis

Widespread throughout Africa, Middle East, parts of India and Mediterranean. Single base change in β globin gene, amino acid 6 (glu→val). In UK Afro-Caribbean population gene is found in ~1:10. RBCs containing HbS deform (elongate) under conditions of reduced oxygenation, and form characteristic sickle cells—do not flow well through small vessels, and are more adherent than normal to vascular endothelium, leading to vascular occlusion and sickle cell crises. Patients with SCA are the offspring of parents both of whom are carriers of the β^S gene, i.e. they both have sickle cell trait, and homozygotes for the abnormal β^S gene demonstrate features of chronic red cell haemolysis and tissue infarction.

Clinical features

Highly variable. Many have few symptoms whilst others have severe and frequent crises, marked haemolytic anaemia and chronic organ damage. HbF level plays role in ameliorating symptoms (↑ HbF→fewer and milder crises). History may reveal a +ve family history or past history of crises.

- ***Infancy***—newborns have higher HbF level than normal adult, protected during first 8–20 weeks of life. Symptoms start when HbF level falls. SCA often diagnosed <1 year.
- ***Infection***—high morbidity and mortality due to bacterial and viral infection. Pneumococcal septicaemia (*Streptococcus pneumoniae*) well recognised. Other infecting organisms: meningococcus (*Neisseria meningitidis*), *Escherichia coli* and *Haemophilus influenzae* (hyposplenic).
- ***Anaemia***—children and adults often severely anaemic (Hb ~6.0–9.0 g/dL). Anaemia is chronic and patients generally well-adapted until episode of decompensation (e.g. severe infection) occurs.

Sickle crises

- ***Vaso-occlusive***—dactylitis, chest syndrome and girdle syndrome. Patients complain of severe bone, joint and abdominal pain. Bone pain affects long bones and spine, and is due to occlusion of small vessels. *Triggers:* infection, dehydration, alcohol, menstruation, cold and temperature changes – often no cause found.
- ***Dactylitis***—mainly children. Metacarpals, metatarsals, backs of hands and feet swollen and tender (small vessel occlusion and infarction). Recurrent, can result in permanent radiological abnormalities in bones of the hands and feet (rare).
- ***Acute chest syndrome***—common cause of death. Chest wall pain, sometimes with pleurisy, fever and SOB. Resembles infection, infarction or embolism. Requires prompt and vigorous treatment. Transfer to ITU if pO_2 cannot be kept >70 mmHg on air. 10% mortality. Treat infection vigorously, often due to *S pneumoniae, H influenzae, Mycoplasma, Legionella.*

- ***Aplastic crises***—sudden ↓ in marrow production (esp. red cells). Parvovirus B19 infection is cause (invades developing RBCs). Mostly self-limiting and after 1–2 weeks the marrow begins to function normally. Top-up transfusion may be needed.
- ***Haemolytic crises***—uncommon; markedly reduced red cell lifespan. May be drug-induced, 2° to infection (e.g. malaria) or associated G6PD deficiency.
- ***Sequestration crises***—mainly children (30%). Pooling of large volumes of blood in spleen and/or liver. Severe hypotension and profound anaemia may result in death.
- ***Other problems***
  - ***Growth retardation:*** common in children, but adult may have normal height (weight tends to be lower than normal). Sexual maturation delayed.
  - ***Locomotor:*** Avascular necrosis of the head of the femur or humerus, arthritis and osteomyelitis (*Salmonella* infection). Chronic leg ulceration is complication of many haemoglobinopathies including sickle cell anaemia. Ischaemia is main cause.
  - ***Genitourinary:*** Renal papillary necrosis⟶haematuria and renal tubular defects. Inability to concentrate urine. Priapism in ~60% males. Less common if HbF↑. Frequent UTIs in women, CRF in adults.
  - ***Spleen:*** Severe pain (infarction of splenic vessels). Spleen may enlarge in early life but after repeated infarcts diminishes in size (⟶hyposplenism by 9–12 months of age). Splenic function is impaired.
  - ***Gastrointestinal:*** Gallstones common (2° to chronic haemolysis). Derangement of LFTs (multifactorial).
  - ***CVS:*** Murmurs (anaemia), tachycardia.
  - ***Eye:*** Proliferative retinopathy (in 30%), blindness (esp. HbSC), retinal artery occlusion, retinal detachment.
  - ***CNS:*** Convulsions, TIAs or strokes, sensory hearing loss (usually temporary).
  - ***Psychosocial:*** Depression, socially withdrawn.

Laboratory features

Anaemia usual (Hb ~6.0–9.0 g/dL in HbSS although may be much lower; HbSC have higher Hb). Reticulocytes may be ↑ (to ~10–20%) reflecting intense bone marrow production of RBCs. Anaemic symptoms usually mild since HbS has reduced O_2 affinity. MCV and MCH are normal, unless also thalassaemia trait (25% cases). Blood film shows marked variation in red cell size with prominent sickle cells and target cells; basophilic stippling, Howell–Jolly bodies and P appenheimer bodies (hyposplenic features after infancy). Sickle cell test (e.g. sodium dithionate) will be positive. Does **not** discriminate between sickle cell *trait* and *homozygous disease*. Serum bilirubin often ↑ (due to excess red cell breakdown).

Blood film in homozygous sickle cell disease. Note the elongated (sickled) red cells.

Confirmatory tests

Haemoglobin electrophoresis shows 80–99% HbS with no normal HbA. HbF may be elevated to about 15%. Parents will have features of sickle cell trait.

Screening

In at-risk groups pregnant woman should be screened early in pregnancy. If both parents of fetus are carriers offer prenatal/neonatal diagnosis. Affected babies should be given penicillin daily and be immunised against *S. pneumoniae, H influenzae* type b, and *Neisseria meningitidis*.

Prenatal diagnosis

May be carried out from first trimester (chorionic villus sampling from 10 weeks gestation) or second trimester (fetal blood sampling from umbilical cord or trophoblast DNA from amniotic fluid). DNA may be analysed using restriction enzyme digestion with Mst II and Southern blotting, RFLP analysis assessing both parental and fetal DNA haplotypes, oligonucleotide probes specific for sickle globin point mutation, or PCR amplification followed by restriction enzyme digestion of amplified DNA. ARMS (amplification refractory mutation system) PCR is useful in ambiguous cases. In late pregnancy fetal blood sampling may be used to confirm diagnosis.

Management

General

Lifelong prophylactic penicillin 250mg bd PO with folate replacement. Pneumovax II vaccination advisable.

Management during pregnancy and anaesthesia

Anaesthesia should be carried out by experienced anaesthetist who is aware of complications of SCA. If the patient is unwell consider transfusion to Hb of 10g/dL, but generally transfusion not necessary.

Management of crises

▶▶ 📖 ***Haematological Emergencies: Sickle Crisis*** p532.

www.bcshguidelines.com/pdf/SICKLE.V4_0802.pdf

Red cell disorders

HbS—new therapies

Agents that elevate HbF levels

It has been recognised for some time that ↑ HbF levels ameliorate β thalassaemia and sickle cell disease. HbF reduces HbS polymerisation and hence sickling. HbF level of >10% reduces episodes of aseptic necrosis; levels >20% HbF are associated with fewer painful crises.

Hydroxyurea—several studies have shown that baboons treated with cytosine arabinoside showed ↑ HbF. Similar results obtained with hydroxyurea which has advantages over other cytotoxics e.g. low risk of secondary malignancy with prolonged use. Hydroxyurea has been evaluated in a large number of clinical trials. Effects are dose-dependent and the highest elevation of HbF is seen at myelosuppressive doses.

Erythropoietin—leads to ↑ HbF but not widely used in the management of haemoglobinopathies. Evidence suggests that rHuEPO provides an additive effect when alternated with hydroxyurea. Dose required is high (1000–3000iu/kg × 3d/week) with co-administration of Fe supplements.

5-azacytidine—inhibitor of methyltransferase, enzyme responsible for methylation of newly incorporated cytosines in DNA. Preventing methylation of the γ globin gene leads to ↑ HbF. ▶▶ Risk of developing 2° malignancy.

Short chain fatty acids—butyrate analogues are potent inducers of haematopoietic differentiation. Elevated concentrations of butyrate and other fatty acids in diabetic mothers is responsible for the persistently elevated HbF in the neonates born to such mothers. Initial studies involving the use of butyrate to increase HbF levels in patients with sickle cell anaemia appeared promising but subsequent studies have been disappointing.

Bone marrow transplantation—sibling donor transplants for sickle cell disease have been carried out in a number of centres. Since the mortality from sickle cell disease has dropped over recent years from 15%→1%, and with the advent of hydroxyurea therapy, there is a less compelling argument for BMT in sickle cell disease.

Gene therapy—potentially curative but experimental. Globin gene transfer has been attempted with variable results. Expression of exogenous gene has been at levels too low to be of benefit.

Charache, S. *et al* (1995) Effect of hydroxyurea on the frequency of painful crises in sickle cell anemia. Investigators of the Multicenter Study of Hydroxyurea in Sickle Cell Anemia. *N Engl J Med*, **332**, 1317–1322; Platt, O.S. *et al.* (1994) Mortality in sickle cell disease. Life expectancy and risk factors for early death. *N Engl J Med*, **330**, 1639–1644.

Red cell disorders

Sickle cell trait (HbAS)

Asymptomatic carriers have one abnormal β^S gene and one normal β gene (with 30 million carriers worldwide).

Clinical features

- Carriers are not anaemic and have no abnormal clinical features.
- Sickling rare unless O_2 saturation falls <40%. Crises have been reported with severe hypoxia (anaesthesia, unpressurised aircraft).
- Occasional renal papillary necrosis, haematuria and inability to concentrate the urine in adults.

Laboratory features

- Hb, MCV, MCH and MCHC normal (unless also α thalassaemia trait).
- HbS level 40–55% (if <40% then also α thalassaemia trait).
- Film may be normal or show microcytes and target cells.
- Sickle cell test will be +ve (HbSS and HbAS).

Carrier detection

Neither FBC nor film can be used for diagnostic purposes. Detection of the carrier state relies on haemoglobin electrophoresis (HbA ~50%; HbS ~50%).

▶ Care needed during anaesthesia (*avoid hypoxia*).

Red cell disorders

Other sickling disorders

HbSC

Milder than sickle cell anaemia but resembles it. Patients have fewer and milder crises. Retinal damage (microvascular, proliferative retinopathy) and blindness are major complications (30–35%). Arrange regular ophthalmological review by specialist. Aseptic necrosis of femoral head and recurrent haematuria are common. Increased risk of splenic infarcts and abscesses.

▶ Beware thrombosis and PE especially in pregnancy.

Clinical

Mild anaemia (Hb 8–14g/dL) and splenomegaly common. Less haemolysis, fewer painful crises, fewer infections and less vaso-occlusive disease than SCA. Growth and development normal. Lifespan normal.

▶ *Pregnancy may be hazardous.*

Film

Prominent target cells with fewer NRBC than seen in SCA. Howell–Jolly and Pappenheimer bodies (hyposplenism). Occasional C crystals may be seen.

Diagnosis

Hb electrophoresis and family studies. MCV and MCH are much lower than in HbSS.

HbSD, $HbSO_{Arab}$

Milder than HbSS. Both rare. Interactions of these globins with HbS results in reduced polymerisation. HbD_{Punjab} $^{(\beta 121\ glu \rightarrow gln)}$ and HbO_{Arab} $^{(\beta 121\ glu \rightarrow lys)}$ cause little disease on their own although there may be mild haemolysis in the homozygote. These haemoglobins cause sickle cell disease when present with HbS.

HbSα thalassaemia

Common in Black individuals. Lessens severity of SCA by reducing the concentration of Hb in red cells.

HbSβ thalassaemia

Caused by inheritance of β^S from one parent and β thalassaemia from the other. Sickle/β° thalassaemia is severe since no normal β globin chains are produced. Sickle/β^+ thalassaemia is much milder having β globin in 5–15% of their Hb. Microcytosis and splenomegaly are characteristic. Family screening will confirm microcytosis and ↑ HbA_2 in one of the parents.

Management

Essentially as for HbSS with prompt treatment of crises (*see above*).

Red cell disorders

Other haemoglobinopathies

HbC disease ($\beta^{6\ glu\rightarrow lys}$)

West Africa. Patients have benign compensated haemolysis. Development is normal, splenomegaly is common. Gallstones are recognised complication. The Hb may be mildly ↓. MCV and MCH ↓ and reticulocytes ↑. Blood film shows prominent target cells and occasional HbC crystals. Hb electrophoresis shows mainly HbC with some HbF. HbA is absent. Red cells said to be 'stiff'. Care with anaesthesia.

HbC trait ($\beta^{6\ glu\rightarrow lys}$)

Asymptomatic. Hb is ↔. Film may be normal or show presence of target cells. HbC 30–40%.

HbD disease (e.g. D_{Punjab} $\beta^{121\ glu\rightarrow gln}$)

Found in North West India, Pakistan and Iran. Film shows target cells.

HbD trait (e.g. D_{Punjab} $\beta^{121\ glu\rightarrow gln}$)

Of little consequence other than interaction with HbS. Hb and MCV ↔. Film normal or shows target cells.

HbE disease ($\beta^{26\ glu\rightarrow lys}$)

South East Asia (commonest Hb variant), India, Burma and Thailand. This Hb is moderately unstable when exposed to oxidants. May produce thalassaemic syndrome when mRNA splice mutants. There is mild anaemia, MCV and MCH ↓, reticulocytes ↔. Film shows target cells, hypochromic and microcytic red cells. There are few symptoms; underlying compensated haemolysis, mild jaundice. Liver and spleen size are normal. Treatment is not usually required.

HbE trait ($\beta^{26\ glu\rightarrow lys}$)

Asymptomatic. Indices similar to β thalassaemia trait. Hb usually ↔.

Red cell disorders

Unstable haemoglobins

Congenital Heinz body haemolytic anaemia caused by point mutations in globin genes. Hb precipitates in red blood cells⟶Heinz bodies. In normal Hb there are non-covalent bonds maintaining the Hb structure; loss of bonds leads to Hb denaturation and precipitation. Production of Heinz bodies leads to less deformable red cells with reduced lifespan.

Predominantly autosomal dominant; most patients are heterozygotes. Mainly affects β globin chain e.g. HbHammersmith (mutation involves amino acid in contact with haem pocket); HbBristol (replacement of non-polar by polar amino acid with distortion of protein).

Clinical features

- Well compensated haemolysis.
- Hb may be ↔ if unstable Hb has high O_2 affinity.
- Haemolysis exacerbated by infection and oxidant drugs.
- Jaundice and splenomegaly are common.
- Some Hbs are unstable *in vitro* but show little haemolysis *in vivo*.

Investigation

- Hb ↔ or ↓.
- MCV often ↓.
- Film shows hypochromic RBCs, polychromatic RBCs, basophilic stippling.
- Heinz bodies seen post-splenectomy.
- Reticulocytes are ↑.
- Demonstrate unstable Hb using e.g. heat or isopropanol stability tests.
- Brilliant cresyl blue will stain Heinz bodies.
- Estimation of P_{50} may be helpful.
- DNA analysis of value in some cases.

Management

Most cases run benign course. Treatment seldom required. Gallstones common. Recommend regular folic acid supplementation. Splenectomy of value in some patients. Avoidance of precipitants of haemolysis advised.

Red cell disorders

Thalassaemias

Arise as a result of diminished or absent production of one or more globin chains. Net result is imbalanced globin chain production. Globin chains in excess precipitate within RBCs leading to chronic haemolysis in bone marrow and peripheral blood. Occur at high frequency in parts of Africa, the Mediterranean, Middle East, India and Asia. Found in high frequency in areas where malaria is endemic and thalassaemia trait probably offers some protection.

Named after affected gene e.g. in α thalassaemia the α globin gene is altered in such a way that either α globin synthesis is *reduced* (α^+) or *abolished* (α°) from RBCs. Severity varies depending on type of mutation or deletion of the α or β globin gene.

α thalassaemia

Two α globin genes on each chromosome 16, with total of 4 α globin genes per cell (normal person is designated αα/αα). Like sickle cell anaemia, patients can either have mild α thalassaemia (*α thalassaemia trait*) where one or two α globin genes are affected or may have severe α thalassaemia if three or four of the genes are affected. α thalassaemia is generally the result of large deletions within α globin complex.

Silent α thalassaemia (–α/αα)

One gene deleted. Asymptomatic. ↓ MCV and MCH in minority.

α thalassaemia trait (αα/–– or –α/–α)

Asymptomatic carrier—recognised once other causes of microcytic anaemia are excluded (e.g. iron deficiency). Hb may be ↔ or minimally ↓. MCV and MCH are ↓. Absence of splenomegaly or other clinical findings. Requires no therapy.

Haemoglobin H disease (––/– α)

Three α genes deleted; only one functioning copy of the α globin gene/cell. Clinical features variable. May be moderate anaemia with Hb 8.0–9.0g/dL. MCV and MCH are ↓. Hepatosplenomegaly, chronic leg ulceration and jaundice (reflecting underlying haemolysis). Infection, drug treatment and pregnancy may worsen anaemia.

Blood film shows hypochromia, target cells, NRBC and increased reticulocytes. Brilliant cresyl blue stain will show HbH inclusions (tetramers of β globin, β_4, that have polymerised due to lack of α chains). Hb pattern consists of 2–40% HbH (β_4) with some HbA, A_2 and F.

Treatment

Not usually required but prompt treatment of infection advisable. Give regular folic acid especially when pregnant. Splenectomy of value in some patients with HbH disease. Needs monitoring and may require blood transfusion.

Haemoglobin Bart's hydrops fetalis (−−/−−)

Common cause of stillbirth in South East Asia. All 4 α globin genes affected. γ chains form tetramers (HbBart's, γ_4) which bind oxygen very tightly, with resultant poor tissue oxygenation. Fetus is either stillborn (at 34–40 weeks gestation) or dies soon after birth. They are pale, distended, jaundiced and have marked hepatosplenomegaly and ascites. Haemoglobin is ~6.0g/dL and the film shows hypochromic red cells, target cells, increased reticulocytes and nucleated red cells. Haemoglobin analysis shows mainly HbBart's (γ_4) with a small amount of HbH (β_4); HbA, A_2 and F are absent.

β thalassaemia

There are only 2 copies of β globin gene per cell. Abnormality in one β globin gene results in *β thalassaemia trait;* if both β globin genes are affected the patient has *β thalassaemia major* or *β thalassaemia intermedia.* Unlike α thalassaemia, most β thalassaemias are due to single point mutations. Results in reduced β globin synthesis (β^+) or absent β globin production (β°). In β thalassaemia major, patients have severe anaemia requiring lifelong support with blood transfusion (with resultant iron overload). There is ineffective erythropoiesis. Not obvious at birth due to presence of HbF ($\alpha_2\gamma_2$) but as γ chain production diminishes and β globin production increases effects of the mutation become obvious. Children fail to thrive, and development is affected. Hepatosplenomegaly (due to production and destruction of red cells by these organs) is typical. Children also develop facial abnormalities as the flat bones of the skull and other bones attempt to produce red cells to overcome the genetic defect. Skull radiographs show 'hair on end' appearances reflecting the intense marrow activity in the skull bones.

Investigation and management

β thalassaemia trait

- Carrier state.
- Hb may be ↓ but is not usually <10.0g/dL.
- MCV ↓ to ~63–77fL.
- Blood film: microcytic, hypochromic RBCs; target cells often present. Basophilic stippling especially in Mediterraneans.
- RCC ↑.
- HbA_2 ($\alpha_2\delta_2$) ↑—provides useful diagnostic test for β thalassaemia trait.
- Occasionally confused with iron deficiency anaemia, however, in thalassaemia trait the serum iron and ferritin are normal (or ↑) whereas in IDA they are ↓.

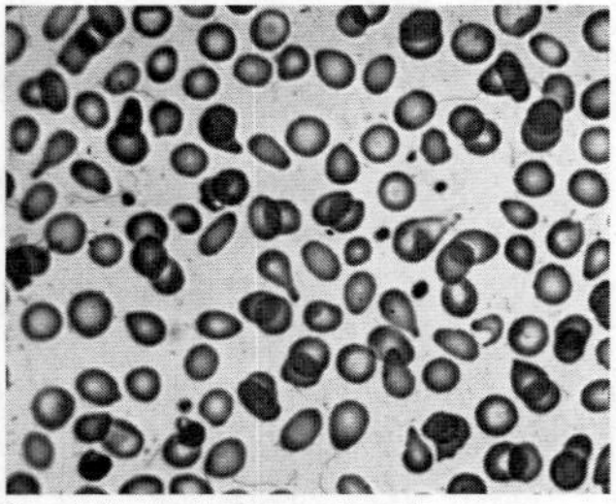

Blood film in thalassaemia trait

Treatment

Not usually required. Usually detected antenatally or on routine FBC pre-op.

β thalassaemia intermedia

- Denotes thalassaemia major not requiring regular blood transfusion; more severe than β thalassaemia trait but milder than β thalassaemia major.
- May arise through several mechanisms e.g.
  - *Inheritance of mild β thalassaemia mutations* (e.g. homozygous β^+ thalassaemia alleles, compound heterozygote for two mild β^+ thalassaemia alleles, compound heterozygotes for mild *plus* severe β^+ thalassaemia alleles).
  - *Elevation of HbF.*
  - *Coinheritance of α thalassaemia.*
  - *Coinheritance of β thalassaemia trait with e.g. HbLepore.*
  - *Severe β thalassaemia trait.*

Clinical

- Present with symptoms similar to β thalassaemia major but with only moderate degree of anaemia.
- Hepatosplenomegaly.
- Iron overload is a feature.
- Some patients are severely anaemic (Hb ~6g/dL) although not requiring regular blood transfusion, have impaired growth and development, skeletal deformities and chronic leg ulceration.
- Others have higher Hb (e.g. 10–12g/dL) with few symptoms.

Management

Depends on severity. May require intermittent blood transfusion, iron chelation, folic acid supplementation, prompt treatment of infection, as for β thalassaemia major.

β thalassaemia major (Cooley's anaemia)

Patients have abnormalities of both β globin genes. Presents in childhood with anaemia and recurrent bacterial infection. There is extramedullary haemopoiesis with hepatosplenomegaly and skeletal deformities.

Clinical

- Moderate/severe anaemia (Hb ~3.0–9.0g/dL).
- MCV and MCHC ↓.
- Reticulocytes ↑.
- Blood film: marked anisopoikilocytosis, target cells and nucleated red cells.
- Methyl violet stain shows RBC inclusions containing precipitated α globin.
- Hb electrophoresis shows mainly HbF ($\alpha_2\gamma_2$). In some β thalassaemias there may be a little HbA ($\alpha_2\beta_2$) if some β globin is produced.
- HbA_2 may be ↔ or mildly elevated.

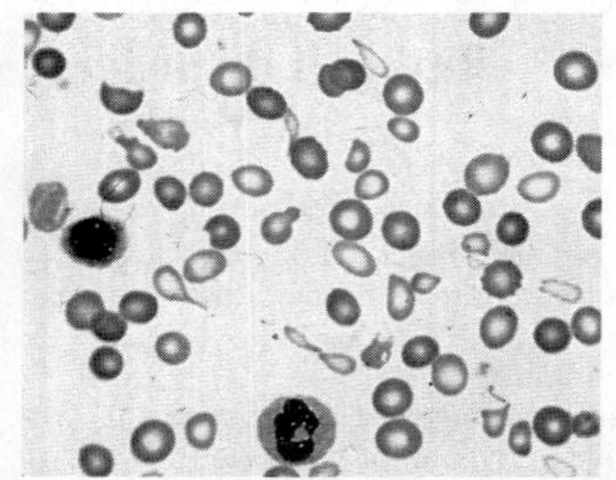

β thalassaemia major: note bizarre red cells with marked anisopoikilocytosis

Management

- Regular lifelong blood transfusion (every 2–4 weeks) to *suppress* ineffective erythropoiesis and allow normal growth and development in childhood.
- Iron overload (*transfusion haemosiderosis*) is major problem—damages heart, endocrine glands, pancreas and liver. Desferrioxamine reduces iron overload (by promoting iron excretion in the urine and stool), and is given for 8–12h per day SC for 5 days/week. Compliance may be difficult, especially in younger patients. Complications of desferrioxamine include retinal damage, cataract and infection with *Yersinia* spp.
- Splenectomy may be of value (e.g. if massive splenomegaly or increasing transfusion requirements) but best avoided until after the age of 5 years due to ↑ risk of infection. Infective episodes should be treated promptly with intravenous antibiotics.
- Bone marrow transplantation has been carried out using sibling donor HLA-matched transplants with good results in young patients with β thalassaemia major. The procedure carries a significant procedure-related morbidity and mortality, along with GvHD (📖 *BMT section p324–326*).

Screening

Screen mothers at first antenatal visit. If mother is thalassaemic carrier, screen father. If both carriers for severe thalassaemia offer prenatal diagnostic testing. Fetal blood sampling can be carried out at 18 weeks gestation and globin chain synthesis analysed. Chorionic villus sampling at 10+ weeks gestation provides a source of fetal DNA that can be analysed in a variety of methods: Southern blotting, oligonucleotide probes or RFLP analysis may determine genotype of fetus. Moving towards PCR based techniques; likely to improve carrier detection.

Weatherall, D.J. & Provan, A.B. (2000) Red cells I: inherited anaemias. *Lancet*, **355**, 1169–1175.

Other thalassaemias

Heterozygous δβ thalassaemia

Produces a picture similar to β thalassaemia trait with ↑ HbF (5–20%) and microcytic RBCs; HbA_2 is ↔ or ↓.

Homozygous δβ thalassaemia

Homozygous condition is uncommon. There is failure of production of both δ and β globins. Milder than β thalassaemia major, i.e. β thalassaemia intermedia. Represents a form of thalassaemia intermedia. Hb 8–11g/dL. Absence of HbA and HbA_2; only HbF is present (100%).

Heterozygous β thalassaemia/δβ thalassaemia

Similar to β thalassaemia major (but less severe). Hb produced is mainly HbF with small amount of HbA_2.

γδβ thalassaemia

Homozygote is not viable. Heterozygous condition is associated with haemolysis in neonatal period and thalassaemia trait in adults with ↔ HbF and HbA_2.

HbLepore

This abnormal Hb is the result of unequal crossing over of chromosomes. Affects β and δ globin genes with generation of a chimeric globin with δ sequences at NH_2 terminal and β globin at COOH terminal. Production of δβ globin is inefficient; there is absence of normal δ and β globins. The phenotype of the heterozygote is thalassaemia trait; the homozygote picture is thalassaemia intermedia.

BCSH haemoglobinopathy diagnosis guidelines
🖰 www.bcshguidelines.com/pdf/bjh809.pdf

Hereditary persistence of fetal haemoglobin

Heterogeneous groups of disorders caused by deletions or cross-overs involving β and γ chain production, or non-deletional forms due to point mutations upstream of the γ globin gene, with high levels of HbF production in adult life. There is ↓ δ and β chain production with enhanced γ chain production. Globin chain imbalance is much less marked than in β thalassaemia, resulting in milder disorder. There are few clinical effects.

May be *pancellular* (very high levels of HbF haemoglobin synthesis with uniform distribution in RBCs) or *heterocellular* (increased numbers of F cells).

Mechanism

Like δβ thalassaemia, HPFH frequently arises from deletions of DNA, which remove or inactivate the β globin gene (*note*: heterocellular HPFH may be result of mutations outside the β globin gene).

Heterozygous HPFH

Anaemia may be mild or absent. Haematological indices are normal. There is balanced α/non-α globin chain synthesis. HbF level ~25%.

Hb patterns in haemoglobin disorders

% Haemoglobin	A	F	A_2	S	Other
Normal	**97**	**<1**	**2–3**		
β thalassaemia trait	80–95	1–5	3–7		
β thalassaemia intermedia	30–50	50–70	0–5		
β thalassaemia major	0–20	80–100	0–13		
HPFH (Black heterozygote)	60–85	15–35	1–3		
HPFH (Black homozygote)		100			
α thalassaemia trait	85–95				Bart's 0–10% at birth
HbH disease	60–95				H 5–30% Bart's 20–30% at birth
HbBart's hydrops					Bart's 80–90%
HbE trait	60–65	1–2	2–3		E 30–35
HbE disease	0	5–10	5		E 95
HbE/β thalassaemia	0	30–40	–		E 60–70
HbE/α thalassaemia	13				E 80
HbD trait	50–65	1-5	1–3		D 45–50
HbD disease	1-5	1-3			D 90–95
HbD/β thalassaemia	0-7	1-7			D 80–90
HbC trait	60–70				C 30–40
HbC disease		slight ↑			C 95
Sickle trait	55–70	1	3	30–45	
Sickle cell anaemia	0	7	3	90	
Sickle/β^+ thalassaemia	5–30	5–15	–	60–85	
Sickle/β° thalassaemia	0	5–30	4–8	70–90	
Sickle/D	0	1–5		50	D 50%
Sickle/C	0	1	*	50–65	C 50%
HbLepore trait 80–90	1–3	2–2.5			Lepore 9–11%
HbLepore disease	0	70–90	0		Lepore 8–30%
HbLepore/β thalassaemia		70–90	2.5		Lepore 5–15%

Red cell disorders

Non-immune haemolysis

4 major groups

- Infections.
- Vascular (mechanical damage).
- Chemical damage.
- Physical damage.

Infection

Malaria—especially falciparum. Causes anaemia through marrow suppression, hypersplenism and RBC sequestration. In addition there is haemolysis due to destruction of parasitised RBCs by RES and intravascular haemolysis when sporozoites released from infected RBCs. Blackwater fever refers to severe acute intravascular haemolysis with haemoglobinaemia, ↓ Hb, haemoglobinuria and ARF.

Babesiosis—*Babesia* (RBC protozoan). Rapid onset of vomiting, diarrhoea, rigors, jaundice, ↑T°. Haemoglobinaemia, haemoglobinuria, ARF and death.

Clostridium perfringens—septicaemia and acute intravascular haemolysis.

Viral—especially viral haemorrhagic fevers e.g. dengue, yellow fever.

Mechanical

Cardiac—turbulence and shear stress following mechanical valve replacement. General feature of haemolysis: ↑ reticulocytes, LDH, plasma Hb, with ↓ haptoglobins ± platelets. Urinary haemosiderin +ve.

MAHA—*see p112.*

HUS/TTP—*see p530.*

March haemoglobinuria—with severe strenuous exercise e.g. running. Destruction of RBCs in soles of feet. Worse with hard soles and uneven hard ground. Mild anaemia. No specific features on film. May be associated GIT bleeding and ↓ ferritin (lost in sweat).

Chemical & physical

Oxidative haemolysis—chronic Heinz body intravascular haemolysis with dapsone or salazopyrine in G6PD deficient people or unstable Hb (and normals if dose high enough). Film: bite cells (RBC). Heinz bodies not prominent if intact spleen. Haemolysis well compensated.

MetHb—*see p110.*

Lead poisoning—moderate ↓ RBC lifespan. Anaemia mainly due to block in haem synthesis although lead also inhibits 5' nucleotidase (NT). Basophilic stippling on film. Ring sideroblasts in BM.

O_2—haemolysis in patients treated with hyperbaric O_2.

Insect bites—e.g. spider, bee-sting (not common with snake bites).

Heat—e.g. burns→severe haemolysis due to direct RBC damage.

Liver disease—reduced RBC lifespan in acute hepatitis, cirrhosis, Zieve's syndrome is an uncommon form of haemolysis—intravascular associated with acute abdominal pain (📖 *p54*).

Wilson's disease—autosomally inherited disorder of copper metabolism, with hepatolenticular, hepatocerebral degeneration.

PNH—see *p124*.

Hereditary acanthocytosis—a-β-lipoproteinaemia. Rare, inherited. Associated with retinitis pigmentosa, steatorrhoea, ataxia and mental retardation.

Hereditary spherocytosis

Most common inherited RBC membrane defect characterised by variable degrees of haemolysis, spherocytic RBCs with ↑ osmotic fragility.

Pathophysiology

Abnormal RBC cytoskeleton: partial deficiency of spectrin, ankyrin, band 3 or protein 4.2 (leads to ↓ binding to band 4.1 protein and ankyrin). Loss of lipid from RBC membrane⟶spherical (*cf.* biconcave) RBCs with reduced surface area⟶get trapped in splenic cords and have reduced lifespan. RBCs use more energy than normal in attempt to maintain cell shape. RBC membrane has ↑ Na^+ permeability (loses intracellular Na^+) and energy required to restore Na^+ balance. Red cells are less deformable than normal.

Epidemiology

In Northern Europeans 1:5000 people are affected. In most cases inheritance is autosomal dominant although autosomal recessive inheritance has been reported.

Clinical features

Presents at any age. Highly variable from asymptomatic to severely anaemic, but usually there are few symptoms. Well-compensated haemolysis; other features of haemolytic anaemia may be present e.g. splenomegaly, gallstones, mild jaundice. Occasional aplastic crises occur, e.g. with parvovirus B19 infection.

Diagnosis

- Positive family history of HS in many cases.
- Blood film shows ↑↑ spherocytic RBCs.
- Anaemia, ↑ reticulocytes, ↑ LDH, unconjugated bilirubin, urinary urobilinogen with ↓ haptoglobins. DAT –ve.

Osmotic fragility test—RBCs incubated in saline at various concentrations. Results in cell expansion and eventually rupture. Normal RBCs can withstand greater volume increases than spherocytic RBCs. Positive result (i.e. confirms HS) when RBCs lyse in saline at near to isotonic concentration, i.e. 0.6–0.8g/dL (whereas normal RBCs will simply show swelling with little lysis). Osmotic fragility more marked in patients who have not undergone splenectomy, and if the RBCs are incubated at 37°C for 24h before performing the test.

Autohaemolysis test—since spherocytic RBCs use more glucose than normal RBCs (to maintain normal shape) red cells incubated in buffer or serum for 48h show lysis and release of Hb into solution, which can be measured. In HS RBCs release greater amounts of Hb *cf.* normal RBCs (3% *vs.* 1% in normal).

Complications

- Aplastic crisis (e.g. parvovirus B19 infection, but may be any virus); see temporary ↓↓ reticulocytes, Hb and Hct.
- Megaloblastic changes in folate deficiency.
- ↑ haemolysis during intercurrent illness e.g. infections.
- Gallstones (in 50% patients; occur even in mild disease).

- Leg ulceration.
- Extramedullary haemopoiesis.
- Iron overload if multiply transfused.

Exclude

Other causes of haemolytic anaemia e.g. immune-mediated, unstable Hbs and MAHA, which can give rise to spherocytic RBCs.

Treatment

Supportive treatment is usually all that is required, e.g. folic acid (5mg/d). In parvovirus crisis Hb drops significantly and blood transfusion may be required. Splenectomy is 'curative' but is reserved for patients who are severely anaemic or who have symptomatic moderate anaemia. Best avoided in patients <10 years old due to risk of ↑ fatal infection post-splenectomy.

▶ Remember pre-splenectomy vaccines and post-splenectomy antibiotics (📖 p582).

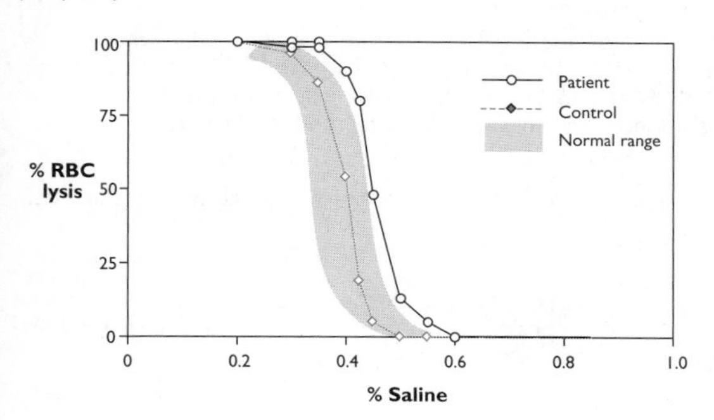

Osmotic fragility assay: note control red cells (red) lyse at lower % saline since they are able to take up more water than spherocytic red cells before lysis occurs.

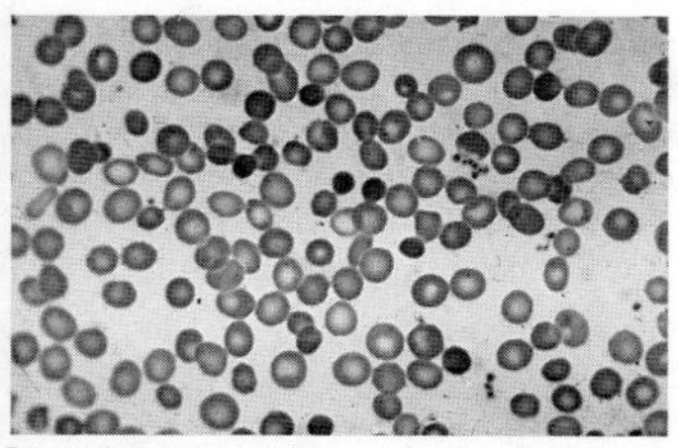

Blood film in hereditary spherocytosis: note large numbers of dark spherical red cells.

Hereditary elliptocytosis

Heterogeneous group of disorders with elliptical RBCs.

3 major groups

- Hereditary elliptocytosis.
- Spherocytic HE.
- South East Asian ovalocytosis.

Pathophysiology

Mutations in α or β spectrin. There may be partial, complete deficiency, or structural abnormality of protein 4.1, or absence of glycophorin C.

Epidemiology

In Northern Europeans 1:2500 are affected. Inheritance is autosomal dominant. More common in areas where malaria is endemic.

Clinical features

Most are asymptomatic. Well-compensated haemolysis. A few patients have chronic symptomatic anaemia. Homozygote more severely affected.

Diagnosis

- May have positive family history.
- Blood film shows ↑↑ elliptical or oval RBCs.
- Anaemia, ↑ reticulocytes, ↑ LDH, unconjugated bilirubin, urinary urobilinogen with ↓ haptoglobins. DAT is –ve.
- Osmotic fragility usually normal (unless spherocytic HE).
- Transient increase in haemolysis if intercurrent infection.

Complications

Usual complications of haemolytic anaemia e.g. gallstones, folate deficiency, etc.

Treatment

Supportive care: folic acid (5mg/d). Most patients require no treatment. In more severe cases consider splenectomy. Remember pre-splenectomy vaccines and post-splenectomy antibiotics (📖 p582).

Spherocytic HE

Elliptical and spherical 'sphero-ovalocytes' in peripheral blood. Haemolysis and ↑ osmotic fragility distinguish it from common hereditary elliptocytosis. Molecular basis is unknown.

Southeast Asian ovalocytosis

Caused by abnormal band 3 protein. RBCs are oval with 1–2 transverse ridges. Cells have ↑ rigidity and ↓ osmotic fragility. RBCs are more resistant to malaria than normal RBCs.

Red cell disorders

Glucose-6-phosphate dehydrogenase deficiency

G6PD is involved in pentose phosphate shunt→generates NADP, NADPH and glutathione (for maintenance of Hb and RBC membrane integrity, and reverse oxidant damage to RBC membrane and RBC components). G6PD deficiency is X-linked and clinically important cause of oxidant haemolysis. Affects ♂ predominantly; ♀ carriers have 50% normal G6PD activity. Occurs in West Africa, Southern Europe, Middle East and South East Asia.

Features:

- Haemolysis after exposure to oxidants or infection.
- Chronic non-spherocytic haemolytic anaemia.
- Acute episodes of haemolysis with fava beans (termed favism).
- Methaemoglobinaemia.
- Neonatal jaundice.

Mechanism Oxidants→denatured Hb→methaemoglobin→Heinz bodies→RBC less deformable→destroyed by spleen.

2 main forms of the enzyme: normal enzyme is G6PD-B, most prevalent form worldwide; 20% of Africans are type A. A and B differ by one amino acid. Mutant enzyme with normal activity = G6PD A(+), find only in Black individuals. G6PD A(–) is main defect in African origin; ↓ stability of enzyme *in vivo*; 5–15% normal activity. 400+ variants but only 2 are relevant clinically: type A(–) = Africans (10% enzyme activity) and Mediterranean (with 1–3% activity).

Drug-induced haemolysis in G6PD deficiency

- Begins 1–3d after ingestion of drug.
- Anaemia most severe 7–10d after ingestion.
- Associated with low back and abdominal pain.
- Urine becomes dark (black sometimes).
- Red cells develop Heinz body inclusions (cleared later by spleen).
- Haemolysis is typically self-limiting.
- Implicated drugs shown in table (*next page*).
- But heterogeneous; variable sensitivity to drugs.
- Risk and severity are *dose related*.

Haemolysis due to infection and fever

- 1–2d after onset of fever.
- Mild anaemia develops.
- Commonly seen in pneumonic illnesses.

Favism

- Hours/days after ingestion of fava beans (broad beans).
- Beans contain oxidants vicine and convicine→free radicals→oxidise glutathione.
- Urine becomes red or very dark.
- Shock may develop—***may be fatal.***

Risk of haemolysis in G6PD deficient individuals

Definite risk	Possible risk
Antimalarial drugs	Aspirin (1g/d acceptable in most cases)
Primaquine	Chloroquine
Pamaquine (not available in UK)	Probenecid
	Quinine & quinidine (acceptable in acute malaria)
Analgesic drugs	
Aspirin	
Phenacetin	
Others	
Dapsone	
Methylthioninium chloride (methylene blue)	
Nitrofurantoin	
4-quinolones (e.g. ciprofloxacin, nalidixic acid)	
Sulphonamides (e.g. cotrimoxazole)	

Neonatal jaundice

- May develop kernicterus (*possible permanent brain damage*).
- Rare in A(–) variants.
- More common in Mediterranean and Chinese variants.

Laboratory investigation

- In steady state (i.e. no haemolysis) the RBCs appear normal.
- Heinz bodies in drug-induced haemolysis (methyl violet stain).
- Spherocytes and RBC fragments on blood film if severe haemolysis.
- ↑ reticulocytes.
- ↑ unconjugated bilirubin, LDH and urinary urobilinogen.
- ↓ haptoglobins.
- DAT –ve.

Diagnosis

Demonstrate enzyme deficiency. In suspected RBC enzymopathy, assay G6PD and PK first, then look for unstable Hb. Diagnosis is difficult during haemolytic episode since reticulocytes have ↑↑ levels of enzyme and may get erroneously normal result; wait until steady state (~6 weeks after episode of haemolysis). Family studies are helpful.

Management

- Avoid oxidant drugs—*see BNF*.
- Transfuse in severe haemolysis or symptomatic anaemia.
- IV fluids to maintain good urine output.
- ± exchange transfusion in infants.
- Splenectomy may be of value in severe recurrent haemolysis.
- Folic acid supplements (?proven value).
- Avoid iron unless definite iron deficiency.

Pyruvate kinase deficiency

Congenital non-spherocytic haemolytic anaemia, caused by deficiency of PK enzyme (involved in glycolytic pathway), leading to unstable enzyme with reduction in ATP generation in RBCs. O_2 curve is shifted to the right due to ↑ 2,3-DPG production.

Epidemiology
Autosomal recessive. Affected persons are homozygous or double heterozygotes.

Clinical features
Variable, with chronic haemolytic syndrome. May be apparent in neonate (if severe) or may present in later life.

Diagnosis
- Variable anaemia.
- Reticulocytes ↑↑.
- DAT –ve.
- LDH ↑.
- Serum haptoglobin ↓.
- Definitive diagnosis requires assay of PK level.

Complications
Aplastic crisis may be seen in viral infection (e.g. parvovirus B19).

Treatment
Dependent on severity. General supportive measures include daily folic acid (5mg/d). Transfusion may be required. Splenectomy may be of value if high transfusion requirements. In aplastic crisis (e.g. viral infection) support measures should be used.

Zanella, A. & Bianchi, P. (2000) Red cell pyruvate kinase deficiency: from genetics to clinical manifestations. *Baillieres Best Pract Res Clin Haematol*, **13**, 57–81.

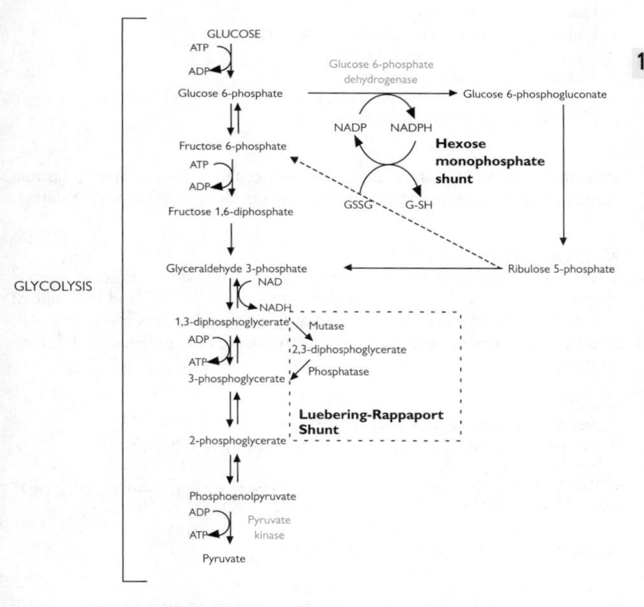

Glycolytic pathway showing key enzymes in red

Other red cell enzymopathies

Glycolytic pathway
- Hexokinase deficiency.
- Glucose phosphate isomerase deficiency.
- Phosphofructokinase deficiency.
- Aldolase deficiency.
- Triosephosphate isomerase deficiency.
- Phosphoglycerate kinase deficiency.

Epidemiology
Incidence <1 in 10^6. Inheritance is autosomal recessive (most double heterozygote) except for phosphoglycerate kinase deficiency (X-linked recessive).

Clinical features
Similar to PK deficiency although most are more severely affected for the degree of anaemia (glycolytic block results in ↓ 2,3-DPG and left shift of O_2 dissociation curve). PFK deficiency is associated with myopathy. TPI and PGK deficiencies are associated with progressive neurological deterioration.

Diagnosis
- *See pyruvate kinase deficiency* (p104).
- Non-specific morphology with anisocytosis, macrocytosis and polychromasia.
- Definitive diagnosis requires assay of deficient enzyme (→reference lab).

Complications
- *See pyruvate kinase deficiency* (p104).

Treatment
Folic acid (5mg/d). Transfusion may be required (beware Fe overload if high transfusion requirement). Role of splenectomy controversial.

Natural history
Similar to pyruvate kinase except TPI and PGK–TPI present in childhood and cause progressive paraparesis, most die <5 years old due to cardiac arrhythmias. PGK can cause exertional rhabdomyolysis and consequential renal failure. Those affected show progressive neurological deterioration.

Nucleotide metabolism—pyrimidine 5' nucleotidase deficiency

Epidemiology
Autosomal recessive. *Note:* lead poisoning causes *acquired* pyrimidine 5' nucleotidase deficiency.

Clinical features
- Moderate anaemia (Hb ~10g/dL).
- ↑ Reticulocytes.
- ↑ bilirubin.
- Splenomegaly.

Diagnosis

- RBCs show prominent basophilic stippling.
- Pyrimidine 5′ nucleotidase assay.

Treatment

Symptomatic, splenectomy is of limited value.

Drug-induced haemolytic anaemia

Large number of drugs shown to cause haemolysis of RBCs. Mechanisms variable. May be immune or non-immune.

- Some drugs interfere with lipid component of RBC membrane.
- Oxidation and denaturation of Hb: seen with e.g. sulphonamides, especially in G6PD deficient subjects, but may occur in normal subjects if drugs given in large doses e.g.
  - *Dapsone.*
  - *Sulfasalazine.*
- ***Hapten mechanism*** describes the interaction between certain drugs and the RBC membrane components generating antigens that stimulate antibody production. DAT +ve.
  - *Penicillins.*
  - *Cephalosporins.*
  - *Tetracyclines.*
  - *Tolbutamide.*
- ***Autoantibody mediated haemolysis*** is associated with warm antibody mediated AIHA. DAT +ve.
  - *Cephalosporins.*
  - *Mefenamic acid.*
  - *Methyldopa.*
  - *Procainamide.*
  - *Ibuprofen.*
  - *Diclofenac.*
  - *IFN-α.*
- ***Innocent bystander mechanism*** occurs when drugs form immune complexes with antibody (IgM commonest) which then attach to RBC membrane. Complement fixation and RBC destruction occurs.
  - *Quinine.*
  - *Quinidine.*
  - *Rifampicin.*
  - *Antihistamines.*
  - *Chlorpromazine.*
  - *Melphalan.*
  - *Tetracycline.*
  - *Probenecid.*
  - *Cefotaxime.*

Laboratory features

As for autoimmune haemolytic anaemia, Hb ↓, reticulocytes ↑, etc.

Differential diagnosis

- Warm/cold autoimmune haemolytic anaemia.
- Congenital haemolytic disorders, e.g. HS, G6PD deficiency, etc.

Treatment

- Discontinue offending drug.
- Choose alternative if necessary.
- If DAT +ve with methyldopa no need to stop unless haemolysis.
- Corticosteroids generally unnecessary and of doubtful value.
- Transfuse in severe or symptomatic cases only.
- Outlook good with complete recovery usual.

Red cell disorders

Methaemoglobinaemia

The normal O_2 dissociation curve requires iron to be in the ferrous form (i.e. reduced, Fe^{2+}). Hb containing the ferric (oxidised, Fe^{3+}) form is termed methaemoglobin (MetHb). MetHb binds O_2 tightly leading to poor tissue oxygenation. May be congenital or acquired.

Methaemoglobinaemia	
Congenital	
HbM	α or β globin mutation in vicinity of Fe Fe becomes stabilised in Fe^{3+} form Heterozygote has 25% HbM
MetHb reductase def.	Due to deficiency of NADH-cytochrome b_5 reductase. Autosomal recessive inheritance; symptoms mainly in homozygote
Clinical features	Cyanosis from infancy. PaO_2 is normal General health is good
Acquired	Occurs when RBCs are exposed to oxidising agents, producing HbM. Implicated agents include: phenacetin, local anaesthetics (e.g. lignocaine), inorganic nitrates (NO_2). Patients may experience severe tissue hypoxia. HbM binds O_2 tightly and fails to release to tissues
	▶▶ HbM ≥60% requires urgent medical attention.

Diagnosis

May be history of exposure to oxidant drugs or chemicals. Spectrophotometry or haemoglobin electrophoresis will demonstrate HbM. Assays for MetHb reductase are available.

Treatment

In patients with congenital symptomatic HbM give ascorbate or methylthioninium chloride (methylene blue). In acquired disorder remove oxidant, if present, and administer methylthioninium chloride (methylene blue).

▶ If severely affected consider exchange blood transfusion.

Red cell disorders

Microangiopathic haemolytic anaemia (MAHA)

Definition

Increased RBC destruction caused by mechanical red cell deformation. Caused by trauma or vascular endothelial abnormalities.

Causes

- TTP/HUS *see p468, 530.*
- PET/HELLP (haemolysis, elevated liver enzymes and low platelets).
- Malignant tumour circulations.
- Renal abnormalities e.g. acute glomerulonephritis, transplant rejection, cyclosporin.
- Vasculitides e.g. Wegener's, PAN, SLE.
- DIC.
- Prosthetic heart valves.
- March haemoglobinuria.
- A-V malformations.
- Burns.

Clinical

- Varying degree of anaemia—most severe in DIC, TTP/HUS and HELLP.
- Often associated with ↓ platelets.
- Blood film shows marked RBC fragmentation, stomatocytes and spherocytes.
- Reticulocytosis often very marked.
- Signs of underlying disease should be sought.

Treatment

- Diagnose and treat underlying disease.
- Give folic acid and iron supplements if deficient.

Antman, K.H. *et al.* (1979) Microangiopathic hemolytic anemia and cancer: a review. *Medicine* (Baltimore), **58**, 377–384.

Red cell disorders

Acanthocytosis

Abnormal RBC shape (thorn-like surface protrusions) seen in a number of conditions, inherited or acquired, affecting RBC membrane lipid structure. RBCs develop normally in marrow but once in plasma adopt characteristic shape. RBCs lose membrane and become progressively less elastic.

Inherited conditions resulting in significant acanthocytosis
- A-β-lipoproteinaemia.
- McLeod phenotype (lacking Kell antigen).
- In(Lu) phenotype.
- In association with abnormalities of band 3 protein.
- Hereditary hypo-β-lipoproteinaemia.

Acquired conditions resulting in significant acanthocytosis
- Severe liver disease.
- Myelodysplastic syndromes.
- Neonatal vitamin E deficiency.

Inherited conditions resulting in mild acanthocytosis
- McLeod phenotype heterozygote.
- Pyruvate kinase deficiency.

Acquired conditions resulting in mild acanthocytosis
- Post-splenectomy and hyposplenic states.
- Starvation including anorexia nervosa.
- Hypothyroidism.
- Panhypopituitarism.

A-β-lipoproteinaemia
Autosomal recessive. Congenital absence of β apolipoprotein. Cholesterol:phospholipid ratio ↑. RBC precursors normal. Usually obvious in early life with associated malabsorption of fat (including vitamins A, D, E and K). Sphingomyelin accumulates.

Haematological abnormalities
- Mild haemolytic anaemia.
- 50–90% circulating RBCs are acanthocytic.
- Reticulocytes mildly ↑.

McLeod phenotype
- ↓ expression of Kell antigen on RBC.
- Mild (compensated) haemolytic anaemia.
- 10–85% acanthocytic RBCs in peripheral blood.

Red cell disorders

Autoimmune haemolytic anaemia

RBCs react with autoantibody ± complement⟶premature destruction of RBCs by reticuloendothelial system.

Mechanism

RBCs opsonised by IgG, recognized by Fc receptors on RES macrophages⟶phagocytosis. If phagocytosis incomplete remaining portion of RBC continues to circulate as ***spherocyte*** (*note:* phagocytosis usually complete if complement involved).

Seen in

- Haemolytic blood transfusion reactions.
- Autoimmune haemolytic anaemia.
- Drug-induced haemolysis (some).

Warm antibody induced	Idiopathic 2° to lymphoproliferative disease e.g. CLL, NHL 2° to other autoimmune diseases e.g. SLE
Cold antibody induced	Idiopathic Cold haemagglutinin disease (CHAD) 2° to *Mycoplasma* infection Infectious mononucleosis Lymphoma
Paroxysmal cold haemoglobinuria	Idiopathic 2° to viral infection Congenital or tertiary syphilis

Warm antibody induced haemolysis

Extravascular RBC destruction by RES mediated by warm-reacting antibody. Most cases are idiopathic with no underlying pathology, but may be 2° to lymphoid malignancies e.g. CLL, or autoimmune disease such as SLE.

Epidemiology

Affects predominantly individuals >50 years of age.

Clinical features

- Highly variable symptoms, asymptomatic or severely anaemic.
- Chronic compensated haemolysis.
- Mild jaundice common.
- Splenomegaly usual.

Diagnosis

- Anaemia.
- Spherocytes on peripheral blood film.
- Reticulocytes are ↑↑.
- Neutrophilia common.
- RBC coated with IgG, complement or both (detect using DAT).
- Autoantibody—often pan-reacting but specificity in 10–15% (Rh, mainly anti-e, anti-D or anti-c).

- LDH ↑.
- Serum haptoglobin ↓.
- Exclude underlying lymphoma (BM, blood and marrow cell markers).
- Autoimmune profile—to exclude SLE or other connective tissue disorder.

Treatment

Prednisolone 1mg/kg/d PO tailing off after response noted (usually 1–2 weeks). If no response consider immunosuppression e.g. azathioprine (suitable for elderly but not younger patients—risk of 2° leukaemia) or cyclophosphamide. Splenectomy should be considered in selected cases. IVIg (0.4g/kg/d for 5d) useful in refractory cases, or where rapid response required. Rituximab (anti-CD20) is emerging as a useful agent for a range of refractory autoimmune disorders, including AIHA. Regular folic acid (5mg/d) is advised.

Gehrs, B.C. & Friedberg, R.C. (2002) Autoimmune hemolytic anemia. *Am J Hematol*, **69**, 258–271.

Cold haemagglutinin disease (CHAD)

Describes syndrome associated with acrocyanosis in cold weather due to RBC agglutinates in blood vessels of skin. Caused by RBC antibody that reacts most strongly at temperatures <32°C. Complement is activated→RBC lysis→haemoglobinaemia and haemoglobinuria. May be idiopathic (1°) or 2° to infection with *Mycoplasma* or EBV (infectious mononucleosis).

Clinical features

- Elderly.
- Acrocyanosis (blue discoloration of extremities e.g. fingers, toes) in cold conditions.
- Chronic compensated haemolysis.
- Splenomegaly usual.

Diagnosis

- Anaemia.
- Reticulocytes are ↑↑.
- Neutrophilia common.
- Positive DAT—C_3 only.
- ± Autoantibodies—IgG or IgM
  - Monoclonal in NHL.
  - Polyclonal in infection-related CHAD.
- IgM antibodies react best at 4°C (thermal amplitude 4–32°C).
- Specificity
  - Anti-I (*Mycoplasma*).
  - Anti-i (infectious mononucleosis)—causes little haemolysis in adults since RBCs have little anti-i (*cf.* newborn i >> I).
- LDH ↑.
- Serum haptoglobin ↓.
- ***Exclude underlying lymphoma*** (BM, blood and marrow cell markers).
- Autoimmune profile to exclude SLE or other connective tissue disorder.

Treatment

- Keep warm.
- Corticosteroids generally of little value.
- Chlorambucil or cyclophosphamide (greatest value when there is underlying B-cell lymphoma, occasionally helpful in 1° CHAD).
- Plasma exchange may help in some cases.
- If blood transfusion required use in-line blood warmer.
- Splenectomy occasionally useful (*note:* liver is main site of RBC sequestration of C3b-coated RBCs).
- Infectious CHAD generally self-limiting.

Natural history

Prolonged survival, spontaneous remissions not unusual, with periodic relapses.

Red cell disorders

Leucoerythroblastic anaemia

Definition

A form of anaemia characterised by the presence of immature white and red blood cells in the peripheral blood. Mature white cells and platelets are also often reduced.

Causes

Marrow infiltration by

- 2° malignancy: commonly breast, lung, prostate, thyroid, kidney, colon.
- Myelofibrosis (a primary myeloproliferative disorder, *see p256*).
- Other haematological malignancy e.g. myeloma and Hodgkin's disease.
- Rarely, severe haemolytic or megaloblastic anaemia.
- Gaucher's disease.

Marrow stimulation by

- Infection, inflammation, hypoxia, trauma (common in ITU patients).
- Massive blood loss.

When due to marrow infiltration, there is often associated neutropenia ± thrombocytopenia. Marrow stimulative causes often have neutrophilia and thrombocytosis.

Investigations

- FBC and blood film. Typical film appearances are of increased polychromasia due to reticulocytosis, nucleated RBCs, poikilocytosis (tear drop forms common in infiltrative causes), myelocytes and band forms, occasionally even promyelocytes and blast cells.
- Clotting screen—where cause is 2° malignancy or infective, DIC may occur.

Bone marrow is usually diagnostic

- Hypercellular BM with normal cell maturation, typical of marrow stimulation causes.
- Infiltration with neoplastic cells of a 2° malignancy may be identified as abnormal clumps with characteristic morphology—immunohistochemistry may identify the primary source e.g. PSA for prostate.
- Increase in reticulin fibres running in parallel bundles identifies fibrotic infiltrative cause—usually myelofibrosis, but may occur with other haematological malignancy.

Treatment

- Diagnose and treat underlying cause if possible.
- Supportive transfusions as required, management of bone marrow failure (*see p562*).

Oster, W. *et al.* (1990) Erythropoietin for the treatment of anemia of malignancy associated with neoplastic bone marrow infiltration. *J Clin Oncol*, **8**, 956–962.

Red cell disorders

Aplastic anaemia

Definition

A gross reduction or absence of haemopoietic precursors in all 3 cell lineages in bone marrow resulting in pancytopenia in peripheral blood. Although this encompasses all situations in which there is myelosuppression, the term is generally used to describe those in which spontaneous marrow recovery is unusual.

Incidence

Rare ~5 cases per million population annually. Wide age range, slight increase around age 25 years and >65 years. 10× more common in Orientals.

Causes

Divided into categories where aplasia is regarded as:

- **Inevitable**
  - TBI dose of >1.5Gy (*note*: >8Gy always fatal in absence of graft rescue).
  - Chemotherapy e.g. high dose busulfan.
- **Hereditary**
  - Fanconi syndrome—stem cell repair defect resulting in abnormalities of skin, facies, musculo-skeletal system and urogenital systems.
  - BM failure often delayed until adulthood.
- **Idiosyncratic**
  - Chronic benzene exposure.
  - Drug-induced, but not dose related—mainly gold, chloramphenicol, phenylbutazone, NSAIDs, carbamazepine, phenytoin, mesalazine.
  - Genetic predisposition demonstrated for chloramphenicol.
- **Post-viral**
  - Parvoviral infections—classically red cell aplasia but may be all elements. Devastating in conjunction with chronic haemolytic anaemia e.g. aplastic sickle crisis.
  - Hepatitis viruses A, B and C, CMV and EBV.
- **Idiopathic**
  - Constitute the majority of cases.

Classification

- According to severity most clinically useful.
- Defines highest risk groups.

Classification of severity in aplastic anaemia

Severe	2 of the following:	neutrophils platelets reticulocytes	$<0.5 \times 10^9$/L $<20 \times 10^9$/L <1%
Very severe		neutrophils and infection present	$<0.2 \times 10^9$/L,

Clinical features
Reflects the pancytopenia. Bleeding from mucosal sites common, with purpura, ecchymoses. Infections, particularly upper and lower respiratory tracts, skin, mouth, peri-anal. Bacterial and fungal infections common. Anaemic symptoms usually less severe due to chronic onset.

Diagnosis and investigation
- FBC and blood film show pancytopenia, MCV may be ↑, film morphology unremarkable.
- Reticulocytes usually absent.
- BM aspirate and trephine show gross reduction in all haemopoietic tissue replaced by fat spaces—important to exclude hypocellular MDS or leukaemia—the main differential diagnoses.
- Flow cytometry using anti-CD55 and anti-CD59 will show lack of both membrane proteins. Ham's acid lysis test is now largely obsolete.
- Specialised cytogenetics on blood to exclude Fanconi syndrome (*see p456*).

Complications
- Progression to more severe disease.
- Evolution to PNH—occurs in 7%.
- Transformation to acute leukaemia occurs in 5–10%.

Treatment
- Mild cases need careful observation only. More severe will need supportive treatment with red cell and platelet transfusions and antibiotics as needed. Blood products should be CMV –ve, and preferably leucodepleted to reduce risk of sensitisation.
- Specific treatment options are between allogeneic transplant and immunosuppression.
- Sibling allogeneic transplant treatment of choice for those <50 with sibling donor. Should go straight to transplant avoiding immunosuppression and blood products if possible.
- Matched unrelated donor transplant should be considered in <25 age group.
- Immunosuppressive options include anti-lymphocyte globulin (ALG) ± cyclosporin. Response to ALG may take 3 months. Refractory or relapsing patients may respond to a second course of ALG from another animal.
- Cyclosporin post-ALG looks promising.
- Androgens or danazol may be useful in some cases.

Abkowitz, J.L. (2001) Aplastic anemia: which treatment? *Ann Intern Med*, **135**, 524–526; Young, N.S. & Barrett, A.J. (1995) The treatment of severe acquired aplastic anemia. *Blood*, **85**, 3367–3377.

Paroxysmal nocturnal haemoglobinuria

Definition
Acquired clonal abnormality of cell membranes rendering them more sensitive to complement-mediated lysis, most noticeable in RBCs. Cells lack phosphatidylinositol glycoproteins (PIG) transmembrane anchors.

Incidence
Rare. Aplastic anaemia is closely related.

Clinical features
- Chronic intravascular haemolytic anaemia particularly overnight (?due to lower blood pH). Infections trigger acceleration of haemolysis.
- WBC and platelet production also often ↓.
- Chronic haemolysis may induce nephropathy.
- Haemoglobinuria usually results in iron deficiency.
- ↑↑ tendency to venous thrombosis particularly at atypical sites e.g. hepatic vein (Budd–Chiari syndrome), sagittal sinus thrombosis.
- Fatigue, dysphagia and impotence occasionally seen.

Diagnosis and treatment
- FBC, blood film—polychromasia and reticulocytosis (*cf.* AA).
- BM aspirate and trephine biopsy—usually hypoplastic with increased fat space but with erythropoietic nests or islands distinct from AA.
- Ham's test (acidified serum lysis) is invariably +ve though seldom used now.
- Cellular immunophenotype shows altered PIG proteins, CD55 and CD59.
- Urinary haemosiderin +ve.

Complications
- May progress to more severe aplasia.
- Transforms to acute leukaemia in 5%.
- Serious thromboses in up to 20%.

Treatment:
- Chronic disease—supportive care may be satisfactory in mild cases.
- Iron replacement usually required.
- Trial of steroid/androgens/danazol may ↓ symptoms and transfusion need.
- ALG/cyclosporin may be indicated for more severe cases as for aplastic anaemia.
- Acute major thromboses should be treated aggressively with urgent thrombolysis and 10 days heparin. Long-term warfarin mandatory. Consider warfarin prophylaxis after any one clotting episode.
- Severe cases <50 years should be considered for sibling allogeneic transplant if they have a donor—consider MUD in <25 age group if no sibling donor.

Prognosis:
Median survival from diagnosis is 9 years. Major cause of mortality is thrombosis and marrow failure. Molecular genetic basis now established—could be a candidate disease for gene transplantation.

Hillmen, P. *et al.* (1995) Natural history of paroxysmal nocturnal hemoglobinuria. *N Engl J Med*, **333**, 1253–1258; Rosse, W.F. (1997) Paroxysmal nocturnal hemoglobinuria as a molecular disease. *Medicine* (Baltimore), **76**, 63–93.

Pure red cell aplasia

Definition
A severe anaemia characterised by reticulocytes <1% in PB, <0.5% mature erythroblasts in BM but with normal WBC and platelets.

Incidence
Rare.

Classification of red cell aplasia		
Congenital	Diamond–Blackfan anaemia (DBA), *see p452*	
Acquired	*Childhood:*	Transient erythroblastopenia of childhood (TEC)
	Adults:	Primary: autoimmune or idiopathic Secondary chronic: thymoma, haematological malignancies especially CLL, pernicious anaemia, some solid tumours, SLE, RA, malnutrition with riboflavin deficiency Secondary transient: infections especially Parvovirus B19, CMV, HIV, many drugs Recent interest following red cell aplasia in renal patients treated with subcutaneous Epo

Clinical features
- Lethargy usually only symptom of the anaemia since slow onset.
- No abnormal physical signs except of any underlying disease.

Diagnosis and investigations
- FBC shows severe normochromic, normocytic anaemia with retics <1%. WBC and platelets normal.
- BM shows absence of erythroblasts but is normocellular (distinguishes from aplastic anaemia).

Treatment
- Treat underlying cause first if identified.
- Remove thymoma.
- If due to parvovirus B19, try IVIg.
- Assume immune origin if no other cause found and give prednisolone 60mg od PO as starter dose ~40% response. Failure of response, try cyclosporin or ALG or azathioprine.

Prognosis
- 15% have spontaneous remission. 65% will respond to immunosuppression.
- 50% will relapse but 80% of relapsers will respond again.
- A few progress to AA or AML.

Red cell disorders

Iron overload

Iron is an essential metal but overload occurs when intake of iron exceeds requirements and occurs due to the absence in humans of a physiological mechanism to excrete excess iron. Sustained ↑ Fe intake (dietary or parenteral) may result in iron accumulation, overload and potentially fatal tissue damage.

Timing and pattern of tissue damage is determined by rate of accumulation, the quantity of total body iron and distribution of iron between reticuloendothelial (RE) storage sites and vulnerable parenchymal tissue. Iron accumulation in parenchymal cells of the liver, heart, pancreas and other organs is the major determinant of clinical sequelae.

Haemochromatosis

- Inherited (autosomal recessive) occurring in up to 0.5% population (N. Europe).
- Haemochromatosis locus is tightly linked to the HLA locus on chromosome 6p and up to 10% population are heterozygous.
- Single missense mutation found in the homozygous state in 80% of patients.
- The gene designated *HFE* is an MHC class Ib gene.
- Homozygotes develop symptomatic iron overload.

Caused by failure to regulate iron absorption from bowel causing progressive increase in total body iron. Parenchymal accumulation occurs initially in liver then pancreas, heart, skin and other organs rather than RE sites. Symptoms do not usually develop until middle age when body iron stores of ≥15–20g have accumulated. Environmental factors (e.g. alcohol use in males and menstruation in females) affect rate of accumulation and age at presentation. Clinical expression of haemochromatosis is seen 10× more commonly in ♂. Only 25% of heterozygotes show evidence of minor increases in iron stores and clinical problems do not occur.

Clinical manifestations of iron overload only occur in homozygotes and presentation as 'bronze diabetes' is characteristic.

Clinical features of Fe overload (homozygous haemochromatosis)

• Skin pigmentation	Slate grey or bronze discolouration
• Hepatic dysfunction	Hepatomegaly, chronic hepatitis, fibrosis, cirrhosis, hepatocellular carcinoma (20–30%)
• Diabetes mellitus	Retinopathy, nephropathy, neuropathy, vascular complications
• Gonadal dysfunction	Hypogonadism, impotence
• Other endocrine dysfunction	Hypothyroidism, hypoparathyroidism, adrenal insufficiency
• Abdominal pain	Unknown aetiology (25%)
• Cardiac dysfunction	Cardiomyopathy, heart failure, dysrhythmias (10–15%)
• Chondrocalcinosis	Arthropathy

Evaluation of iron status

Most useful indirect measure of iron stores is serum ferritin estimation. Rises to maximum concentration of 4000μg/L and may underestimate extent of iron overload in some patients. *Note:* may be spuriously increased by infection, inflammation or neoplasia. The % transferrin saturation provides confirmatory evidence but no measure of the extent of iron overload. Liver biopsy provides a direct albeit invasive measure of iron stores (% iron concentration by weight) and visual assessment of iron distribution, and the extent of tissue damage.

Diagnosis

May be difficult to differentiate haemochromatosis from iron overload 2° to other causes, particularly that associated with chronic liver disease. Recent identification of *HFE* gene will provide a tool for more definitive diagnosis and screening of relatives (previously performed by serum ferritin estimation).

Management

- Aim to reduce iron stores to <50μg/L and prevent complications of overload.
- Achieved by regular venesection (500mL blood) on weekly basis until iron deficiency develops (may take many months).
- Hb should be measured prior to each venesection and response to therapy can be monitored by intermittent measurement of the serum ferritin.
- Once iron deficiency develops a maintenance regimen can be commenced with venesection every 3–4 months.

Natural history

Cirrhosis and hepatocellular carcinoma are the most common causes of death in patients with haemochromatosis and are due to hepatic iron accumulation. Cirrhosis does not usually develop until the hepatic iron concentration reaches 4000–5000μg/g of liver (normal 50–500μg/g). Hepatocellular carcinoma is the cause of death in 20–30% but does not occur in the absence of cirrhosis which increases the risk over 200×. If venesection can be commenced prior to the development of cirrhosis and other complications of haemosiderosis the life expectancy is that of a normal individual. Reduction of iron overload by venesection has only a small effect on symptomatology which has already developed: skin pigmentation diminishes, liver function may improve, cardiac abnormalities may resolve, diabetes and other endocrine abnormalities may improve slightly, arthropathy is unaffected.

Olynyk, J.K. *et al.* (1999) A population-based study of the clinical expression of the hemochromatosis gene. *N Engl J Med*, **341**, 718–724; Sanchez, A.M. *et al.* (2001) Prevalence, donation practices, and risk assessment of blood donors with hemochromatosis. *JAMA*, **286**, 1475–1481.

Transfusion haemosiderosis

Iron overload occurs in patients with transfusion dependent anaemia, notably thalassaemia major, Diamond–Blackfan syndrome, aplastic anaemia and acquired refractory anaemia. In many of these conditions iron overload is aggravated by physiological mechanisms which promote increased dietary absorption of iron in response to ineffective erythropoiesis. Each unit of blood contains 250mg iron and average transfusion dependent adult receives 6–10g of iron/year. Distribution of iron is similar to haemochromatosis with primarily liver parenchymal cell accumulation followed by pancreas, heart and other organs. Cardiac deposition occurs in patients who have received 100 units of blood (20g iron) without chelation, and is followed by damage to the liver, pancreas and endocrine glands.

Clinical features of iron overload in children who require transfusion support for hereditary anaemia are listed. Similar problems excluding those related to growth and sexual maturation develop in patients who commence a transfusion programme for acquired refractory anaemia in later life.

Features of transfusion haemosiderosis in hereditary anaemia

- Growth retardation in second decade.
- Hypogonadism—delayed or absent sexual maturation.
- Skin pigmentation—slate grey or bronze discolouration.
- Hepatic dysfunction—hepatomegaly, chronic hepatitis, fibrosis, cirrhosis, hepatocellular carcinoma.
- Diabetes mellitus.
- Other endocrine dysfunction—rarely hypothyroidism, hypoparathyroidism, adrenal insufficiency.
- Cardiac dysfunction—cardiomyopathy, heart failure, dysrhythmias (main cause of death).
- Death from heart disease in adolescence.

Management

- Iron chelation therapy by parenteral desferrioxamine is the only treatment for patients with transfusion haemosiderosis, who remain anaemic. Haemosiderosis due to previous transfusions in conditions where Hb now normal e.g. treated AML, may be venesected to remove iron.
- Regular treatment is required in transfusion dependent children if they are to avoid the consequences of iron overload in the second decade of life.
- SC administration of desferrioxamine by portable syringe pump over 9–12h on 5–7 nights/week is a common regimen.
- Ascorbic acid supplementation may help mobilise iron and increase excretion with desferrioxamine but can cause hazardous redistribution of storage iron.
- Early and regular desferrioxamine infusion ↓ hepatic iron and improves hepatic function, promotes growth and sexual development and protects against heart disease and early death.

- Much work has been expended in the search for an effective non-toxic oral chelator and deferiprone is currently under evaluation in clinical trials.

Natural history

The prognosis of the underlying haematological condition in transfusion dependent elderly patients may eliminate the need for iron chelation. In others with a longer life expectancy, IV infusion of desferrioxamine with each blood transfusion may adequately delay the rate of iron accumulation.

Other causes of haemosiderosis

Dietary iron overload may also occur as a result of chronic over-ingestion of iron-containing traditional home-brewed fermented maize beverages peculiar to sub-Saharan Africa, which overwhelms physiological controls on iron absorption. Iron stores may >50g and iron is initially deposited in both hepatocytes and Kupffer cells but when cirrhosis develops, accumulates in the pancreas, heart and other organs. Over-ingestion of medicinal iron may possibly have a similar though less dramatic effect but is certainly harmful to patients with iron-loading disorders. The excessive iron absorption seen in patients with chronic liver disease is associated with accumulation in Kupffer cells rather than hepatic parenchyma. Rare congenital defects associated with iron overload have been reported.

White blood cell abnormalities 3

Neutrophilia

Neutrophils are derived from same precursor as monocytes. Cytoplasm contains granules; the nucleus has 3–4 segments. Functions include chemotaxis—neutrophils migrate to sites of inflammation by chemotactic factors e.g. complement components (C5a and C3), and cytokines. Cytotoxic activity is via phagocytosis and destruction of particles/invading microorganisms (latter often antibody coated = *opsonised*). Granules contain cationic proteins⟶lyse Gram –ve bacteria, 'defensins', myeloperoxidase—interacts with H_2O_2 and HCl⟶hypochlorous acid (HOCl); lysozyme (hydrolyses bacterial cell walls); superoxide (O_2^-) and hydroxyl (OH^-) radicals. Neutrophil lifespan is ~1–2d in tissues.

Normal neutrophil count 2.0–7.5 × 10^9/L (neonate differs from adult; see *Normal ranges p690*).

Neutrophilia is defined as an absolute neutrophil count >7.5 × 10^9/L.

Mechanisms
- Increased production.
- Accelerated/early release from marrow⟶blood.
- Demargination (marginal pool⟶circulating pool).

Causes
- Infection (bacterial, viral, fungal, spirochaetal, rickettsial).
- Inflammation (trauma, infarction, vasculitis, rheumatoid disease, burns).
- Chemicals e.g. drugs, hormones, toxins, haemopoietic growth factors e.g. G-CSF, GM-CSF, adrenaline, corticosteroids, venoms.
- Physical agents e.g. cold, heat, burns, labour, surgery, anaesthesia.
- Haematological e.g. myeloproliferative disease, CML, PPP (primary proliferative polycythaemia), myelofibrosis, chronic neutrophilic leukaemia.
- Other malignancies.
- Cigarette smoking.
- Post-splenectomy.
- Chronic bleeding.
- Idiopathic.

Investigation
History and examination. Ask about cigarette smoking, symptoms suggesting occult malignancy.

Other investigations
ESR, CRP.

Treatment
Usually treatment of underlying disorder is all that is required.

Leukaemoid reaction
May resemble leukaemia (hence name); see ↑ WBC (myeloblasts and promyelocytes prominent). Occurs in severe and/or chronic infection, metastatic malignancy.

White blood cell abnormalities

Neutropenia

Defined as absolute peripheral blood neutrophil count of $<2.0 \times 10^9$/L. Racial variation: Black and Middle Eastern people may have neutrophil count of $<1.5 \times 10^9$/L normally.

Congenital neutropenia syndromes

Kostmann's syndrome: 📖 *Paediatric haematology, p459.*

Chediak–Higashi: 📖 *Paediatric haematology, p465.*

Shwachman–Diamond syndrome: 📖 *Paediatric haematology, p459.*

Cyclical neutropenia: 3–4 week periodicity; often 21d cycle, lasts 3–6d.

Miscellaneous: transcobalamin II deficiency, reticular dysgenesis, dyskeratosis congenita.

Acquired neutropenia

Acquired neutropenia: commonest causes	
Infection	Viral, e.g. influenza, HIV, hepatitis, overwhelming bacterial sepsis
Drugs	Anticonvulsants (e.g. phenytoin) Antithyroid (e.g. carbimazole) Phenothiazines (e.g. chlorpromazine) Antiinflammatory agents (e.g. phenylbutazone) Antibacterial agents (e.g. cotrimoxazole) Others (gold, penicillamine, tolbutamide, mianserin, imipramine, cytotoxics)
Immune mediated	Autoimmune (antineutrophil antibodies) SLE Felty's syndrome (rheumatoid arthritis + neutropenia + splenomegaly; no correlation between spleen size and degree of neutropenia)
As part of pancytopenia	
Bone marrow failure	Leukaemia, lymphoma, LGLL, haematinic deficiency, anorexia
Splenomegaly	Any cause

Clinical features—when severe neutropenia: throat/mouth infection, oral ulceration, septicaemia.

Diagnosis—examine peripheral blood film, check haematinics, autoimmune profile, anti-neutrophil antibodies, haematinics, bone marrow aspirate and trephine biopsy if indicated (e.g. severe or prolonged neutropenia, or features suggestive of infiltration of marrow failure syndrome).

Treatment—consists of prompt antibiotic therapy if infection, IVIg and corticosteroids may be helpful but effects unpredictable. In seriously ill patients consider use of G-CSF (need to exclude underlying leukaemia before starting therapy with growth factors). Consider prophylaxis with low dose antibiotics (e.g. ciprofloxacin 250mg bd) and antifungal (e.g. fluconazole 100mg od) agents. Drug-induced neutropenia usually recovers on stopping suspected agent (may take 1–2 weeks).

Bux, J. *et al.* (1998) Diagnosis and clinical course of autoimmune neutropenia in infancy: analysis of 240 cases. *Blood*, **91**, 181–186; Dale, D.C., Bolyard, A.A. & Aprikyan, A. (2002) Cyclic neutropenia. *Semin Hematol*, **39**, 89–94.

Lymphocytosis and lymphopenia

Lymphocytes are small cells with a high N:C ratio; some (e.g. natural killer cells) have prominent cytoplasmic granules. Two principal types: B and T lymphocyte. B-cells express monoclonal surface (not cytoplasmic) IgM and often IgD. B-cell stimulation through cross linkage of surface Ig molecules or via effector T cells causes their differentiation into plasma cells. Predominant role is humoral immunity via Ig secretion.

T cells are derived from stem cells that undergo maturation in thymus and express T-cell receptor molecule (CD3) on cell surface. Responsible for cell-mediated immunity e.g. delayed hypersensitivity, graft rejection, contact allergy and cytotoxic reactions against other cells.

Lymphocytosis (peripheral blood lymphocytes >4.5×10^9/L)

- Leukaemias and lymphomas including: CLL, NHL, Hodgkin's disease, acute lymphoblastic leukaemia, hairy cell leukaemia, Waldenström's macroglobulinaemia, heavy chain disease, mycosis fungoides, Sézary syndrome, large granular lymphocyte leukaemia, adult T-cell leukaemia lymphoma (ATLL).
- Infections e.g. EBV, CMV, *Toxoplasma gondii*, rickettsial infection, *Bordetella pertussis*, mumps, varicella, coxsackievirus, rubella, hepatitis virus, adenovirus.
- 'Stress' e.g. myocardial infarction, sickle crisis.
- Trauma.
- Rheumatoid disease (occasionally).
- Adrenaline.
- Vigorous exercise.
- Post-splenectomy.
- β thalassaemia intermedia.

Lymphopenia (peripheral blood lymphocytes <1.5×10^9/L)

- Malignant disease e.g. Hodgkin's disease, some NHL, non-haematopoietic cancers, angioimmunoblastic lymphadenopathy.
- MDS.
- Collagen vascular disease e.g. rheumatoid, SLE, GvHD.
- Infections e.g. HIV.
- Chemotherapy.
- Surgery.
- Burns.
- Liver failure.
- Renal failure (acute and chronic).
- Anorexia nervosa.
- Iron deficiency (uncommon).
- Aplastic anaemia.
- Cushing's disease.
- Sarcoidosis.
- Congenital disorders (rare) such as SCID, reticular dysgenesis, agammaglobulinaemia (Swiss type), thymic aplasia (DiGeorge's syndrome), ataxia telangiectasia.

White blood cell abnormalities

Eosinophilia

Differential diagnosis

Common

- Drugs (huge list e.g. gold, sulphonamides, penicillin); erythema multiforme (Stevens–Johnson syndrome).
- Parasitic infections: hookworm, *Ascaris,* tapeworms, filariasis, amoebiasis, schistosomiasis.
- Allergic syndromes—asthma, eczema, urticaria.

Less common

- Pemphigus.
- Dermatitis herpetiformis (DH).
- Polyarteritis nodosa (PAN).
- Sarcoid.
- Tumours esp. Hodgkin's.
- Irradiation.

Rare

- Hypereosinophilic (Loeffler's) syndrome.
- Eosinophilic leukaemia.
- AML with eosinophilia esp. M4Eo (*see p151*).

Discriminating clinical features

- Drugs: history of exposure, time course of eosinophilia with resolution on cessation of drug.
- Allergic conditions: history of eczema, urticaria or typical rashes. Symptoms and signs of asthma.
- Parasites: history of exposure from foreign travel, symptoms and signs of iron deficiency anaemia (hookworm is commonest cause worldwide). Blood film may show filariasis. Stool microscopy and culture for ova, cysts and parasites for amoebiasis, *Ascaris*, *Taenia*, schistosomiasis.
- Skin diseases: typical appearances confirmed by biopsy e.g. dermatitis herpetiformis and pemphigus.
- PAN: renal failure, neuropathy, angiography and ANCA positivity.
- Sarcoid: multi-system features with non-caseating granulomata in biopsy of affected tissue or on BM biopsy; high serum ACE.
- Hodgkin's: lymphadenopathy, hepatosplenomegaly—BM or node biopsy.
- Hypereosinophilic syndrome: history of allergy, cough, fever and pulmonary infiltrates on CXR, may be cardiac involvement. Eosinophils on blood film have normal morphology and granulation. Diagnosis on exclusion of similar causes.
- Eosinophilic leukaemia: eosinophils on blood film have abnormal morphology with hyperlobular and hypergranular forms. BM heavily infiltrated with same abnormal cells. Other signs of myeloproliferative disease may be present.
- AML M4Eo: blasts with myelomonoblastic features on BM and blood film (*see p151*).

White blood cell abnormalities

Basophilia and basopenia

Basophils are found in peripheral blood and marrow (≡ mast cells in tissues). Short lifespan (1–2d), cannot replicate. Degranulation results in hypersensitivity reactions (IgE F_c receptors trigger), flushing, etc.

Basophilia (peripheral blood basophils >0.1 × 10^9/L)

- Myeloproliferative disorders
  - CGL.
  - Other chronic myeloid leukaemias.
  - PRV.
  - Myelofibrosis.
  - Essential thrombocythaemia.
  - Basophilic leukaemia.
- AML (rare).
- Hypothyroidism.
- IgE-mediated hypersensitivity reactions.
- Inflammatory disorders e.g. rheumatoid disease, ulcerative colitis.
- Drugs e.g. oestrogens.
- Infection e.g. viral.
- Irradiation.
- Hyperlipidaemia.

Basopenia (peripheral blood basophils <0.1 × 10^9/L)

- As part of generalised leucocytosis e.g. infection, inflammation.
- Thyrotoxicosis.
- Haemorrhage.
- Cushing's syndrome.
- Allergic reaction.
- Drugs e.g. progesterone.

White blood cell abnormalities

Monocytosis and monocytopenia

Bone marrow monocytes give rise to blood monocytes and tissue macrophages. Part of reticuloendothelial system (RES). Other components of RES: lung alveolar macrophages; pleural and peritoneal macrophages; Kupffer cells in liver; histiocytes; renal mesangial cells; macrophages in lymph node, spleen and marrow.

Contain 2 sets of granules (1) lysosomal (acid phosphatase, arylsulphatase and peroxidase), and (2) function of second set unknown.

Monocytosis (peripheral blood monocytes >0.8 $\times$ 10^9/L)

Common
- Malaria, trypanosomiasis, typhoid (commonest world-wide causes).
- Post-chemotherapy or stem cell transplant esp. if GM-CSF used.
- Tuberculosis.
- Myelodysplasia (MDS).

Less common
- Infective endocarditis.
- Brucellosis.
- Hodgkin's lymphoma.
- AML (M4 or M5).

Discriminating clinical features
- Malaria: identification of parasites on thick and thin blood films.
- Trypanosomiasis: parasites seen on blood film, lymph node biopsy or blood cultures.
- Typhoid: blood culture, faecal and urine culture and BM culture.
- Infective endocarditis: cardiac signs and blood cultures.
- Tuberculosis: AFB seen and cultured in sputum, EMU, blood or BM, tuberculin positivity on intradermal challenge, caseating granulomata on biopsy of affected tissue or BM.
- Brucellosis: blood cultures and serology.
- Hodgkin's: lymphadenopathy, hepatosplenomegaly, eosinophilia, biopsy of node or BM.
- MDS: typical dysplastic features on blood film or BM (*see p218*).
- AML (M4 or M5): monoblasts on blood film and BM biopsy. Skin and gum infiltration common, *see p150*.

Monocytopenia (peripheral blood monocytes <0.2 $\times$ 10^9/L)
- Autoimmune disorders e.g. SLE.
- Hairy cell leukaemia.
- Drugs e.g. glucocorticoids, chemotherapy.

White blood cell abnormalities

Mononucleosis syndromes

Definition

Constitutional illness associated with atypical lymphocytes in the blood.

Clinical features

Peak incidence in adolescence: may be subclinical or acute presentation consisting of fever, lethargy, sweats, anorexia, pharyngitis, lymphadenopathy (cervical>axillary>inguinal), tender splenomegaly ± hepatomegaly, palatal petechiae, maculopapular rash especially if given ampicillin. Rarely also pericarditis, myocarditis, encephalitis. Usually self-limiting illness but complications include lethargy persisting for months or years (chronic fatigue syndrome), depression, autoimmune haemolytic anaemia, thrombocytopenia, secondary infection and splenic rupture.

Causes

EBV, CMV, *Toxoplasma, Brucella*, Coxsackie and adenoviruses, HIV sero-conversion illness.

Pathophysiology

In EBV related illness, EBV infection of B lymphocytes results in immortalisation and generates a T cell response (the *atypical lymphocytes*) which controls EBV proliferation. In severe immunodeficiency following prolonged use of cyclosporin, oligoclonal EBV-related lymphoma may develop which usually regresses with reduction of immunosuppressive therapy but may evolve to a monoclonal and aggressive lymphoma e.g. after MUD stem cell transplant. In malarial Africa, EBV infection is associated with an aggressive lymphoma—Burkitt's lymphoma *see p204*.

Diagnosis – haematological features

- Atypical lymphocytes on blood film (recognised by the dark blue cytoplasmic edge to cells and invagination (scalloping) around red blood cells).
- Usually lymphocytosis with mild neutropenia.
- Occasionally anaemia due to cold antibody mediated haemolysis (anti-i)—identify with cold haemagglutinin titre.
- Paul Bunnell/monospot test for presence of heterophile antibody +ve when cause is EBV but only in the first few weeks. False +ves can occur in lymphoma.
- ↑ bilirubin and abnormal LFTs.
- Serological testing should include EBV capsid Ag, CMV IgM, Toxoplasma titre, Brucella titre, HIV 1 and 2 Ag and Ab.
- Immunophenotype of peripheral blood B lymphocytes shows polyclonality (distinguishes from lymphoma and other lymphoproliferative disorders).

Treatment

Rest and symptom relief are mandatory. No other specific treatment has been shown to influence outcome.

White blood cell abnormalities

Leukaemia

4

Acute myeloblastic leukaemia (AML)

Malignant tumour of haemopoietic precursor cells of non-lymphoid lineage, almost certainly arising in the bone marrow.

Incidence

Commonest acute leukaemia in adults. 3 per 100,000 annually. Increasing frequency with age (median 64 years; incidence 35/100,000 at age 90). Infrequent in children under 15 years.

Aetiology

Unclear—association with pre-existing myelodysplasia, previous cytotoxic chemotherapy (particularly alkylating agents and epipodophyllotoxins), ionizing radiation, benzene exposure, constitutional chromosomal abnormalities (e.g. Down's (older patients) and Fanconi's syndromes) and smoking.

Diagnosis

Made by examination of the peripheral blood film and bone marrow (≥20% blasts). Cytochemical stains, immunological markers, cytogenetic analysis and molecular markers are necessary to differentiate AML from ALL and further classify the disease in preparation for therapy.

Morphological classification

The French–American–British (FAB) system is based on predominant differentiation pathway and degree of differentiation:

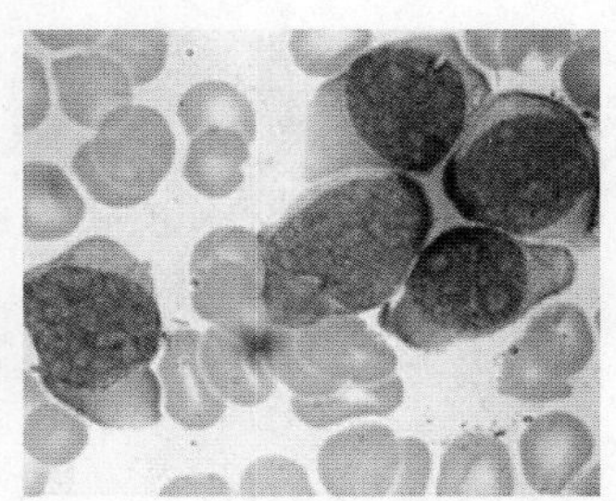

Bone marrow showing myeloblasts in AML

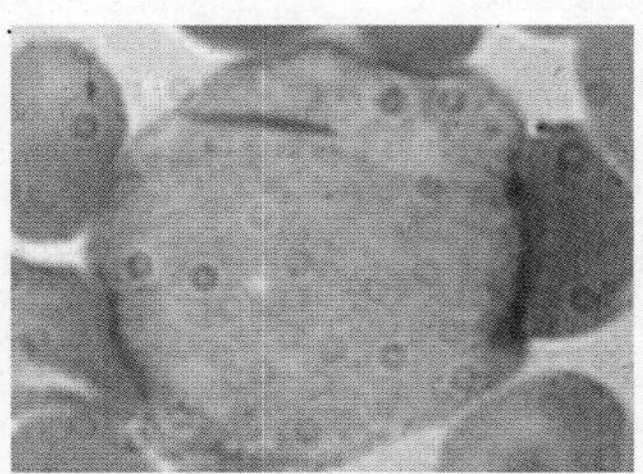

AML: myeloblast with large Auer rod (top left).

M0	AML with minimal differentiation (SB & MPO cytochemistry negative but myeloid immunophenotyping; may also express CD4 & CD7); 3% of cases.
M1	AML without maturation (<10% promyelocytes/myelocytes or monocytes; may have Auer rods) 20% of cases.
M2	AML with maturation (≥10% promyelocytes/myelocytes; < 20% monocytes; may have Auer rods; t(8;21)) commonest subtype: 30% of cases.
M3	Acute promyelocytic leukaemia (>30% promyelocytes; multiple Auer rods (faggot cells); t(15;17)) 10% of cases.
M3v	Microgranular variant of APL (high WBC count; minimal granulation; Auer rods rare; t(15;17)).
M4	Acute myelomonocytic leukaemia (mixed myeloid (>20% blasts & promyelocytes) & monocytic (≥20%) maturation; monocytic cells are non-specific esterase positive; may have Auer rods) 20% of cases.
M4Eo	M4 variant with 5–30% eosinophils; associated with inv(16) chromosome abnormality. 5% of cases
M5a	Acute monoblastic leukaemia (poorly differentiated subtype with ≥80% monocytoid cells of which ≥80% are monoblasts; Auer rods unusual) 10–15% cases are M5a or M5b.
M5b	Acute monocytic leukaemia (differentiated subtype with ≥80% monocytoid cells including NSE-positive cells with typical monocytic appearance; Auer rods rare)
M6	Acute erythroleukaemia (myeloblasts sometimes with Auer rods plus ≥50% bizarre often multinucleated erythroblasts; erythroblasts often PAS-positive) 3–5% of cases but 10–20% of secondary leukaemias.
M7	Acute megakaryoblastic leukaemia (difficult to diagnose morphologically; often dry tap due to fibrosis; requires immunophenotyping with anti-platelet antibodies or electron microscope analysis of platelet peroxidase) rare.

Cytochemistry

Former mainstay of leukaemia diagnosis; Sudan black (SB), myeloperoxidase (MPO) and esterase (chloroacetate and non-specific esterase) stains are positive in AML and negative in ALL (<3% blasts positive). Non-specific esterase (NSE) is positive in monocytic cells.

World Health Organisation (WHO) classification of acute myeloid leukaemia

Although the FAB classification has provided a morphological classification of AML for almost 30 years the correlation between morphology and both genetic and clinical features is imperfect. The WHO classification attempts to correlate morphological, genetic and clinical features to categorise cases of AML into unique clinical and biological subgroups.

In the WHO classification the blast threshold for the diagnosis of AML is reduced from 30% to 20% BM blasts (i.e. most patients previously diagnosed as RAEB-t will be classified as AML with multilineage dysplasia) and patients with clonal recurring abnormalities t(8;21)(q22;q22), inv(16)(q13q22), t(16;16)(p13;q22) or t(15;17)(q22;q12) should be considered to have AML regardless of the blast percentage.

WHO classification of acute myeloid leukaemia

Acute myeloid leukaemia with recurrent genetic abnormalities

- Acute myeloid leukaemia with t(8;21)(q22;q22), (*AML1/ETO*)
- Acute myeloid leukaemia with abnormal BM eosinophils and inv(16)(q13;q22) or t(16;16)(p13;q22), (*CBFβ/MYH11*) (= FAB M4Eo)
- Acute promyelocytic leukaemia with t(15;17)(q22;q12), (*PML/RARα*) and variants (= FAB M3)
- Acute myeloid leukaemia with 11q23 (*MLL*) abnormalities

Acute myeloid leukaemia with multilineage dysplasia

- Following MDS or MDS/MPD
- Without antecedent MDS or MDS/MPD, but with dysplasia in at least 50% of cells in 2 or more myeloid lineages

Acute myeloid leukaemia and myelodysplastic syndromes, therapy-related

- Alkylating agent/radiation-related type
- Topoisomerase II inhibitor-related type (some may be lymphoid)
- Others

Acute myeloid leukaemia, not otherwise categorised

Categorise as:

- Acute myeloid leukaemia, minimally differentiated (= FAB M0)
- Acute myeloid leukaemia, without maturation (= FAB M1)
- Acute myeloid leukaemia with maturation (= FAB M2)
- Acute myelomonocytic leukaemia (= FAB M4)
- Acute monoblastic/ acute monocytic leukaemia (= FAB M5a/5b)
- Acute erythroid leukaemia: erythroid/myeloid (≥ 50% erythroid precursors plus ≥20% blasts; = FAB M6) and pure erythroleukaemia (≥80% immature erythroid precursors)
- Acute megakaryoblastic leukaemia (= FAB M7)
- Acute basophilic leukaemia
- Acute panmyelosis with myelofibrosis (= acute myelofibrosis)
- Myeloid sarcoma

Immunophenotyping

Monoclonal antibodies to cell surface antigens reliably differentiate AML from ALL and confirm the diagnosis of M0, M6 and M7 (📖p153).

Panel of monoclonal antibodies to differentiate AML & ALL	
Myeloid	Anti-MPO; CD13; CD33; CDw65; CD117
B lymphoid	CD19; cytoplasmic CD22; CD79a; CD10
T lymphoid	Cytoplasmic CD3; CD2; CD7
Immunophenotypic patterns in AML subtypes	
Undifferentiated (M0)	Anti-MPO; CD13; CD33; CD34; CDw65; CD117; negative cytochemistry; lymphoid markers
Myelomonocytic (M1-M5):	anti-MPO; CD13; CD33; CDw65; CD117
Monocytic (M4 & M5)	Stronger expression of CD11b & CD14
Erythroid (M6)	Anti-glycophorin A
Megakaryocytic (M7)	CD41; CD61

Bain, B.J. *et al.* (2002) Revised guideline on immunophenotyping in acute leukaemias and chronic lymphoproliferative disorders. *Clin Lab Haematol*, **24**, 1–13.
http://www.bcshguidelines.com/pdf/CLH135.PDF

Lineage infidelity

It is sometimes impossible to define a single lineage for leukaemic blasts on the basis of phenotypic marker expression. The expression of markers of more than one cell lineage by a leukaemic cell is termed lineage infidelity and may reflect abnormal gene expression in the clone or abnormal maturation of an early uncommitted precursor. Blasts can display cytochemical and immunophenotypic markers of both myeloid and lymphoid precursors. Up to 50% of myeloid leukaemias may be positive for lymphoid antigens, most commonly CD2 (34%) and CD7 (42%) and this does not appear to have prognostic significance.

Biphenotypic leukaemias

A minority of acute leukaemias (~7%) have two distinct leukaemic cell populations on phenotyping and are characterised as biphenotypic leukaemias. Most commonly these cell populations express B-lymphoid and myeloid markers and are associated with a high frequency of t(9;22)(q34;q11), the Ph chromosome. These patients have variable response rates. Some may display 'lymphoid' features such as marked lymphadenopathy and high blast counts.

Cytogenetic analysis

Should be performed in all cases of acute leukaemia. It detects translocations and deletions that provide independent prognostic information in AML.

'Favourable risk' cytogenetics

- t(8;21)(q22;q22): FAB M2; 5–8% adults <55 years, rare older; fusion gene *AML1/ETO*.
- inv(16)(p13;q22) or t(16;16)(p13;q22): FAB M4Eo; 10% adults <45 years, rare older; fusion gene *CBFβ/MYH11*.
- t(15;17)(q21;q11): FAB M3; 15% adults <45 years, rare older; fusion gene *PML-RARα*. Variants: t(11;17)(q23;q11) fusion gene *PLZF-RARα*; t(5;17)(q32;q11) fusion gene *NPM-RARα*; t(11;17)(q13;q11) fusion gene *NuMA-RARα*.

'Intermediate risk' cytogenetics

- Normal karyotype: any FAB type; 15–20% adults.
- + 8: any FAB type; 10% adults.
- abnormal 11q23*: >50% infant AML cases; 5–7% adults; fusion gene *MLL*.
- Others: del(9q)*; del(7q)*; +6; +21; +22; –Y and 3–5 complex abnormalities* plus other structural or numerical defects not included in the good risk or poor risk groups.

'Poor risk' cytogenetics

- –5/del(5q): any FAB type; >10% adults >45years.
- –7/del(7q): any FAB type; >10% adults >45 years.
- Complex karyotypes (>5 abnormalities*)
- Others: t(6;9)(p23;q34); t(3;3)(q21;q96); 20q; 21q; t(9;22); abn 17p.

Note: This classification is based on the MRC-UK scheme[1]. Abnormalities marked * are classed as 'unfavourable' i.e. 'poor risk' in the scheme used by US Cooperative Groups[2].

Molecular analysis

Fluorescence *in situ* hybridisation (FISH) and reverse transcriptase-polymerase chain reaction (RT-PCR) methods add sensitivity and precision to the detection of translocations, deletions and aneuploidy in cases where conventional cytogenetics fails or gives normal results. RT-PCR detects minimal residual disease overlooked by conventional methods.

Clinical features

- Acute presentation usual; often critically ill due to effects of bone marrow failure.
- Symptoms of anaemia: weakness, lethargy, breathlessness, lightheadedness and palpitations.
- Infection: particularly chest, mouth, perianal, skin (*Staphylococcus*, *Pseudomonas*, HSV, *Candida*). Fever, malaise, sweats.
- Haemorrhage (especially M3 due to DIC): purpura, menorrhagia and epistaxis, bleeding gums, rectal, retina.
- Gum hypertrophy and skin infiltration (M4, M5).
- Signs of leucostasis e.g. hypoxia, retinal haemorrhage, confusion or diffuse pulmonary shadowing.
- Hepatomegaly occurs in 20%, splenomegaly in 24%; the latter should raise the question of transformed CML; lymphadenopathy is infrequent (17%)
- CNS involvement at presentation is rare in adults with AML.

1 Grimwade, D. *et al.* (2001) The predictive value of hierarchical cytogenetic classification in older adults with acute myeloid leukemia (AML): analysis of 1065 patients entered into the United Kingdom Medical Research Council AML11 trial. *Blood*, **98**, 1312–1320 **2** Smith, M.A. *et al.* (1996) The secondary leukemias: challenges and research directions. *J Natl Cancer Inst*, **88**, 407–418.

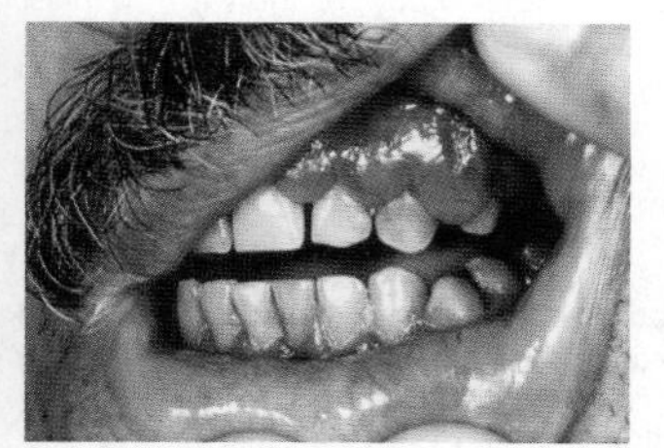

Gum hypertrophy in AML.

Investigations and diagnosis

- FBC and blood film.
- Bone marrow aspirate ± biopsy.
- Bone marrow cytogenetics.
- Immunophenotyping of blood or marrow blasts.
- Total WBC usually increased with blasts on blood film—but WBC may be low.
- Hb, neutrophils and platelets usually ↓.
- Bone marrow heavily infiltrated with blasts (≥20%)
- Further recommended investigations—📖*p544*.

Emergency treatment

- Seek expert help immediately.
- Intensive cardiovascular and respiratory resuscitation may be needed if septic shock or massive haemorrhage.
- Immediate empirical broad spectrum antibiotic treatment for neutropenic sepsis.
- Leucapheresis if peripheral blast count high or signs of leucostasis (retinal haemorrhage, reduced conscious level, diffuse pulmonary shadowing on CXR, or hypoxia).
- Intensive hydration with alkalinisation of the urine to prevent acute tumour lysis syndrome in patients with a high peripheral blast cell count ($>100 \times 10^9$/L).

Supportive treatment

- Explain diagnosis and offer counselling—the word '*leukaemia*' and prospect of prolonged chemotherapy are often distressing.
- RBC and platelet transfusion support will continue through treatment.
- Start neutropenic regimen (📖*p550*) as prophylaxis.
- Start hydration aiming for urine output >100mL/h throughout induction therapy.
- Start allopurinol or Rasburicase to prevent hyperuricaemia.
- Insert tunnelled central venous catheter (📖*p568*).

Specific treatment

Initial aim of therapy is to eliminate the leukaemic cells and achieve a complete haematological remission (CR), defined as normal BM cellularity with blast cells <5% and normal representation of trilineage haematopoiesis, normalisation of peripheral blood count with no blast cells, neutrophils ≥1.5 × 10^9/L, platelets ≥100 × 10^9/L and Hb>10g/dL. Leukaemia is undetectable by conventional morphological techniques but may be demonstrated by more sensitive molecular techniques (when available) and CR is not synonymous with cure. CR may result from a three-log kill from 10^{12} leukaemic cells at diagnosis to 10^9 at CR.

Treatment consists of 3 phases: (1) remission induction to achieve CR (usually 1–2 courses of combination chemotherapy); (2) consolidation therapy to reduce leukaemia burden further and reduce risk of relapse (optimum number unknown, usually 2–4 which may include an 'intensification' phase or an autologous or allogeneic stem cell transplant); (3) maintenance therapy has been abandoned in AML except in some elderly patients where intensive consolidation cannot be tolerated.

- Enter patient into MRC or other high quality trial if possible. MRC randomised studies in acute leukaemia are based on large patient numbers and compare incremental experimental therapy with best treatment arm from previous trials.
- Treatment protocols are age related; patients >60 only tolerate less intensive treatments and very rarely transplantation.
- Supportive treatment alone is a valid treatment option in the >75 age group or if there are coexistent serious general medical problems.
- Outline treatment for patients <60 years is 4–5 courses of intensive combination chemotherapy initially including daunorubicin or another anthracycline and cytosine arabinoside each lasting 5–10 days with a 2–3 week period of profound myelosuppression.
- Major complications are infective episodes which may be bacterial (Gram +ve and Gram –ve), fungal (*Candida* and *Aspergillus*), and less commonly viral (esp. HSV, HZV).
- APML (FABM3) is a distinct category of AML requiring different treatment. The risk of DIC prior to and during initial therapy due to release of thromboplastins from leukaemic cells is an indication for urgent treatment. The use of all-*trans*-retinoic acid (ATRA) with initial therapy reduces the risk of DIC. After this the prognosis is good. ATRA induces differentiation of the abnormal clone by overcoming the molecular block resulting from the t(15;17) translocation. ATRA alone cannot achieve sustained remission but in combination with chemotherapy 70% of patients may be cured. Arsenic trioxide appears to be a useful agent in those patients who relapse. Persistence of the fusion product after therapy detected by RT-PCR predicts relapse.
- Autologous stem cell transplantation is an option for intensive consolidation of younger patients (<60) with intermediate or poor-risk disease who achieve CR. It has lower procedure-related mortality or morbidity than an allograft but lacks a graft-versus-leukaemia effect and has a relapse rate of 40–50%.
- Allogeneic stem cell transplantation from a compatible sibling donor is an option for younger patients (<45) with intermediate or poor-risk disease. Significant mortality (7–13%) and morbidity may be reduced

by non-myeloablative conditioning regimens and increase the age range. Unrelated donor grafts have higher toxicity. Donor lymphocyte infusion (DLI) is used to treat recurrence after an allogeneic transplant.
- In the longer term, relapse is the main complication.

Prognosis

- 70–80% of patients aged <60 years will achieve a CR with a modern regimen and good supportive care; more intensive induction and consolidation regimens reduce the risk of relapse.
- Relapse risk at 5 years in patients <60 with favourable risk cytogenetics is 29–42%; intermediate risk 39–60%; poor risk 68–90%.
- 50–60% of patients aged ≥60 years achieve CR with induction treatment (rate drops with each decade) but relapse occurs in 80–90%; a higher proportion have poor risk karyotype, previous myelodysplasia and co-morbidity; treatment-related morbidity and mortality is high.

Prognostic factors

The most important prognostic factors predicting for achievement of remission and for subsequent relapse are:

1. Advancing patient age; <50 favourable; >60 unfavourable.
2. Presenting leucocyte count; $<25 \times 10^9$/L favourable; $>100 \times 10^9$/L unfavourable.
3. History of antecedent MDS or leukaemogenic therapy: unfavourable.
4. Presence of specific cytogenetic abnormalities (📖*p154*).
5. FAB subtype: M3, M4Eo favourable; M0, M5a, M5b, M6, M7 unfavourable.
6. Failure to achieve CR with first cycle of induction therapy predicts for relapse.

Management of relapse

- Most relapses occur in the first 2–3 years.
- Younger age and longer duration of first CR are good prognostic factors for achieving second CR.
- ~50% of patients achieve second CR with further therapy; under 10% survive over 3 years without a transplant procedure.

Acute lymphoblastic leukaemia (ALL)

Malignant tumour of haemopoietic precursor cells of the lymphoid lineage probably arising from the marrow in most cases.

Incidence

Commonest malignancy in childhood with the majority of cases in the 2–10 age group (median 3.5 years). Five times more frequent in childhood than AML. Rare leukaemia in adults, 0.7 to 1.8/100,000 annually. In adults, there is a peak at 15–24 years and a further peak in old age (2.3/100,000 >80 years).

Aetiology

Unknown. Predisposing factors are ionizing radiation (AML is more common) and congenital predisposition in Down's (20-fold in childhood), Bloom's, Klinefelter's and Fanconi's syndromes. Chemicals, pollution, viruses, urban/rural population movements, father's radiation exposure, radon levels and proximity to power lines have all been postulated.

Morphological Classification (French–American–British, FAB)	
L1	Small monomorphic type—small homogeneous blasts, single inconspicuous nucleolus, regular nuclear outline; commonest subtype.
L2	Large heterogeneous type—larger blasts, more pleomorphic and multinucleolate, irregular frequently clefted nuclei with conspicuous nucleoli.
L3	Burkitt cell type—large homogeneous blasts, abundant strongly basophilic cytoplasm with vacuoles; associated with B-cell phenotype.

Immunophenotyping

A panel of monoclonal antibodies is used to differentiate ALL from AML (📖*p153*). A further panel of B-and T-lineage markers and lymphocyte maturation markers subclassify ALL.

Immunological classification of ALL

B lineage

- *Pro B-ALL*: HLA-DR+,TdT+,CD19+ (5% children; 11% adults).
- *Common ALL*: HLA-DR+,TdT+,CD19+,CD10+ (65% children; 51% adults).
- *Pre B-ALL*: HLA-DR+,TdT+,CD19+,CD10±,cytoplasmic IgM+ (15% children; 10% adults).
- *B-cell ALL*: HLA-DR+,CD19+,CD10±,surface IgM+ (3% children; 4% adults)

T lineage

- *Pre-T ALL*: TdT+,cytoplasmic CD3+,CD7+ (1% children; 7% adults).
- *T-cell ALL*: TdT+,cytoplasmic CD3+, CD1a/2/3+,CD5+ (11% children; 17% adults).

Cytogenetic analysis

- Provides important prognostic information in both childhood and adult ALL. Abnormalities are detected in up to 85%. The major abnormalities are clonal translocations: t(9;22), t(4;11), t(8;14), t(1;19) or t(10;14) and other structural abnormalities (9p, 6q or 12p). If no structural abnormalities are present, the abnormalities can be classified by the modal chromosome number: <46 (hypodiploid); 46 with other structural abnormalities (pseudodiploid); 47–50 (hyperdiploid); >50 (hyper-hyperdiploid). With the exception of t(9;22) each has an incidence in the order of 5–10% or less.
- t(9;22)(q34;q11) produces the Philadelphia chromosome found in 5% of children and 25% of adults with ALL and is a very strong adverse prognostic factor in both; the resultant BCR-ABL hybrid product is the same 210 kDa protein detected in CML in 33% but is a smaller 180 kDa protein in 66%; it can be used for minimal residual disease detection.
- t(8;14) is associated with B-cell ALL (L3 morphology) and occurs in 5% of cases (dysregulates the *myc* proto-oncogene), t(1;19) is associated with B-cell precursor ALL; t(4;11) occurs in 80% of infants with ALL and 6% of adults and fuses the *MLL* gene from 11q23 to the *AF4* gene from 4q21 which can be detected by PCR; all these abnormalities are associated with refractory disease and early relapse
- Hyper-hyperdiploidy (>50 chromosomes) confers a favourable prognosis; combined +4, +10 confers a favourable outcome in B-cell precursor ALL; patients with hypoploidy (<46 chromosomes) and pseudodiploidy fare less well.

Clinical features

- Acute presentation usual; often critically ill due to effects of bone marrow failure.
- Symptoms of anaemia: weakness, lethargy, breathlessness, lightheadedness and palpitations.
- Infection: particularly chest, mouth, perianal, skin (*Staphylococcus*, *Pseudomonas*, HSV, *Candida*). Fever, malaise, sweats.
- Haemorrhage: purpura, menorrhagia and epistaxis, bleeding gums, rectal, retina.
- Signs of leucostasis e.g. hypoxia, retinal haemorrhage, confusion or diffuse pulmonary shadowing.
- Mediastinal involvement occurs in 15% and may cause SVC obstruction
- CNS involvement occurs in 6% at presentation and may cause cranial nerve palsies especially of facial VII nerve, sensory disturbances and meningism.
- Signs include widespread lymphadenopathy in 55%, mild to moderate splenomegaly (49%), hepatomegaly (45%) and orchidomegaly.

Investigations and diagnosis

- FBC and blood film.
- Bone marrow aspirate ± biopsy.
- Bone marrow cytogenetics.

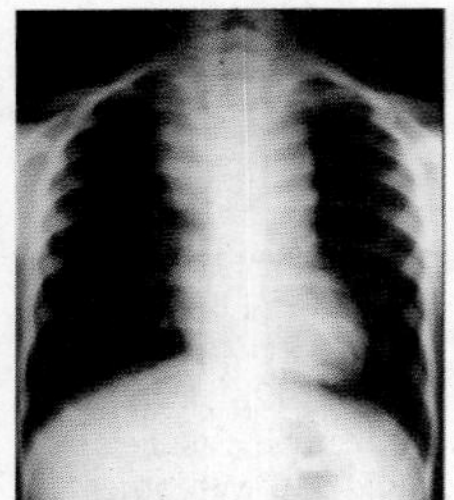

Mediastinal mass in T-ALL.

- Immunophenotyping of blood or marrow blasts.
- Total WBC usually high with blast cells on film but may be low (previously known as aleukaemic leukaemia).
- Hb, neutrophils and platelets often low and clotting may be deranged.
- Bone marrow heavily infiltrated with blasts (≥20%).
- CXR and CT scan needed if ALL has B-cell or T-cell phenotype for abdominal or mediastinal lymphadenopathy respectively.
- Lumbar puncture mandatory to detect occult CNS involvement but may be postponed until treatment reduces high peripheral blast count to prevent seeding (*Note*—fundoscopy, CT head scan and platelet transfusion usually required).

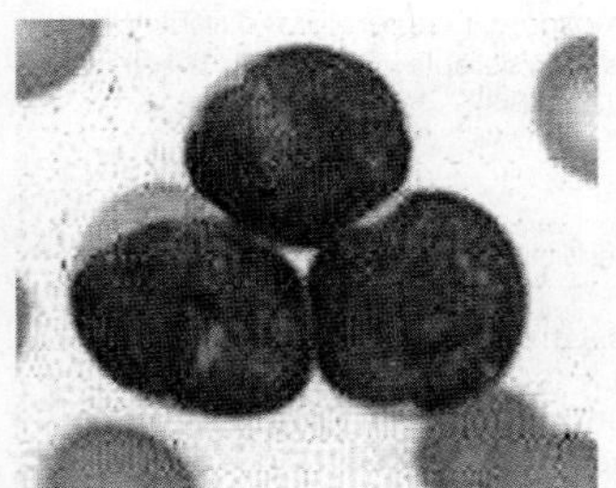

Bone marrow: lymphoblasts in ALL L1.

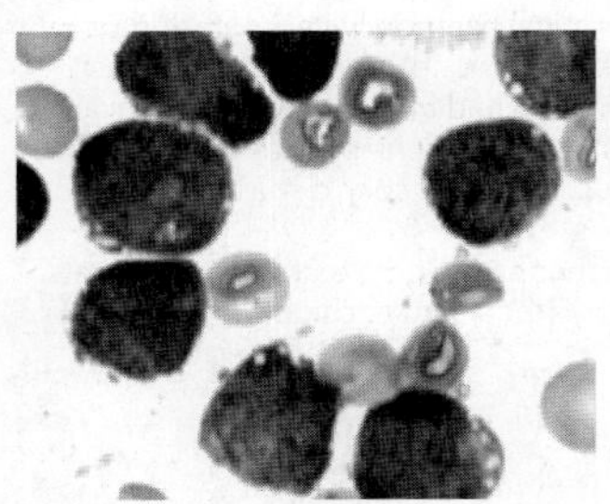

Bone marrow: lymphoblasts in ALL L3.

Emergency treatment

- ►►Seek expert help immediately.
- Cardiovascular and respiratory resuscitation may be needed if septic shock or massive haemorrhage.
- Immediate empirical broad spectrum antibiotic treatment for neutropenic sepsis.
- Leucapheresis may be needed if peripheral blast count high or signs of leucostasis (retinal haemorrhage, reduced conscious level, diffuse pulmonary shadowing on CXR or hypoxia).
- LP if meningism (note precautions above).

Supportive treatment

- Provide explanation and offer counselling—the word '*leukaemia*' and prospect of prolonged chemotherapy are often distressing.
- RBC and platelet transfusion support will continue through treatment.
- Start neutropenic regimen (📖*p550*) as prophylaxis against infections.
- Start hydration aiming for urine output >100mL/h throughout induction therapy (📖*p560 Tumour lysis syndrome*—a special problem in B-cell or T-cell ALL).
- Start allopurinol to prevent hyperuricaemia (*Note*: interaction with 6-mercaptopurine: discontinue allopurinol or reduce dose of 6-MP) or Rasburicase (especially with high counts).
- Insert tunnelled central venous catheter (📖*p568*).

Specific treatment

The aims of treatment are outlined under specific treatment in AML. The regimens used in adult ALL have evolved from successful treatments for childhood ALL.

Treatment for ALL consists of four contiguous phases:

1. Remission induction using vincristine, prednisolone, daunorubicin and asparaginase to achieve complete remission; more intensive induction using more anthracycline improves leukaemia-free survival.
2. CNS prophylaxis generally combines cranial irradiation (18–24 Gy in 12 fractions over 2 weeks) and intrathecal (IT) chemotherapy (methotrexate ± cytarabine or prednisolone) given early in the consolidation phase; IT therapy is continued in the consolidation and maintenance phases; CNS prophylaxis reduces the rate of CNS relapse from 30%⟶5%.
3. Consolidation therapy to reduce tumour burden further and reduce risk of relapse and development of drug-resistant cells; consists of alternating cycles of induction agents and other cytotoxics; usually includes one or two 'intensification' phases; combinations of methotrexate at high dose, cytarabine, etoposide, *m*-amsacrine, mitoxantrone (mitozantrone) and idarubicin are used.
4. Maintenance therapy is necessary for all patients who do not proceed to a stem cell transplant; daily 6-MP and weekly methotrexate for 2–3 years plus cyclical administration of IV vincristine and IT methotrexate.

(▶▶ *simultaneous administration of IV vincristine and IT methotrexate MUST be avoided as errors can be fatal*)

or

Allogeneic stem cell transplantation: an option for adults <50 with a compatible sib; leukaemia-free survival is superior after first remission allograft in patients with high risk disease (40% *vs.* <10% for Ph+ ALL); treatment-related mortality up to 30%; in low risk patients SCT should be reserved for second CR.

Matched unrelated donor transplant: an option in younger patients (<40) with very high risk disease (Ph/BCR-ABL positive ALL) but has up to 48% treatment-related mortality.

or

Autologous stem cell transplantation: an alternative for adults up to 60: lower treatment related mortality (up to 8%); no clear survival advantage over maintenance therapy in first remission for most patients but may improve survival in very high risk disease without option of allograft.

- Enter patient into MRC or other high quality trial if possible.
- Major complications are infective episodes which may be bacterial (Gram +ve and Gram –ve), viral (esp. HSV, HZV) and fungal (*Candida* and *Aspergillus*).
- In the longer term, relapse is the main complication.
- Mature B-cell ALL is treated with shorter more intensive cycles including high dose methotrexate, high dose cytarabine and fractionated cyclophosphamide; it has a higher incidence of CNS disease at diagnosis and relapse.
- CNS leukaemia at diagnosis is treated by adding intensified intrathecal triple therapy to cranial irradiation; IT methotrexate, cytarabine and prednisolone 2–3 × times weekly over 3–4 weeks until 2 consecutive CSF samples are negative; insertion of an Ommaya reservoir facilitates such frequent IT therapy.

Minimal residual disease detection

Flow cytometry for clonal immunophenotypes or FISH or RT-PCR for fusion proteins or clonal Ig/TCR gene rearrangements identified at diagnosis can detect minimal residual disease (MRD) at a sensitivity of 10^{-3}–10^{-6}. Morphological and molecular CR can be distinguished and detection of MRD has strong negative prognostic implications.

Prognosis

Overall ~75% of adults with ALL achieve a CR with a modern regimen and good supportive care; more intensive induction and consolidation reduces relapse risk but adds toxicity; results in patients >50 are less good.

In contrast to the high cure rate in childhood ALL, leukaemia free survival in adult ALL in general is <30% at 5 years (patients > 50 years 10–20%). Leukaemia-free survival (LFS) after chemotherapy in patients without adverse risk factors is >50% whereas that for very high risk Ph/BCR-ABL+ ALL is <10%; hence the latter should have an allograft in CR1 if possible.

Prognostic factors

The most important prognostic factors are listed below. These are useful for risk stratification to identify patients who require transplantation in first CR.

- Patient age (<50y CR >80%, LFS>30%; ≥50y CR <60%, LFS <20%)
- High leucocyte count (>30 × 10^9/L in B precursor-ALL; >100 × 10^9/L in T-ALL) poor risk.
- Immunophenotype: pro-B-ALL and pro-T-ALL have poorer outcomes; common pre-B-ALL still poor; mature B-cell ALL and T-cell ALL had poorer outcomes before the use of more intensive regimens, now better.
- Cytogenetics: Ph+ very poor prognosis: <10% LFS after chemotherapy; for others (📖*p159*).
- Long time to CR (>4–5 weeks)
- High MRD level after induction (>10^{-3}); persistent/increasing MRD during consolidation.

Management of relapse

- Relapse rate is highest within the first 2 years but may occur after 7 years.
- 20% occur outside the bone marrow, generally CNS; testis and other sites occur in 5%.
- Isolated extramedullary relapse is often followed by haematological relapse; these patients require local treatment followed by reinduction therapy.
- Best predictive factor for response is duration of first CR (better >18 months).
- With second-line regimens 50–60% of patients will achieve a short second CR (generally <6 months) and prompt BMT offers the only prospect of LFS and cure.

Chronic myeloid leukaemia (CML)

Malignant tumour of an early haemopoietic progenitor cell. The clonal marker is found in all three myeloid lineages and in some B and T lymphocytes demonstrating a primitive origin.

Incidence

Rare disease with a frequency of 1.25 per 100,000. Rare in children and median age of onset is 50 years with slight ♂ excess. Irradiation is the only known epidemiological factor.

Classification

Classified as a myeloproliferative disorder (📖*p238*) with which it shares a number of clinical features. However, it also has certain unique biological properties:

- Characterised in >80% patients by the presence of the Philadelphia chromosome (Ph). Reciprocal translocation between chromosomes 9 and 22, (t9;22)(q34;q11), involving two genes, *BCR* and *ABL* that form a fusion gene *BCR-ABL* on chromosome 22. This produces an aberrant 210 kDa protein that has greater tyrosine kinase activity than the normal ABL protein. This gene is believed to play a role in the pathogenesis of CML but additional genetic changes appear necessary.
- 10% of patients have variant translocations involving chromosome 22 ± 9 and other chromosomes. A further 8% with typical clinical features lack the Ph chromosome, i.e. have Ph-negative CML; half of these have the hybrid *BCR-ABL* gene: Ph-negative, BCR-ABL-positive CML.

Natural history

- Biphasic or triphasic disease—chronic phase, accelerated phase and blast crisis; 50% transform directly from chronic phase to blast crisis.
- >85% patients present in chronic phase.
- Duration of chronic phase varies (typically 3–6 years; median 4.2 years).
- Transformation is least likely in the 2 years immediately after diagnosis but occurs at an annual rate of 20–25% thereafter.
- Accelerated phase characterised by blood counts and organomegaly becoming increasingly refractory to therapy; some have constitutional symptoms; generally brief.
- Blast crisis resembles acute leukaemia with >20% blasts and promyelocytes in blood or marrow.

Clinical symptoms and signs

- 30% asymptomatic at diagnosis; present after routine FBC.
- Fatigue, lethargy, weight loss, sweats.
- Splenomegaly in >75%; may cause (L) hypochondrial pain, satiety and sensation of abdominal fullness.
- Gout, bruising/bleeding, splenic infarction and occasionally priapism.
- Signs include moderate to large splenomegaly (40% >10cm), hepatomegaly (2%), lymphadenopathy unusual.
- Occasional signs of leucostasis at presentation.

Diagnosis and investigations

- FBC and blood film show ↑ WBC (generally $>25 \times 10^9$/L, often $100–300 \times 10^9$/L): predominantly neutrophils and myelocytes; basophilia; sometimes eosinophilia.
- Anaemia common; platelets typically normal or ↑.
- Neutrophil alkaline phosphatase (NAP) score and ESR ↓ in absence of secondary infection.
- LDH and urate levels ↑.
- Bone marrow shows marked hypercellularity due to myeloid hyperplasia (blasts <10% in chronic phase; >10% in accelerated phase; >20% blasts + promyelocytes = blast crisis); trephine useful to assess marrow fibrosis.
- Cytogenetic examination of blood or marrow for confirmatory t(9;22).

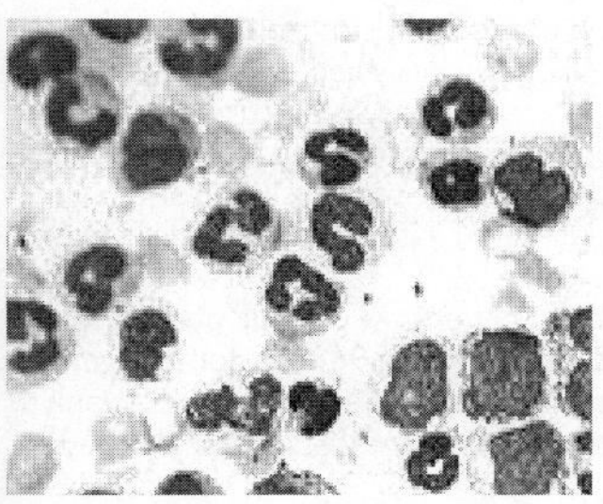

Peripheral blood film in CML: note large numbers of granulocytic cells at all stages of differentiation.

Differential diagnosis

Differentiate chronic phase CML from leukaemoid reaction due to infection, inflammation or carcinoma (NAP ↑ or normal; absent Ph chromosome) and CMML (absolute monocytosis; trilineage myelodysplasia; absent Ph chromosome); 5% present with predominant thrombocytosis and must be differentiated from ET (NAP ↑/normal; absent Ph chromosome).

Prognostic factors

- Sokal score based on age, spleen size, platelet count and % blasts in blood can be used to identify good, moderate and poor prognosis groups; (*see p685*)
- Response to IFN-α therapy is an important prognostic factor.

Treatment of chronic phase

- HLA-type patients aged <50 years and their sibs; 30% have a compatible sibling donor; if no compatible sibling and aged <40, perform preliminary MUD search to determine prospective donor availability.
- Therapeutic decision making in chronic phase is difficult: allogeneic transplantation is the only curative treatment; however, it carries significant morbidity and mortality and many patients find this a difficult

option; it is vital that each patient is aware of treatment options and their risks and benefits.

- Leukapheresis should be performed with cryopreservation of stem cells which may be used for future autologous rescue if required; it may also be necessary for treatment of leucostasis or priapism.
- Allopurinol should be commenced.
- Hydroxyurea has been drug of choice for controlling WBC, 'normalising' the FBC and reducing spleen size in chronic phase. Maintenance 1–1.5g PO od. No effect on cytogenetics or natural history. Side effects: rash, mouth ulcers and diarrhoea.
- Interferon-α (IFN-α) at a target dose of 5 million units/m^2/day SC corrects haematological abnormalities in 75% and produces complete cytogenetic response (CCR) in 10–15% and major cytogenetic response (MCR; <33% Ph+ cells) in 15–30%.
- Treatment with IFN-α is associated with prolonged time to progression and longer survival (57% at 5 years), most significantly in those with complete and major responses; adding cytarabine increases CCRs to 25–35% and improves survival.
- IFN-α side effects (malaise, febrile reactions, anorexia and weight loss, depression) reduce quality of life and not tolerable for many patients.
- Polyethylene glycol-IFN administered once weekly and has a more favourable side effect profile.
- Imatinib (Glivec®) gives better cytogenetic responses and progression free survival with fewer side effects; has changed the therapeutic algorithm in CML; a small molecule signal transduction inhibitor that specifically targets BCR-ABL and some other tyrosine kinases:
  - 400mg PO od in newly diagnosed patients in chronic phase produces complete haematological response in 96%, major cytogenetic response in 83% and complete cytogenetic response in 68%; only 3% achieve a molecular remission (negative RT-PCR for BCR-ABL at 10^{-5}–10^{-6}).
  - Most patients achieve major cytogenetic response (MCR) within first 6 months of therapy; patients with MCR have lower risk of relapse.
  - Commonest side effects are myelosuppression, oedema, nausea, muscle cramps, skin rash, fatigue, diarrhoea, headache and arthralgia; most are mild to moderate and easily manageable.
  - Now approved in both US by FDA, and in UK by NICE for not only IFN-α-resistant patients for all newly diagnosed patients.[1]
  - Imatinib combined with IFN-α or cytarabine are under examination.
  - Uncertainty about long term outcomes, resistance and response duration.
- Sibling-matched allogeneic stem cell transplant is treatment of choice for age <50 unless they develop a major cytogenetic response, but only 30% will have sibling match. Transplant related mortality is approximately 20%. Outcomes best in younger patients (<30) in chronic phase <1 year from diagnosis. RT-PCR for BCR-ABL is used to monitor minimal residual disease once Ph-negative engraftment is achieved.

1 www.nice.org.uk

- MUD allogeneic transplant, if available, should be used for <25 age group and considered <40 years but transplant related mortality rises up to 45%.
- Non-myeloablative conditioning has been used to reduce treatment related toxicity in older patients using donor lymphocyte infusions to produce a graft-versus-leukaemia (GvL) effect; it is too early to assess long term results.

A treatment 'algorithm'

- A young patient (<40) with CML in chronic phase with a matched sibling donor should probably still be allografted within 6–12 months of diagnosis but may prefer a trial of imatinib.
- All other patients should receive imatinib (in the UK if fail to tolerate IFN-α); review BM cytogenetics at 6 months.
- If BM <35% Ph-negative, alternatives should be discussed: i.e. increased Imatinib, trials of combination therapy or stem cell transplantation, if an option.
- If BM ≥35% Ph-neg continue therapy as long as cytogenetics stable or improving (RT-PCR for BCR-ABL if CCR).
- Monitor at least annually; if progression, discuss above options especially BMT.

Complications

- Modest increased infection risk—sometimes atypical organisms.
- Acceleration to blast crisis (75% myeloid, 25% lymphoid).
- Lymphoid blast crisis treatable with modified ALL protocol, may survive >12 months.
- Myeloid blast crisis usually refractory to conventional chemotherapy, survival 2–5 months.

Prognosis

Overall median survival with standard chemotherapy 5.5 years (range 3 months–22 years). Survival improvement with Imatinib not yet quantified. Sibling matched allogeneic transplant (all ages 5 year median survival 60%). MUD transplant (all ages—5 year median survival 40%). Blast crisis overall median survival 6 months.

Treatment of advanced phase CML

- Accelerated phase patients on imatinib 600mg od have haematological and cytogenetic responses, prolongation of time to progression and improved survival. Eligible patients should receive an allograft.
- Blast crisis CML responds to imatinib 600mg od in a high proportion of cases with less toxicity than chemotherapy but response duration is short and where possible an allograft should be performed.
- Allogeneic BMT offers eligible patients with advanced phase CML the only prospect of prolonged survival and possible cure; results are significantly less good than for BMT in chronic phase (0–10% 5 year survival in blast crisis) though achievement of second chronic phase improves the results after blast crisis.
- Relapse after allogeneic BMT has been successfully treated with donor lymphocyte infusions (DLI) (60–80% response in molecular or cytogenetic relapse); GvHD is a side effect but is less frequent with incremental doses of DLI.

Chronic lymphocytic leukaemia (B-CLL)

Progressive accumulation of mature-appearing, functionally incompetent, long-lived B lymphocytes in peripheral blood, bone marrow, lymph nodes, spleen, liver and sometimes other organs.

Incidence

Commonest leukaemia in Western adults (25–30% of all leukaemias). 2.5/100,000 per annum. Predominantly disease of elderly (in over 70s, >20/100,000). Median age at diagnosis 65 years. ♂:♀ ratio ~2:1.

Aetiology

Unknown. No causal relationship with radiation, chemicals or viruses. Small proportion are familial. Genetic factors suggested by low incidence in Japanese even after emigration. Lymphocyte accumulation appears to result from defects in intracellular apoptotic pathways: 90% of CLL cases have high levels of BCL-2 which blocks apoptosis.

Clinical features and presentation

- Often asymptomatic; lymphocytosis ($>5.0 \times 10^9$/L) on routine FBC.
- With more advanced disease: lymphadenopathy: painless, often symmetrical, splenomegaly (66%), hepatomegaly and ultimately BM failure due to infiltration causing anaemia, neutropenia and thrombocytopenia.
- Recurrent infection due to acquired hypogammaglobulinaemia: esp. Herpes zoster.
- Patients with advanced disease: weight loss, night sweats, general malaise.
- Autoimmune phenomena occur; DAT +ve in 10–20% cases, warm antibody AIHA in <50% these cases. Autoimmune thrombocytopenia in 1–2%.

Diagnosis

FBC: lymphocytosis $>5.0 \times 10^9$/L; usually $>20 \times 10^9$/L, occasionally $>400 \times 10^9$/L; anaemia, thrombocytopenia and neutropenia absent in early stage CLL; autoimmune haemolysis ± thrombocytopenia may occur at any stage.

Blood film: lymphocytosis with 'mature' appearance; characteristic artefactual damage to cells in film preparation produces numerous 'smear cells' (*Note*: absence of smear cells should prompt review of diagnosis); spherocytes, polychromasia and ↑ retics if AIHA; ↓ platelets if BM failure or ITP.

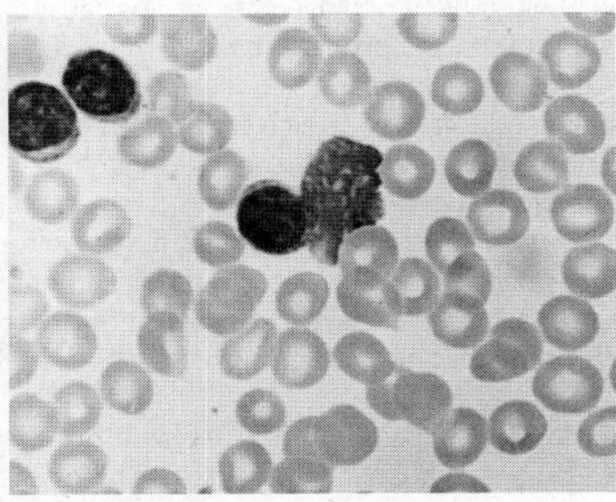

Blood film in CLL: numerous 'mature' lymphocytes with smear cells. From *Oxford Textbook of Oncology*, 2E, with permission.

Immunophenotyping: crucial to differentiation from other lymphocytoses (📖*table p174*). First line panel: CD2; CD5; CD19; CD23; FMC7; SmIg (κ/λ); CD22 or CD79b. CLL characteristically CD2 and FMC7 –ve; CD5, CD19 and CD23 +ve; SmIg, CD22, CD79b weak; κ or λ light chain restricted.

Immunoglobulins: immuneparesis (hypogammaglobulinaemia) common; monoclonal paraprotein (usually IgM) <5%.

Bone marrow: >30% 'mature' lymphocytes.

Trephine biopsy: provides prognostic information: infiltration may be nodular (*favourable*); interstitial; mixed; diffuse (*unfavourable*).

Lymph node biopsy: rarely required; appearances of lymphocytic lymphoma.

Cytogenetics: prognostic value; abnormalities in >80% using FISH: 13q– (55%), 11q– (18%), 12q+ (16%), 17p– (7%), 6q– (7%); 11q–, 17q– very *unfavourable*; sole 13q– or 6q– *favourable*. Clonal evolution occurs over time. 11q– and 17q– associated with advanced disease.

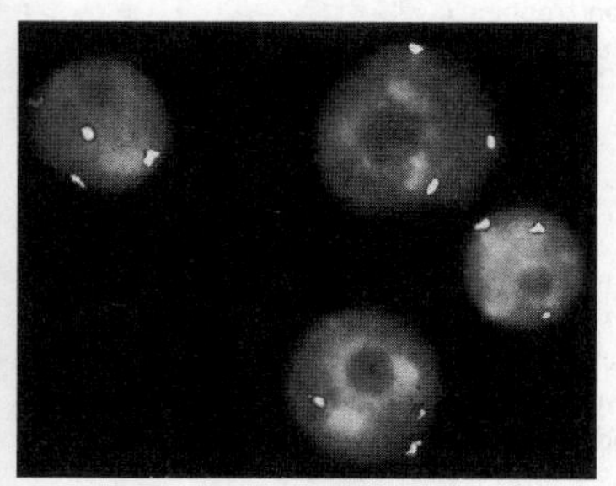

FISH showing trisomy 12 (three bright spots in each nucleus, each of which represents chromosome 12). From *Oxford Textbook of Oncology*, 2E, with permission.

Other tests: U&E; LFTs; LDH; β2-microglobulin; imaging as necessary for symptoms.

Differential diagnosis

Morphology and immunophenotyping (📖*p174*) will differentiate CLL from other chronic lymphoproliferative disorders.

Scoring system in B-cell lymphoproliferative disorders

Devised to facilitate diagnosis based on the antigen profile of CLL using a panel of 5 monoclonal antibodies[1]:

Marker		(Score)		(Score)
SmIg	weak	(1)	moderate/strong	(0)
CD5	positive	(1)	negative	(0)
CD23	positive	(1)	negative	(0)
FMC7	negative	(1)	positive	(0)
CD79b	weak	(1)	strong	(0)

Total scores for CLL range from 3–5 and for non-CLL cases from 0–2.

Poor prognostic factors

- ♂ sex.
- Advanced clinical stage (*see below*).
- Initial lymphocytosis > 50 × 10^9/L.
- >5% prolymphocytes in blood film.
- Diffuse pattern of infiltrate on trephine.
- Blood lymphocyte doubling time <12 months.
- Cytogenetic abnormalities 11q– or 17q–.
- ↑ serum β2-microglobulin.
- ↑ serum LDH.
- ↑ serum thymidine kinase.
- ↑ soluble CD23.
- Unmutated IgV_H genes.
- Poor response to therapy.

'Atypical CLL' includes those with >10% prolymphocytes 'CLL/PLL' which may show an aberrant phenotype (SmIg strong +ve, FMC7/CD79b +ve) is associated with trisomy 12 and p53 abnormalities and a more aggressive course.

Clinical staging

2 systems widely used to classify patients as low, intermediate or high risk:

1 Moreau, E.J. *et al.* (1997) Improvement of the chronic lymphocytic leukemia scoring system with the monoclonal antibody SN8 (CD79b). *Am J Clin Pathol*, **108**, 378–382.

Rai modified staging

Level of risk	Stage		Median survival
Low	0	Lymphocytosis alone	>13 yrs
Intermediate	I	Lymphocytosis & lymphadenopathy	8 yrs
	II	Lymphocytosis, spleno or hepatomegaly	5 yrs
High	III	Lymphocytosis, anaemia (Hb <11.0g/dL)*	2 yrs
	IV	Lymphocytosis, thrombocytopenia (<100 × 10^9/L)*	1 yr

*not due to autoimmune anaemia or thrombocytopenia.

Binet clinical staging

Stage	Clinical features	Median survival
A	No anaemia or thrombocytopenia <3 lymphoid regions enlarged	12 yrs
B	No anaemia or thrombocytopenia 3 or more lymphoid regions enlarged	5 yrs
C	Anaemia (Hb ≤10g/dL) and/or thrombocytopenia (≤100 × 10^9/L)	2 yrs

Clinical management

- Patients with asymptomatic lymphocytosis simply require monitoring.
- *Note*: some patients have very indolent disease (e.g. 'Smouldering CLL': Binet stage A, non-diffuse bone marrow involvement; lymphocytes <30 × 10^9/L, Hb >12g/dL, lymphocyte doubling time >12 months; Binet stage A with somatic mutation of IgV_H gene have median survival 25 years).
  - Chemotherapy reserved for patients with symptomatic or progressive disease: anaemia (Hb <10g/dL) or thrombocytopenia (<100 × 10^9/L), constitutional symptoms due to CLL (>10% weight loss in 6 months, fatigue, fever, night sweats), progressive lymphocytosis >300 × 10^9/L; doubling time <12 months, symptomatic lymphadenopathy/hepatosplenomegaly, autoimmune disease refractory to steroids, repeated infections ± hypogammaglobulinaemia.
  - Advise patients to report infection promptly since immunocompromised ± added effects of hypogammaglobulinaemia.
  - Monthly IVIg reduces recurrent infections but no effect on survival.
  - Manage symptomatic autoimmune complications with corticosteroids.
- First line therapy generally the alkylating agent chlorambucil at a dose of 6–10mg/d (0.1–0.2mg/kg/d) PO for 7–14 days in 28 day cycles until disease stabilised (usually 6–12 cycles). Produces improved FBC and shrinks lymph nodes and spleen in most patients. CR 3%. No effect on

survival. Further responses in most patients if repeated on progression. Side effect myelosuppression. Long-term exposure increases risk of myelodysplasia or 2° leukaemia. Cyclophosphamide is alternative but offers no advantage.

- Higher doses of chlorambucil (15mg/d to maximum response or toxicity) followed by twice weekly maintenance for 3 years improves response rate and survival.
  - Avoid steroids except for autoimmune complications or for 1–2 weeks as preliminary treatment in very cytopenic patients with extensive BM infiltration.
  - Radiotherapy helpful for persistent or bulky lymphadenopathy; splenic irradiation is sometimes helpful in frail patients unfit for splenectomy.
  - Splenectomy is useful therapy for massive splenomegaly or hypersplenism.
- Purine analogue therapy induces apoptosis in CLL. Higher response rate, CR rate (27%) and progression-free survival but not curative. Fludarabine (25mg/m^2/d IV or 40mg/m^2/d PO × 5 days q28) is currently second line treatment in UK. Cladribine is an alternative. Side effects include infection, myelosuppression and autoimmune anaemia or thrombocytopenia.
- *Note*: purine analogues cause profound lymphodepletion with risk of opportunistic infection due to *P carinii*, *M tuberculosis*, H zoster and other organisms. Patients should receive cotrimoxazole prophylaxis (480mg bd tiw) throughout therapy and for 6 months post therapy and all blood products should be irradiated for 2 years post therapy.
- Addition of cyclophosphamide (250mg/m^2 IV or 400mg/m^2 PO × 5 days) concurrently to fludarabine improves response rates in refractory patients 📖*p616*.
- Autologous SCT has been carried out after high dose chemotherapy ± TBI for younger (<55 years) patients who achieve CR with fludarabine. Remains an investigative treatment.
- Allogeneic SCT has been successful in small numbers of younger, symptomatic patients with high risk CLL and HLA-matched siblings.
- Campath-1H is a humanised anti-CD52 monoclonal antibody (administered IV or SC) which preferentially eliminates CLL cells from blood, marrow and spleen. It has been approved in the USA for fludarabine-refractory CLL but its role may be in the treatment of minimal residual disease after fludarabine. Side effects: immunosuppression and virus reactivation (HZV and CMV).
- Rituximab is an anti-CD20 chimeric monoclonal antibody; less effective monotherapy than campath-1H; addition to fludarabine–improves the *de novo* patient CR rate to 47% and addition to fludarabine–cyclophosphamide improves the CR rate to 66% with no evidence of MRD by RT-PCR.

Prognosis

CLL remains an incurable disease with current therapy apart from a few allografted patients but most patients with early stage, asymptomatic CLL die of other, unrelated causes. Infection is major cause of morbidity and mortality in symptomatic patients. Advanced stage patients eventually develop refractory disease and bone marrow failure. Terminally some refractory patients show prolymphocytic transformation.

A minority (<10%) develop high grade NHL (Richter's syndrome): median interval from diagnosis 24 months; associated with all stages; abrupt onset; chemoresistant; median survival 4 months. Second malignancy (skin, colon) occurs in up to 20%.

Cell markers in chronic lymphoproliferative disorders

Mature B-cell lymphoproliferative disorders

Marker	CLL	PLL	HCL	SLVL	FL	MCL
Surface Ig	weak	++	++	++	++	++
CD5	+	–/+	–	–	–	+
CD10	–	–/+	–	–	+	–
CD11c	–/+	–	+	+/–	–	–
CD19	++	++	++	++	++	++
CD20	–/+	+	+	+	+	++
CD22	–/weak	+	+	+	+/–	+/–
CD23	++	–/+	–	+/–	–/+	–
CD25	+/–	–	++	–/+	–	–
CD79b	weak/–	++	+	++	++	++
FMC7	–/+	+	+	++	++	++
CD103	–	–	+	–/+	–	–
HC2	–	–	+	–/+	–	–
Cyclin D1	–	+	–/weak	–	–	++

CLL, chronic lymphocytic leukaemia; PLL, prolymphocytic leukaemia; HCL, hairy cell leukaemia; SLVL, splenic lymphoma with villous lymphocytes; FL, follicular lymphoma; MCL, mantle cell lymphoma.

Mature T-cell lymphoproliferative disorders

Marker	T-LGLL	NK-LGLL	T-PLL	ATLL	SS
TdT*	–	–	–	–	–
CD2	+	+	+	+	+
CD3	++	–	++	++	++
CD4	–	–	+/–	++	++
CD5	+	+	+	+	+
CD7	–/+	–	+++	–	–/+
CD8	++	–	–/+	–	–
CD16	+	+	–	–	–
CD25	–	–	–/+	++	–
CD56	–/+	+	–	–	–
Other		CD11b+ CD16+ CD57+		HTLV1+	

T-LGLL, T-cell large granular lymphocyte leukaemia; NK-LGLL, NK-cell large granular lymphocyte leukaemia; T-PLL, T cell prolymphocytic leukaemia; ATLL, adult T cell leukaemia/lymphoma; SS, Sézary syndrome. *TdT: terminal deoxynucleotidyl transferase differentiates these cells from lymphoblasts of ALL.

Leukaemia

Prolymphocytic leukaemia (PLL)

Uncommon aggressive clinicopathological variant of CLL with characteristic morphology and clinical features. B-cell and rare T-cell forms recognised.

Epidemiology

Median age at presentation is 67 years; ♂:♀ ratio 2:1. Accounts for <2% cases of 'CLL'. B-PLL 75%, T-PLL 25%.

Clinical features

- Symptoms of bone marrow failure and constitutional symptoms: lethargy, weight loss, fatigue, etc.
- Massive splenomegaly, typically >10cm below costal margin may cause abdominal pain. Hepatomegaly common.
- Minimal lymphadenopathy in B-PLL, generalised lymphadenopathy more common in T-PLL.
- Skin lesions occur in 25% T-PLL as do serous effusions.

Investigation and diagnosis

- FBC : high WBC (typically $>100 \times 10^9$/L; commonly $>200 \times 10^9$/L in T-PLL); anaemia and thrombocytopenia usually present.
- Differential shows >55% (often >90%) prolymphocytes.
- Morphology: large lymphoid cells, abundant cytoplasm (B-PLL mainly), prominent single central nucleolus.
- Bone marrow diffusely infiltrated.
- Immunophenotype: 📖*table p174*.
- Cytogenetics—B-PLL: 14q+ in 60%; t(11;14)(q13;q32)in 20%; *p53* gene abnormalities in 75%; T-PLL chromosome 14 abnormalities in >70%; +8 in 50%.

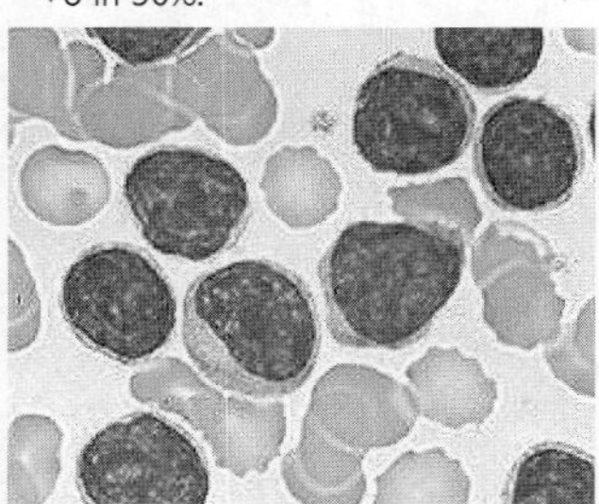

Blood film in PLL: cells are larger than those seen in CLL but have similar 'mature' nucleus.

Differential diagnosis

B-PLL and CLL are not always easily distinguished and mixed 'CLL/PLL' recognised (>10%, <55% prolymphocytes). Clinical features, morphology and notably markers (📖*p174*) used to distinguish PLL from other lymphoproliferative disorders.

Management

- PLL is typically resistant to chlorambucil.

- *Splenectomy*: may be symptomatically helpful, 'debulking', follow up with other therapy.
- *Splenic irradiation*: offers symptomatic relief if unfit for splenectomy.
- *Combination chemotherapy*: CHOP may achieve responses in about 33% and prolong survival in younger patients.
- *Purine analogue therapy*: Fludarabine, 2-CDA or deoxycoformycin may produce responses in some patients.
- *Campath-1H*: anti-CD52 monoclonal antibody produces responses in both B-PLL and T-PLL. In T-PLL CR rates of 40–60% have been achieved lasting several months and permitting subsequent high dose therapy with autologous or allogeneic SCT and prolonged survival.
- *Rituximab*: anti-CD20 monoclonal antibody: there are reports of responses in B-PLL.
- *Stem cell transplantation*: in view of the poor prognosis of PLL, younger patients who achieve a CR should be considered for allogeneic SCT where possible or autologous SCT.

Natural history

PLL is a relentlessly progressive disease and treatment is unsatisfactory. T-PLL carries poor prognosis with median survival 6–7 months. Median survival in B-PLL is 3 years.

Hairy cell leukaemia and variant

Uncommon low grade B-cell lymphoproliferative disorder associated with splenomegaly, pancytopenia and typical 'hairy cells' in blood and bone marrow.

Epidemiology

Accounts for 2% of leukaemias, 8% of chronic lymphoproliferative disorders. No known aetiological factors. Presents in middle age (>45 years) with ♂:♀ ratio of 4:1

Clinical features

- Typically non-specific symptoms: lethargy, malaise, fatigue, weight loss and dyspnoea.
- 15% present with infections, often atypical organisms due to monocytopenia.
- ~30% have recurrent infection; 30% bleeding or easy bruising.
- Splenomegaly in 80% (massive in 20–30%), hepatomegaly in 20%.
- Lymphadenopathy rare (<5%).
- Pancytopenia may be an incidental finding on a routine FBC.
- Vasculitic polyarthritis and visceral involvement similar to polyarteritis nodosa occurs in some patients with HCL.

Investigation and diagnosis

- FBC: moderate to severe pancytopenia; Hb <8.5g/dL 35%.
- Blood film: low numbers of 'hairy cells' in 95%; florid leukaemic features unusual
- Hairy cells—kidney shaped nuclei, clear cytoplasm and irregular cytoplasmic projections (more notable on EM).
- WBC differential: neutropenia, $<1.0 \times 10^9$/L in 75%; monocytopenia is a consistent feature.
- Cytochemistry: +ve for tartrate-resistant acid phosphatase (TRAP) in 95%; now identified by flow cytometry using antibody to TRAP.
- Immunophenotyping: typically CD11c, CD25, CD103 & HC2 +ve; differentiates HCL from other chronic lymphoproliferative disorders (📖*table, p174*).
- Bone marrow: aspiration often unsuccessful—'dry tap' due to ↑ BM fibrosis; trephine shows diagnostic features with focal or diffuse infiltration of HCL where cells have characteristic 'halo' of cytoplasm confirmed by immunocytochemistry with anti-CD20/DBA-44 and anti-TRAP.
- Abdominal CT for intra-abdominal lymphadenopathy (15–20%).

Differential diagnosis

Confirmation of diagnosis may be difficult because of low numbers of circulating leukaemic cells and dry tap on marrow aspiration; trephine histology usually diagnostic; differential diagnosis includes myelofibrosis and other low grade lymphomas notably SLVL.

Prognostic factors

No established staging system. Response to therapy is probably the best prognostic indicator. Bulky abdominal lymphadenopathy at diagnosis correlates with poor response to first line therapy.

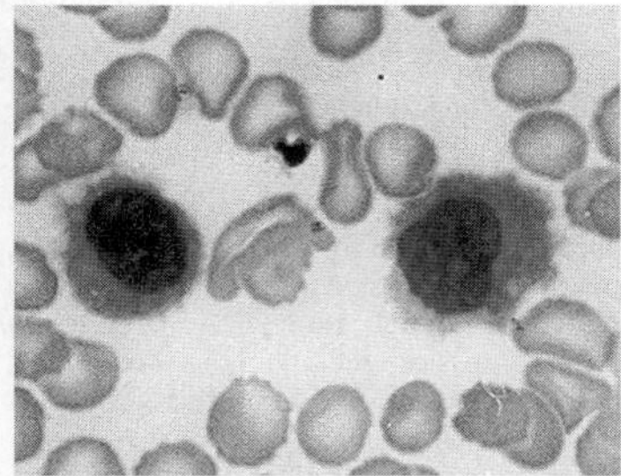

Peripheral blood film in HCL showing typical 'hairy' lymphcytes. From *Oxford Textbook of Oncology*, 2E, with permission.

Management

- In <10% patients, often elderly with minimal or no splenomegaly and cytopenia, the disease remains relatively stable and may be observed.
- Therapy is required in patients with Hb <10g/dL, neutropenia $<1.0 \times 10^9$/L, thrombocytopenia $<100 \times 10^9$/L, symptomatic splenomegaly, recurrent infection, extralymphatic involvement, autoimmune complications, florid leukaemia or progressive disease.
- *Supportive management* is important particularly in the early stages of therapy where cytopenias can worsen: treat infections promptly. *Note*: increased incidence of atypical mycobacterial infections in HCL.
- *Splenectomy*: indicated for massive splenomegaly and beneficial in managing severe pancytopenia in patients with minimal marrow infiltration. Non-curative but 2–15% will normalise FBC for up to 25 years without further therapy. Histology shows characteristic infiltration of red pulp and atrophy of white pulp. Avoid drug therapy for 6 months after splenectomy to assess response.
- *Purine analogues* are the established first line therapy and most patients achieve a durable CR. CD4 lymphodepletion causes immunosuppression: require *P carinii* prophylaxis and irradiated blood products.
- *Deoxycoformycin* 4mg/m^2 IV bolus every 1–2 weeks to maximum response plus 2 cycles (generally 6–10); check creatinine clearance pre-therapy (must be >60mL/min for full dose; half dose >40mL/min) improvement begins after 2 cycles; maximum response generally 4–7 months; 90% objective responses; 75% CR; 15% in continued CR at 8 years; some patients are probably cured.
- *Cladribine*: infusion of 0.1mg/kg/d × 7 days will produce comparable remission rates; remission duration may be shorter; temporarily myelosuppressive, maximum 1 week after infusion; repeat at 6 months if no CR; avoid cotrimoxazole during infusions (causes rash).
- *IFN-α* 3 million units SC daily achieves a partial response in up to 80% but CR in <5%; continue to maximum response then cut to three times weekly for 6–24 months or indefinitely; normalisation of blood

counts generally occurs within 6 months and responses persist 12–15 months after discontinuation.
  - IFN-α may be useful as initial therapy (tiw) for 2–4 months before a purine analogue in patients with profound cytopenias and for HCL refractory to purine analogue therapy. Side effects cause intolerance in some patients.
- *G-CSF* may be useful in patients with severe neutropenia.
- Monitor response by trephine biopsy stained for CD20/DBA-44 and TRAP.

Natural history

Hairy cell leukaemia is associated with prolonged survival (95% at 5 years), with newer agents capable of producing remissions; some patients may achieve long term cure. For others careful application of available treatments at points of disease relapse/progression will still allow prolonged, good quality survival. If a remission of >5 years has been achieved then a further remission with the same agent is likely.

Hairy cell variant

Describes a very rare variant of HCL where the presenting WBC count is high due to circulating leukaemic cells ($40–60 \times 10^9$/L) and monocytopenia is absent. Cells are villous but have a central round nucleus and a distinct nucleolus like PLL. Marrow is aspirated easily due to low reticulin but the trephine appearance is similar to HCL and associated neutropenia. Immunophenotype differs from typical HCL: CD11c+, CD25 & HC2 –ve, CD103 usually –ve. Response to deoxycoformycin or IFN-α is poor but chlorambucil appears active in this form, and the variant generally follows an indolent course.

Leukaemia

Splenic lymphoma with villous lymphocytes (SLVL)

Rare B-cell lymphoproliferative disorder in which marked splenomegaly and moderate lymphocytosis represent the main clinical findings. May correspond histologically to splenic marginal zone lymphoma.

Clinical and laboratory features

- Non-specific symptoms, e.g. fatigue.
- Affects older patients, mean age at diagnosis 72 years.
- Moderate to massive splenomegaly.
- Hepatomegaly in 50%.
- Lymphadenopathy rare.
- Anaemia and thrombocytopenia in 25–30% usually due to hypersplenism. Neutropenia not marked.
- Total WBC not grossly elevated (usually $<40 \times 10^9$/L; *cf.* PLL).
- Monocytopenia not a feature (*cf.* HCL)
- Cell morphology: larger than typical CLL cells, round/oval nuclei, villous cytoplasmic projections at one/both poles of the cells.
- Immunophenotype: CD19+, FMC7+, CD23– usually negative for CD5 & CD25: 20% +ve but fail to co-express CD11c and CD103 differentiating SLVL from HCL; 📖*table p174*.
- Monoclonal IgM or IgG paraprotein; free urinary light chains in 66%.
- BM aspirate may show lymphocytosis (some plasmacytoid) with typical immunophenotype; biopsy may be normal but usually shows patchy/nodular lymphoid infiltration.
- Spleen histology: characteristic with nodular infiltration involving the white pulp (*cf.* HCL).

Differential diagnosis

Main differentials are mantle cell lymphoma (especially 20% CD5+ SLVL) CLL, PLL, HCL and hairy cell variant. Diagnosis requires careful morphological and immunophenotypic assessment (📖*p174*).

Prognosis and treatment

Generally follows an indolent course. ≥10% may require no treatment. Splenectomy recommended for bulky organ enlargement or hypersplenism (and/or to confirm diagnosis in some cases) and can control most symptoms. Progression after splenectomy may respond to chlorambucil or fludarabine given as for CLL. Toxic effects may be marked with purine analogues in this elderly group of patients. Median survival over 6 years.

Leukaemia

Mantle cell lymphoma (MCL)

B-cell derived lymphoid neoplasm defined in the WHO/REAL classification (*p195*) by clinical, morphological, immunophenotypic, cytogenetic and molecular criteria.

Incidence and aetiology

4–8% of cases of adult NHL. Aetiology unknown. t(11;14) causes dysregulation of BCL-1 and overexpression of cyclin D1, a protein involved in cell proliferation.

Clinical features and presentation

- Most common in ♂ >50 years (median age 63).
- 36% have lymphocytosis in peripheral blood which may cause presentation as ?CLL.
- Commonly advanced disease at presentation (87%) with generalised lymphadenopathy (57%); splenomegaly (47%); hepatomegaly (18%).
- Extranodal involvement, particularly in GI tract is common (18%).

Diagnosis and investigation

- FBC: lymphocytosis in 36%; anaemia and mild thrombocytopenia only in very advanced disease.
- Blood film: intermediate size lymphocytes; nucleus often has clefts and indentations; smear cells unusual (*cf.* CLL).
- Immunophenotype: critical to diagnosis (📖*p174*); SmIg strongly+ CD5+, CD10–, CD19+, CD23–, CD79b+, cyclin D1+.
- Cytogenetics: t(11;14) in 50–90% by FISH techniques.
- Bone marrow: trephine biopsy demonstrates involvement in >70% with nodular, interstitial or diffuse patterns similar to CLL.
- Lymph node biopsy: mantle zone expansion or diffuse effacement of nodal architecture by uniform 'centrocytes'; characteristic immunochemistry pattern: CD5+, CD10–, CD79b+, cyclin-D1+.
- Up to 30% have detectable paraprotein band, usually IgM.

Differential diagnosis

In patients with lymphocytosis differentiation from CLL by immunophenotype, notably strong SmIg+, CD23– and cyclin-D1+; from PLL when CD5+ by morphology; from follicular lymphoma by CD5+, CD10– and cyclin D1.

Prognostic factors

Stage using Ann Arbor system (*p210*). Use International Prognostic Index (*p200*) to assess prognosis. Age >70, HB <12g/dL, poor performance status and blood involvement are unfavourable features.

Management and prognosis

There is no evidence that MCL has been cured by either conventional chemotherapy or autologous SCT. Response rates of 50–90% have been achieved with COP or CHOP including CR rates of 30–50%. Median freedom from progression is <1 year. There is no survival advantage for anthracycline containing regimens.

- Fludarabine–cyclophosphamide regimens (📖*p616*) appear to have a high response rate in previously treated patients.

- Rituximab, the anti-CD20 monoclonal antibody produces responses as a single agent and is under examination in combination with fludarabine–cyclophosphamide.
- MCL is generally an aggressive disease with a median survival of 3 years. Most patients develop progressive refractory disease. A small number follow a more indolent course.

Large granular lymphocyte leukaemia (LGLL)

Uncommon lymphoproliferative disorder, characterised by an increase in LGLs in blood. Heterogeneous—may be T-cell or NK-cell phenotype; not all cases are clonal.

Clinical features

- Any age group; median age at diagnosis 55 years.
- Asymptomatic, modest lymphocytosis with large granular lymphocytes on routine FBC.
- Occasional presentation with fatigue or recurrent bacterial infections.
- Arthralgia, itching, rash (25%), mouth ulcers; association with seropositive rheumatoid arthritis in 20% and Felty's syndrome (neutropenia + splenomegaly + rheumatoid arthritis).
- Splenomegaly recorded in 50–80% cases. Lymphadenopathy rare.

Laboratory findings

- Hb and platelets usually normal; chronic neutropenia and mild anaemia may be present.
- Mild/moderate lymphocytosis (usually $<10 \times 10^9$/L); large cells with abundant cytoplasm and distinct granules.
- Most type as 'cytotoxic' T cells (CD3+ CD8+ CD16+ CD56– CD57+); others as NK cells (CD3– CD8– CD16+ CD56+ CD57+/-).
- Clonal rearrangement of T-cell receptor genes in T-LGLL.
- Polyclonal hypergammaglobulinaemia, rheumatoid factor and antinuclear antibodies occur in 50% even without joint disease.
- Bone marrow involvement is often subtle; may be diffuse or nodular pattern usually non-paratrabecular.
- No characteristic cytogenetic pattern.

Differential diagnosis

Reactive lymphocytosis (screen for infection especially EBV); other T-cell lymphoproliferative disorders (immunophenotype; 📖*p174*).

Prognosis and management

- Incurable but generally stable benign disease. Patients with NK phenotype (more common in Japan) or a CD3+ CD56+ clonal disorder established by TCR rearrangements, i.e. a true leukaemia, may have a more aggressive course. Patients with polyclonal disease associated with rheumatoid factor and modest neutropenia may run a more benign course.
- Care is essentially supportive with prompt treatment of infection with appropriate broad spectrum antibiotics.
- G-CSF may be of value in symptomatic chronic neutropenia. Corticosteroids in modest dosage may improve neutropenia but can predispose to infection, including fungal infections.
- Immunosuppression with low dose methotrexate (10mg/m^2 PO weekly), cyclosporin (2mg/kg PO bd) or cyclophosphamide (100mg PO od) has been effective in ~50% of patients with persistent severe neutropenia.

- The rare patient with an aggressive course has a poor prognosis and lymphoma-type regimens show little benefit.

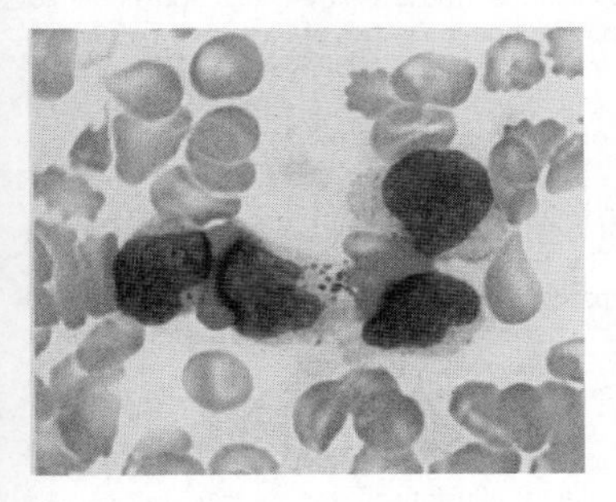

Blood film showing large granular lymphocytes in LGL leukaemia.

Adult T-cell leukaemia-lymphoma (ATLL)

Aggressive lymphoid neoplasm with viral pathogenesis and distinct geographical distribution.

Incidence

Highest incidence among populations where HTLV-I infection endemic: Kyushi district of SW Japan, Caribbean, parts of Central and South America, Central and West Africa. Incidence 2/1000 males and 0.5–1/1000 females seropositive for HTLV-I (37% males >40) in SW Japan. Risk 2.5% at 70 years. Non-endemic cases generally originate from these areas.

Aetiology

HTLV-I provirus demonstrated in ATLL cells and all patients with ATLL are seropositive for previous HTLV-I infection. HTLV-I clearly involved in pathogenesis. Not all infected patients develop ATLL and long latent period suggests that further event(s) are necessary for neoplastic transformation.

Clinical features and presentation

- Median age at diagnosis 58 (range 20–90); ♂:♀ ratio 1:4.
- Usually short history of rapidly increasing ill health.
- Abdominal pain, diarrhoea, pleural effusion, ascites and respiratory symptoms (often due to leukaemic infiltration of lungs).
- History of residence or origin in HTLV-I endemic area usual.
- Lymphadenopathy 60%; hepatomegaly 26%, splenomegaly 22%; skin lesions 39%.

Diagnosis and investigation

- FBC: WBC usually markedly ↑ (up to 500×10^9/L) but may be normal; anaemia and thrombocytopenia common.
- Blood film: large numbers of lymphoid cells with marked nuclear irregularity occasionally multilobulated with 'floral' or 'clover leaf' appearance.
- Immunophenotyping: generally CD4+, CD8–, CD25+, HLA-DR+ T cells (📖 *p174*).
- Cytogenetics: multiple abnormalities described; no consistent pattern.
- Serum chemistry: hypercalcaemia in 33–50% of patients at diagnosis.
- Bone marrow: diffuse infiltration by ATLL cells.
- Serology: positive for HTLV-I.

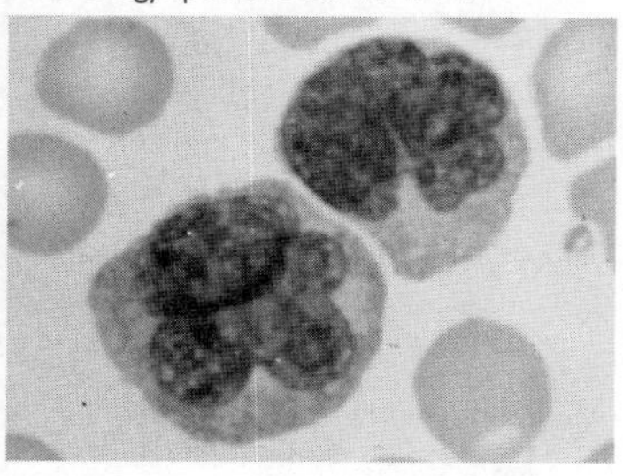

Blood film in ATLL: note clover-leaf cell (centre). From *Oxford Textbook of Oncology*, 2E, with permission.

Prognostic factors and staging

Poor prognostic features are

- ↑ LDH.
- Hypercalcaemia.
- Hyperbilirubinaemia.
- ↑ WBC.

Four clinical subtypes are described: acute, chronic, smouldering and lymphomatous forms. Acute subtype most common (66%), median survival 6 months despite therapy. Other forms have longer survival but often progress to the acute form after several months. The smouldering form is most indolent and is associated with few circulating cells, skin lesions and occasional pulmonary involvement and survival >24 months.

Management and prognosis

Treatment of ATLL is unsatisfactory. Short responses including CRs (6–12 months) have been achieved with combination chemotherapy (e.g. CHOP) for acute and lymphomatous forms. Infectious complications are frequent with this and more intensive therapy. Single agent deoxycoformycin has produced responses in relapsed or refractory patients.
Patients with acute ATLL or lymphomatous ATLL have median survivals of 6 and 10 months respectively. Death is usually due to opportunistic infection.

Sézary syndrome (SS)

Leukaemic phase of a low grade cutaneous mature T-cell lymphoma (mycosis fungoides; MF).

Incidence

Occurs in up to 20% of cases of cutaneous T-cell lymphoma; median age 52; ♂:♀ ratio 2:1.

Clinical features

- Generally diagnosed as a result of blood film report in a patient with exfoliative erythroderma; but not necessarily end-stage and may present *de novo*.
- MF classically progresses through eczematoid plaque stage, infiltrative plaque stage and overt tumour stage and has characteristic histology on skin biopsy (epidermotropism and Pautrier microabscesses).

Investigations and diagnosis

- FBC: generally moderate leucocytosis (WBC rarely >20 × 10^9/L); Hb and platelets usually normal.
- Blood film: typically reveals large numbers of large lymphoid cells with characteristic 'cerebriform' folded nucleus.
- Immunophenotyping: CD3+, CD4+, CD7–, CD8–, CD25– T cells.
- Cytogenetics: no typical pattern.

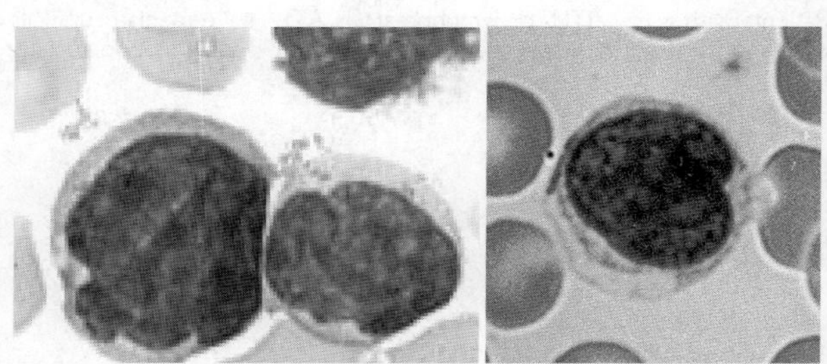

Blood film in Sézary syndrome showing typical cerebriform nuclei. Image on right is from *The Oxford Textbook of Oncology*, 2E, with permission.

Management and prognosis

Patients with SS have a poor prognosis. There is no evidence that single agent or combination chemotherapy improves survival. Median survival 6–8 months.

Leukaemia

Lymphoma

Non-Hodgkin's lymphoma (NHL)

NHL is a diagnosis applied to a group of histologically and biologically heterogeneous clonal malignant diseases arising from the lymphoid system.

Epidemiology

The annual incidence in Western countries is 14–19 cases per 100,000 (i.e. 4% of all cancers) and has increased at a rate of 3–4% per annum since the 1970s. Incidence increases with age. ♂:♀ ratio 3:2. The increased incidence is only in part due to increased mean age of the population, improvements in diagnosis, the HIV pandemic and immunosuppressive therapy.

Aetiology

The rearrangement and mutation of immunoglobulin genes that occur in B-cell differentiation and the response to antigen offers an opportunity for genetic accidents such as translocations or mutations involving immunoglobulin gene loci that have been characterised in many lymphomas. Most translocations involve genes associated with either proliferation (e.g. *c-MYC*) or apoptosis (e.g. *BCL-2*). Factors associated with NHL are:

- Congenital immunodeficiency: ataxia telangiectasia, Wiskott–Aldrich syndrome, X-linked combined immunodeficiency (?EBV infection important).
- Acquired immunodeficiency: immunosuppressive drugs, transplantation, HIV infection (typically high grade and often occur in extranodal sites e.g. brain).
- Infection: HTLV-I (ATLL); EBV (Burkitt lymphoma and immunodeficiency related high grade lymphomas); *Helicobacter pylori* (gastric MALT lymphomas).
- Environmental toxins: association with exposure to agricultural pesticides, herbicides and fertilisers, solvents and hair dyes.
- Familial: risk increased 2–3 fold in close relatives (?genetic or environmental).

Classification

The World Health Organisation (WHO) classification of lymphoid neoplasms (*p195*) has refined the Revised European American Lymphoma (REAL) classification producing a list of clinico-pathologically well characterised lymphomas using morphology, immunophenotype, genotype, the normal cell counterpart and clinical behaviour. Inter- and intraobserver reproducibility is 85–95%. In Europe and the USA 85% of lymphomas are B-cell type.

The clinical behaviour of lymphomas informs management strategies in clinical practice and current treatment protocols are still based on classification systems that group histological diagnoses into indolent (low grade) and aggressive (intermediate and high grade or simply high grade) NHL. More biologically relevant classification of lymphoma diagnosis using the WHO system and emerging therapeutic options based on immunological and molecular characteristics may increase the diagnosis-specific nature of therapy in the future.

WHO classification of lymphoid neoplasms

B-cell neoplasms

Precursor B-cell neoplasms

- Precursor B-lymphoblastic leukaemia/lymphoma (precursor B-cell acute lymphoblastic leukaemia)

Mature (peripheral B-cell) neoplasms

- Chronic lymphocytic leukaemia/B-cell small lymphocytic lymphoma
- B-cell prolymphocytic leukaemia
- Lymphoplasmacytic lymphoma
- Splenic marginal zone B-cell lymphoma (splenic lymphoma with villous lymphocytes)
- Hairy cell leukaemia
- Plasma cell myeloma/plasmacytoma
- Extranodal marginal zone B-cell lymphoma (MALT lymphoma)
- Nodal marginal zone B-cell lymphoma
- Follicular lymphoma
- Mantle cell lymphoma
- Diffuse large B-cell lymphomas
- Burkitt lymphoma/leukaemia

T-cell neoplasms

Precursor T-cell neoplasms

- Precursor T-lymphoblastic leukaemia/lymphoma (precursor T-cell acute lymphoblastic leukaemia)
- Blastoid NK-cell lymphoma

Mature (peripheral) T-cell neoplasms

- T-cell prolymphocytic leukaemia
- T-cell large granular lymphocytic leukaemia
- Aggressive NK-cell leukaemia
- Adult T-cell leukaemia/lymphoma
- Extranodal NK/T-cell lymphoma (nasal type)
- Enteropathy type T-cell lymphoma
- Hepatosplenic T-cell lymphoma
- Subcutaneous panniculitis-like T-cell lymphoma
- Mycosis fungoides/Sézary syndrome
- Primary cutaneous anaplastic large cell lymphoma
- Peripheral T-cell lymphoma (not otherwise specified)
- Angioimmunoblastic T-cell lymphoma
- Primary systemic anaplastic large cell lymphoma

Hodgkin lymphoma

- Nodular lymphocyte predominant Hodgkin lymphoma
- Classical Hodgkin lymphoma
  - *Nodular sclerosis Hodgkin lymphoma (Grades 1 & 2)*
  - *Lymphocyte-rich classical Hodgkin lymphoma*
  - *Mixed cellularity Hodgkin lymphoma*
  - *Lymphocyte depleted Hodgkin lymphoma*

Harris, N.L. *et al.* (1994) A revised European-American classification of lymphoid neoplasms: a proposal from the International Lymphoma Study Group. *Blood*, **84**, 1361–1392; Jaffe ES *et al* (2001). *In* Kleihues P, Sobin L eds. *WHO Classification of Tumours*. Lyon: ARC Press.

'Clinical grade' & frequency of lymphomas in the REAL classification

Diagnosis	% of all cases
Indolent lymphomas (low risk)	
Follicular lymphoma (*Note*: grade I & II; grade III intermediate risk)	22%
Marginal zone B-cell, MALT lymphoma	8%
Chronic lymphocytic leukaemia/small lymphocytic lymphoma	7%
Marginal zone B-cell, nodal	2%
Lymphoplasmacytic lymphoma	1%
Aggressive lymphomas (intermediate risk)	
Diffuse large B-cell lymphoma	31%
Mature (peripheral) T-cell lymphomas	8%
Mantle cell lymphoma	7%
Mediastinal large B-cell lymphoma	2%
Anaplastic large cell lymphoma	2%
Very aggressive lymphomas (high risk)	
Burkitt lymphoma	2%
Precursor T-lymphoblastic	2%
Other lymphomas	7%

A clinical evaluation of the International Lymphoma Study Group classification of non-Hodgkin's lymphoma. The Non-Hodgkin's Lymphoma Classification Project. (1997) *Blood*, **89**, 3909–3918.

Presentation

The features at presentation reflect a spectrum from low grade lymphoma (widely disseminated at diagnosis but with an indolent course; non-destructive growth patterns) to high grade lymphoma (short history of localised rapidly enlarging lymphadenopathy ± constitutional upset with drenching night sweats, >10% weight loss and/or fever; destructive growth patterns).

In Europe and the USA almost 75% of adults present with nodal disease, usually superficial painless lymphadenopathy. 25% are extranodal (~50% in the Far East) and may present with oropharyngeal involvement (5–10%), GI involvement (15%), CNS involvement (5–10%, esp. high grade NHL) skin involvement (esp. T-cell lymphomas) or autoimmune cytopenias. Patients with GI involvement have a higher frequency of oropharyngeal involvement (Waldeyer's ring) and vice versa. Hepatosplenomegaly is common in advanced disease.

Clinical features of indolent lymphomas:

Up to 40% of cases; slowly progressive disorders.

Follicular lymphoma: most common in middle and old age (median age 55 years); presents with painless lymphadenopathy at ≥1 sites, effects of BM infiltration, constitutional symptoms (15–20%) or pressure effects of bulky nodes (ureter, spinal cord or orbit); LN may fluctuate in size; at diagnosis, 66% stage III or IV, 70% BM involvement, 15–20% localised stage I or II disease; median survival ~8–10 years; ~30% may transform to high grade DLBCL (often resistant to treatment; median survival 12 months). Note:

cases of FL with a high proportion of centroblasts (>50%) on histology follow a more aggressive clinical course and are treated as aggressive lymphomas.

Marginal zone lymphomas take 3 forms:

- Mucosa-associated lymphoid tissue (MALT) lymphomas—associated with local invasion at site of origin, e.g. stomach, small bowel, salivary gland or lung; gastric MALT lymphomas present with long history of abdominal pain; diagnosis by endoscopic biopsy; localised in 80–90% and respond to antibiotic treatment for *H pylori*; good prognosis (>80% 5 year survival).
- Nodal marginal zone lymphoma (MZL) or monocytoid B-cell lymphoma rare; associated with Sjögren's syndrome—usually localised to head, neck and parotid gland.
- Spleen MZL related to SLVL (*p182*); elderly patients with marked splenomegaly ± hypersplenism, BM involvement ± villous lymphocytosis, lymphadenopathy absent.

Small lymphocytic lymphoma: nodal form of CLL (*p168*); generally age >60 years; disseminated peripheral lymphadenopathy and splenomegaly; lymphocyte count <4.5 × 10^9/L; BM involvement in 80%; constitutional symptoms <20%; serum paraprotein, usually IgM in 30%; median survival 8–10 years; some patients evolve into CLL, others to DLBCL.

Lymphoplasmacytic lymphoma: occurs in older patients; usually isolated lymphadenopathy ± serum paraprotein; usually IgM, symptoms of hyperviscosity if markedly ↑ (📖*Waldenström's macroglobulinaemia, p284*).

Clinical features of aggressive lymphomas

~50% of cases; rapidly progressive if untreated.

Diffuse large B-cell lymphoma: most common lymphoma diagnosis; occurs at all ages, generally >40 years; presents with localised stage I or II disease in 50% of patients but disseminated extranodal disease is not uncommon; constitutional symptoms in 33%; extranodal sites in 30-40% most commonly GI. Ascites and pleural effusions are common end-stage symptoms.

T-cell rich B-cell lymphoma: subtype of DLBCL; occurs in younger patients; more aggressive with early BM involvement.

Mature (or peripheral) T-cell lymphomas: a number of different conditions; most common T-cell NHL in the West but more common in Far East; median age 56; ♂:♀ ratio 2:1; variable clinical behaviour; nodal form generally more aggressive and less responsive to therapy than DLBCL; heterogeneous group of extranodal forms; 80% stage III–IV at diagnosis; constitutional symptoms, BM and skin involvement common; 41% 5 year survival with combination therapy.

Mycosis fungoides: mature T-cell lymphoma; presents as localised or generalised plaque or erythroderma; lymphadenopathy in 50%; median survival 10 years but prognosis poor with lymphadenopathy, blood (📖*Sézary syndrome p190*) or visceral involvement .

Angio-immunoblastic lymphadenopathy: constitutional symptoms, generalised lymphadenopathy, hepatosplenomegaly, skin rash, polyclonal hypergammaglobulinaemia, DAT+ve haemolytic anaemia and eosinophilia; 33% of patients progress to immunoblastic lymphoma; poor prognosis.

Mantle cell lymphoma: usually elderly; median 63 years; B symptoms 50%; usually disseminated at diagnosis: BM involvement 75%, GI involvement 15–20%; poor therapeutic outcome: partial responses and eventual chemoresistance; median survival 3–4 years (📖*p184*).

Mediastinal large B-cell lymphoma: typically occurs in women <30 years; anterior mediastinal mass sometimes causes superior vena caval obstruction; tendency to disseminate to other extranodal sites including CNS; cure rate with therapy similar to LBCL.

Anaplastic large cell lymphoma: usually occurs in younger patients and children; typically as lymphadenopathy at a single site; favourable prognosis as curable with chemotherapy; 64% overall 5 year survival.

Clinical features of very aggressive lymphomas

~10% cases of NHL; require prompt treatment.

Burkitt lymphoma

- *Endemic BL*: presents in childhood/adolescence in Africa with large extranodal tumours in jaw or abdominal viscera; 90% associated with EBV infection; aggressive but curable disease.
- *Sporadic BL*: often children, rare in adults (median age 31); presents with rapidly growing lymphadenopathy, often intra-abdominal mass arising from a Peyer's patch or mesenteric node; BM, CNS and blood involvement frequent; 30% associated with EBV infection; also associated with HIV infection; aggressive but curable disease in non-HIV-associated cases.

Lymphoblastic lymphomas:

- Young patients (median age 15 years; >50% of childhood lymphomas); share features with ALL; T-cell LBL more frequent (85%) and usually associated with thymic mass; 33-50% present with BM involvement; CNS involvement common; commonly progresses to ALL; aggressive but potentially curable in children.

Laboratory features

- Normochromic normocytic anaemia common.
- Leucoerythroblastic film if extensive BM infiltration ± pancytopenia.
- Hypersplenism (occasionally).
- PB may show lymphoma cells in some patients: moderate lymphocytosis in MCL; cleaved 'buttock' cells in FL and blasts in high grade disease.
- LFTs abnormal in hepatic infiltration.
- Serum LDH and β2-microglobulin are useful prognostic factors (📖*p200*).
- Lymph node biopsy provides the best material for classification and …cise diagnosis using morphology, immunophenotype and genetic

features e.g. translocations or immunoglobulin and T-cell receptor gene rearrangement.
- ~20% of patients with SLL or FL have a serum paraprotein, usually IgM.

Diagnostic immunohistochemical and cytogenetic features

Indolent lymphomas

Follicular lymphomas: Pan-B markers; CD5–, CD10+, BCL–2+. t(14;18)(q32;q21) in 90% (*cf.* reactive lymphoid hyperplasia with normal follicles BCL-2–).

Small lymphocytic lymphoma: Pan-B markers (CD20+, CD79a+); CD5+, weak SmIg, CD23+, cyclin-D1– (*cf.* MCL).

Marginal zone lymphomas: Pan-B markers; CD5–, CD10–, BCL-2–. t(11,19)(q21;q21) 50%, t(1;14)(p22;q32) rare, overexpress bcl-10 and poor response to *H pylori* eradication.

Aggressive lymphomas

Diffuse large B-cell lymphoma: Pan-B markers (CD20+, CD79a+), generally Ig+; Ki67 <90% favours DLBCL (*cf.* Burkitt >99%); probably multiple unrecognised entities; two subgroups delineated by gene expression profiling using DNA microarrays: germinal centre-B-cell profile (favourable) and activated B-cell profile (unfavourable). Der(3)(q27) involving *BCL-6* gene mutations 35%; t(14;18) 25%; t(8;14) 15%.

Mature T-cell lymphomas: Pan-T markers (CD3+, CD2+); TdT– (*cf.* precursor T-lymphoblastic TdT+).

Mantle cell lymphoma: Pan-B markers; CD5+, strong SIg, CD23–, cyclin-D1+. t(11;14)(q13;q32) in 70%.

Anaplastic large cell lymphoma: Pan-T markers, TdT–, CD30+, ALK+. t(2;5)(p23;q35) in 60%.

Very aggressive lymphomas

Burkitt lymphoma: Pan-B markers, Ig+, Ki67 >99% favours BL (*cf.* DLBCL <90%). 80% t(8;14)(q24;q32), 15% t(2;8)(q11;q24), 5% t(8;22)(q24;q11) juxtapose *c-MYC* with Ig gene loci and cause MYC overexpression but this is not diagnostically useful as expressed in normal cells and other lymphomas. Endemic cases have raised antibody titres to EBV antigens and multiple copies of EBV DNA in the tumour (unusual in sporadic cases).

Precursor B-lymphoblastic: Pan-B markers, Ig–, CD10+, TdT+.

Precursor T-lymphoblastic: Pan-T markers, TdT+.

Staging investigations

- Histological diagnosis by expert haematopathologist: biopsy of lymph node or extranodal mass with immunophenotyping ± molecular analysis.
- Detailed history and physical examination including Waldeyer's ring

- FBC, plasma viscosity/ESR and blood film.
- U&E, uric acid, LFTs, LDH, serum β2-microglobulin.
- Serum protein electrophoresis
- Bone marrow trephine biopsy.
- CXR.
- CT of chest, abdomen and pelvis to define areas of nodal and extranodal disease.
- Others as necessary e.g. LP and CT head/spine for patients with overt CNS symptoms: LP also for high grade disease with marrow, testicular or paranasal sinus involvement, lymphoblastic or Burkitt histology; MRI spine, bone scan, gallium scan, PET scan etc

Staging helps to define prognosis and select appropriate therapy. Also helps assess response to therapy. The Ann Arbor staging system developed for Hodgkin's disease is widely used in NHL (📖*Hodgkin's disease p210*).

Prognostic factors
- Histologic grade.
- Performance status.
- Constitutional (B) symptoms unfavourable.
- Age (unfavourable >60 years).
- Disseminated disease (stage III–IV) unfavourable.
- Extranodal disease (poorer ≥2 extranodal sites).
- Bulky disease (poorer if >10 cm).
- Raised serum LDH (poorer if ↑).
- Raised serum β2-microglobulin.
- High proliferation rate measured by Ki-67 immunochemistry.
- BCL-2 protein expression.
- *P53* mutations.
- T-cell phenotype.
- High grade transformation from low grade NHL.

The International Prognostic Index (IPI) was developed for aggressive NHL and validated in all clinical grades of NHL as a predictor of response to therapy, relapse and survival. One point is awarded for each of the following characteristics: age >60, stage III or IV, ≥2 extranodal sites of disease, performance status ≥2 and raised serum LDH to identify 4 risk groups. An age-adjusted IPI has also been developed.

Score	Risk group	%CR	5yr CR-DFS	5yr overall survival
0 or 1	Low	87%	70%	73%
2	Low/intermediate	67%	50%	51%
3	Intermediate/high	55%	49%	43%
4 or 5	High	44%	40%	26%

A predictive model for aggressive non-Hodgkin's lymphoma. The International Non-Hodgkin's Lymphoma Prognostic Factors Project. (1993) *N Engl J Med*, **329**, 987–994.

Treatment of indolent lymphomas

FL and SLL comprise the majority of patients and are treated in a similar way. These diseases are usually responsive to chemotherapy and radiotherapy but unless truly localised, inevitably recur. There is no firm evidence of a curative therapy for advanced disease. Many patients have few or no symptoms; the decision to initiate treatment and choice of treatment must take account of individual quality of life issues. At each stage, the pros and cons of treatment options should be shared with the patient to reach an agreed treatment decision.

Initial treatment of localised FL and SLL

Involved field radiotherapy (35–40Gy) may be curative in the few patients with localised disease. 5-year DFS >50% may be expected. Recurrence generally outside radiation field. Late relapses occur. Addition of chemotherapy improves DFS but not overall survival.

Initial treatment of advanced FL and SLL

Three options are available: (1) watch and wait; (2) conventional chemotherapy and/or radiotherapy; (3) intensive chemotherapy and/or radiotherapy.

Watch-and-wait: therapy may be deferred for many months/years after diagnosis until clinical symptoms develop. Patients may have better quality of life and avoid exposure to cytotoxic agents but must be monitored closely to prevent or identify insidious complications promptly. Overall survival >80% at 5 years.

Conventional therapy: generally involves one of the following approaches:

- *Chlorambucil* (0.1–0.2mg/kg/d x 7–14 days, q28 or 0.4–0.6mg/kg every 2 weeks) or cyclophosphamide (50–150mg/d PO) as single agents or with prednisolone; response rates of 50–80% after 12–18 months' treatment; most relapse within 5 years; convenient oral regimen; well tolerated.
- *'Simple' combination chemotherapy e.g. CVP:* more rapid response than chlorambucil (useful with bulky disease or symptomatic patients) but otherwise similar: response rates 80–90%; median response 1.5–3 years; few durable remissions; IV and oral regimen; causes alopecia.
- *'High grade' regimens:* high 'CR' rates (~60%) with CHOP-type regimens but continuous pattern of relapse and overall survival not convincingly improved in indolent FL (histological grades I and II). In histological 'grade III' FL CHOP produces results equivalent to those in DLBCL (*see below*).
- *Radiotherapy* for treatment of local problems e.g. cord compression.

Intensive therapy: patients with high tumour burden and high LDH who achieve CR have significantly longer survival (63% at 10 years). To improve the CR rate high dose chemotherapy ± TBI followed by autologous SCT (with monoclonal antibody purging of the 'graft' in some centres) has been utilised in younger patients with advanced FL and/or poor prognostic features after initial response to chlorambucil or CHOP. ~80% CR rate; 66% overall survival and up to 40% DFS at 8 years. Still largely investigational; continuing risk of relapse; too early to assess effect on long term survival. Myelodysplasia develops in up to 15% of heavily pre-treated long-term survivors.

Relatively few allografts have been undertaken. Most use TBI-containing conditioning. CR rate >80% and relapse rates are clearly lower than after autograft (12% *vs.* 55% at 5 years) and very few after 2 years. Curative potential requires longer follow-up. The benefit of better disease control is offset by a higher treatment-related mortality (15–30%). Non-myeloablative regimens may reduce toxicity, preserve the GvL effect and widen the availability of this treatment. AlloSCT should be considered in appropriate patients with poor prognosis disease. Total lymphoid (or nodal) irradiation may achieve very high CR rates with 5-year DFS rates >60% but is rarely utilised due to toxicity.

Further treatment of indolent lymphomas

When indolent lymphoma progresses after a partial or complete response to initial therapy, it is important to rule out transformation to DLBCL (esp. if LDH ↑, LN rapidly enlarging, constitutional symptoms, extranodal disease). In recurrent indolent NHL, further responses can be achieved with the prior therapy in most patients who have achieved a durable response (>12 months). However, chemoresistance to alkylating agents ultimately develops.

Interferon-α maintenance: several large randomised trials demonstrate a beneficial effect on survival for patients treated with ≥9 million units/week administered with and after intensive chemotherapy for >18 months or until progression; side effects reduce quality of life and the attraction of this therapy.

Purine analogues: fludarabine has a response rate of 70% (38% CRs) in untreated patients and ~50% (15% CRs) in previously treated patients. Responses to cladribine are similar for previously treated patients but less in *de novo* treatment and responses are less durable. Neither convincingly improve disease free or overall survival. Fludarabine achieves responses in most patients with FL or SLL refractory to chlorambucil. Combinations of fludarabine with cyclophosphamide or with mitoxantrone (mitozantrone) and dexamethasone (FMD) increase response rates and are widely used. Prophylaxis of *P carinii* by cotrimoxazole in all patients and HZV by acyclovir in some is required during and for 6 months after therapy. Cellular blood products must be irradiated for 2 years after therapy.

Monoclonal antibody therapy:

- Rituximab (MabThera, Rituxan) is a humanised anti-CD20 monoclonal antibody. As a single agent 375mg/m^2 infusion weekly × 4 weeks achieves a response rate ~50% (6% CRs) in previously treated patients; median duration 13 months[1]. On relapse 40% will respond again. In newly diagnosed patients 4 further doses given over 9 months as maintenance therapy enhances EFS (22 *vs.* 13 months). Toxicity is mild though there is a risk of anaphylaxis with the first course. Combination with chemotherapy enhances the response rate. In newly diagnosed patients: CHOP-R 100% responses, 66% CRs, >50% progression-free survival (PFS) with median follow up of 6 years. It has been used for '*in vivo* purging' prior to stem cell harvest to improve the prospect of a PCR-negative harvest. In the UK, NICE recommends its use in chemoresistant disease.

- Tositumomab, (Bexaar) a ^{131}I-radiolabelled murine anti-CD20 monoclonal antibody; beta and gamma emission; due to the targeted radiation a single infusion achieves higher response rates (97% OR and 76% CR in untreated patients; 74% OR & 30% CRs in treated patients) and a higher response rate and more prolonged responses in advanced disease than the prior chemotherapy had achieved; transient mild to moderate myelosuppression; antimurine antibodies develop especially in untreated patients.
- Ipritumomab (Zevalin) a ^{90}Yt-labelled murine anti-CD20 monoclonal antibody; beta emission only; also achieves superior response rates (80%) to rituximab in relapsed FL.

Treatment of marginal zone lymphomas

Gastric MALT lymphoma: eradication of *H. pylori* by 2 week course of clarithromycin, amoxicillin with omeprazole achieves CR in up to 80% of patients. Local radiotherapy or single agent chlorambucil can achieve CR in non-responders. *Non-gastric MALT lymphomas*: single agent chlorambucil, simple combination regimens or local radiotherapy achieve good responses.

Initial treatment of aggressive lymphomas

Many patients can be cured by combination chemotherapy or by radiotherapy.

Localised DLBCL: patients with stage I and non-bulky stage II (mass <10 cm) disease without adverse prognostic factors treated with 3 cycles of CHOP followed by involved field radiotherapy (45–50Gy) achieve a 99% response rate 77% PFS and 85% long term survival. This is superior to radiotherapy alone (15% relapse in irradiation field) and to 8 cycles of CHOP.

Advanced stage DLBCL: several chemotherapy regimens have curative potential. CR rates 50% to >80%. Although CR rates to CHOP regimen have been bettered by some multi-agent regimens, long-term follow-up reveals comparable or inferior long-term PFS rates and greater treatment related toxicity. A prospective randomised trial comparing CHOP, m-BACOD, ProMACE-CytaBOM, and MACOP-B revealed no significant difference in response rates, time to treatment failure or survival. Several trials failed to demonstrate the superiority of any particular chemotherapy regimen for NHL. The CHOP regimen (*p604*) has been widely used because of ease of administration and relative tolerability. Some 30% of patients are cured using CHOP alone. The addition of Rituximab to CHOP improves responses and survival (see below).[2] R-CHOP has been endorsed by NICE[5] for use as first line therapy in CD20+ DLBCL stage II, III or IV. Evaluate response to therapy after 3–4 courses and complete 6 courses if complete remission has been achieved.

Consolidation therapy in DLBCL: in future different protocols may be appropriate for different risk groups of patients (risk-adapted therapy). Consolidation of 1st CR by high dose therapy and autologous SCT has been examined in randomised trials. Improved DFS (and overall survival in one of three studies) was demonstrated for patients with ≥2 adverse factors on IPI. Further studies are in progress. It seems likely that a group of poor prognosis patients may benefit from intensive consolidation and the option should be discussed with eligible high risk patients in first remission.

Monoclonal antibody therapy: rituximab produces responses in ~30% relapsed DLBCL. More promising role in combination with initial chemotherapy: addition of Rituximab to CHOP initial therapy improved the CR rate (76% *vs.* 63%) and EFS (57% *vs.* 38%) and overall survival (70% *vs.* 57%) at 2 years with no added toxicity in a randomised study of 400 elderly patients with DLBCL[2]. Confirms Phase II data and further Phase III studies in progress has been endorsed by NICE[5] R-CHOP for use as first line therapy for DLBCL.

Tositusimab: under examination in combination with BEAM high dose therapy to enhance tumour cell kill in autologous SCT for aggressive lymphoma.

Mantle cell lymphoma: CHOP produces response rate ~80% (CR ~50%) with PFS <18 months and overall survival of 3 years and is not markedly different from results obtained with CVP. Regimens such as fludarabine and cyclophosphamide can achieve further responses. Rituximab alone achieves response rate ~35% (14% CR) with a median duration <1 year. Combination of rituximab with CHOP achieved a high rate of 'molecular remissions' as initial therapy but a disappointing median PFS of 16 months. The combination of rituximab with several salvage regimens (e.g. FCM) improves responses. Relapsed patients with MCL who respond to salvage therapy achieve further remissions with high dose therapy and autologous SCT but further relapse is usual. Rituximab pre-harvest acts as *in vivo* purge increasing the proportion of PCR –ve collections. High dose therapy and ASCT in first remission prolongs response duration and probably survival but is probably not curative[3]. Suitable patients with a sibling allogeneic SCT option should receive an allograft.

Initial treatment of very aggressive lymphomas

Non-endemic Burkitt lymphoma: successful treatment of BL in children has informed adult treatment. High remission rates and long-term DFS achieved with intensive short duration (3–6 months) multi-agent chemotherapy regimens including high dose methotrexate, high dose cytarabine, etoposide, ifosfamide and CNS prophylaxis. Protocols designed for lymphoblastic lymphoma or ALL clearly inferior to specific BL protocols. 90% EFS rates in childhood BL. Treatment of adults with BL with intensive regimens including intrathecal therapy such as CODOX-M/IVAC (Vincristine, doxorubicin, cyclophosphamide, methotrexate, folinic acid, G-CSF plus IT cytarabine and IT methotrexate/etoposide, ifosfamide, mesna, cytarabine, folinic acid, G-CSF plus IT methotrexate) improves response and survival rates (~50% curable) though not to childhood results. The role of high dose therapy is uncertain. Meningeal involvement still carries poor prognosis.

Lymphoblastic lymphoma: management in adults has also followed more successful intensive regimens in childhood based on ALL treatment (including CNS prophylaxis). High CR rates (~85%) and 5 year DFS up to 45% reported. The poor outlook for patients has led to evaluation of high-dose therapy with autologous or allogeneic BMT early in its management.

Adult T-leukaemia/lymphoma: 📖p188.

Salvage therapy in aggressive and very aggressive lymphoma
Patients who relapse or fail to achieve remission with initial therapy have a poor prognosis. Without effective second-line (salvage) therapy, almost all die of progressive lymphoma in a median period of 3–4 months.

Conventional chemotherapy: although relatively high CR rates have been reported with several salvage regimens, <10% patients with relapsed or refractory NHL will achieve long-term DFS. The addition of rituximab to EPOCH and ICE salvage regimens improves response rates.

High dose therapy and SCT: high dose therapy (generally BEAM, BEAC or CBV) and autologous SCT is used to treat patients with relapsed or refractory aggressive or very aggressive NHL. A significant proportion of patients with DLBCL are cured (5 year EFS 46%; overall survival 53%) and its superiority to conventional dosage salvage therapy (5 year EFS 12%; overall survival 32%) was demonstrated in a randomised trial[4]. Best results are obtained when lymphoma still responsive to conventional dosage therapy and SCT performed in a state of minimal residual disease. HDT is generally preceded by 1-2 cycles of combination therapy e.g. mini-BEAM, DHAP, ESHAP with aim of testing chemo-responsiveness, inducing minimal residual disease and harvesting PBSCs. Syngeneic and allogeneic transplants have been used less frequently but are associated with cures.

1 McLaughlin, P. *et al.* (1998) Rituximab chimeric anti-CD20 monoclonal antibody therapy for relapsed indolent lymphoma: half of patients respond to a four-dose treatment program. *J Clin Oncol*, **16**, 2825–2833 **2** Coiffier, B. *et al.* (2002) CHOP chemotherapy plus rituximab compared with CHOP alone in elderly patients with diffuse large-B-cell lymphoma. *N Engl J Med*, **346**, 235–242 **3** Vandenberghe, E. *et al.* (2003) Outcome of autologous transplantation for mantle cell lymphoma: a study by the European Blood and Bone Marrow Transplant and Autologous Blood and Marrow Transplant Registries. *Br J Haematol*, **120**, 793–800. **4** Philip, T. *et al.* (1995) Autologous bone marrow transplantation as compared with salvage chemotherapy in relapses of chemotherapy-sensitive non-Hodgkin's lymphoma. *N Engl J Med*, **333**, 1540–1545. **5** NICE Technology Appraisal 65, September 2003

CNS lymphoma

Primary CNS lymphoma

2% of NHL cases; incidence increased partly by HIV pandemic; non-HIV related aged 55–70; commonly involves frontal lobes, corpus callosum or deep periventricular structures; cognitive or personality change common; 10% seizures; 40% evidence of leptomeningeal spread; diagnosis by gadolinium-enhanced magnetic resonance and stereotactic needle biopsy; systemic lymphoma uncommon; poor prognosis improved by addition of systemic chemotherapy with high dose methotrexate to whole brain radiotherapy; improves survival with >95% responses and median survival 30–60 months; 50% relapse risk; most relapses in CNS, others mainly leptomeningeal and ocular, <10% systemic; delayed neurotoxicity common, esp. >60 years: dementia, ataxia, urinary dysfunction.

Secondary CNS lymphoma

Usually meningeal involvement; occurs in up to 10% of cases of NHL; intrathecal methotrexate, cytarabine and prednisolone twice weekly until CSF clear then weekly × 6 ± cranial irradiation as for ALL; insertion of Ommaya reservoir facilitates administration; simultaneous systemic therapy including high dose methotrexate and cytarabine (penetrate CNS) normally necessary; poor prognosis; median survival <3 months.

Lymphoma

Hodgkin's lymphoma (Hodgkin's disease)

First described by Thomas Hodgkin in 1832 the lineage of the neoplastic cells remained a subject of debate for over 160 years. Micromanipulation of tissue sections followed by single cell PCR for Ig gene amplification demonstrates that the neoplastic cells in Hodgkin's lymphoma (HL) are clonal B cells originating in a lymph node germinal centre. HL is a germinal centre-derived B-cell lymphoma.

Incidence

- 1% cancer registrations per annum. Annual incidence ~3 per 100,000 in Europe and USA (less common in Japan).
- Bimodal age incidence—major peak between 20 and 29 years and minor peak 60 years.
- Overall higher incidence in ♂.
- Nodular sclerosing (NS) histology is most common subtype in young adults (>75% of NS cases are <40 years) and peak at this age is confined to NS subtype and has a ♀ preponderance.

Risk factors

- Associated with high socioeconomic status in childhood (esp. NS in young adults) and with Caucasian race in the USA.
- Familial aggregations frequently reported: 99× ↑ risk in identical twins; 7× risk for siblings of young adults (no increase for sibs of older adults); ? genetic or environmental effect.
- Considerable evidence linking EBV to HL: ↑ risk of HL in individuals with a history of infectious mononucleosis; EBV encoded nuclear RNAs detected in Reed-Sternberg (RS) cells; 26–50% cases +ve for EBV by molecular analysis (esp. mixed cellularity (MC) subtype).

Histology and classification

Immunological analysis has resulted in reclassification of HL in the REAL and WHO Classifications of Lymphoid Neoplasia (📖*p195*) into 2 major groups:

Nodular lymphocyte-predominant HL (NLPHL): 3–8%; contains large atypical B cells and lymphocytic and histiocytic (L&H) 'popcorn' cells. These cells are CD30–, CD15–, CD20+, CD45+, CD75+, CD79a+.

'Classical' HL: large mononuclear (Hodgkin's cells) or binucleate/multinuclear RS cells make up only 1–2% of the cellularity of the lymph node. These cells are CD30+ and typically CD15+, CD20–, CD45–, CD75–, CD79a–. The predominant cells are an infiltrate of lymphocytes, plasma cells, eosinophils and histiocytes containing scattered neoplastic cells and a variable degree of fibrosis.

Four histological subtypes:

Nodular sclerosing HL (NSHL): ~80%; prominent bands of fibrosis and nodular growth pattern; lacunar Hodgkin's cells; variable numbers of RS cells.

Mixed cellularity HL (MCHL): ~17%; mixed infiltrate of lymphocytes, eosinophils and histiocytes with classical RS cells.

Lymphocyte depleted HL (LDHL): rare; diffuse hypocellular infiltrate with necrosis, fibrosis and sheets of RS cells.

Lymphocyte rich classical HL (LRCHL): uncommon; diffuse predominantly lymphoid infiltrate with scanty RS cells of 'classical' phenotype.

Clinical features

- Presentation commonly with painless 'rubbery' supradiaphragmatic lymph node enlargement: frequently cervical gland(s).
- Initial mode of spread occurs predictably to contiguous nodal chains.
- Often involves supraclavicular and axillary glands and other sites.
- Waldeyer's ring involvement is rare and suggests a diagnosis of NHL.
- Lymphadenopathy in HL may wax and wane during observation.
- Spleen involved in ~30% but palpable splenomegaly only in 10%, hepatomegaly 5%.
- Abdominal lymphadenopathy is unusual without splenic involvement.
- Supradiaphragmatic disease ± intra-abdominal involvement is usual, and regional disease limited to subdiaphragmatic sites is uncommon (except NLPHL).
- Bulky mediastinal and hilar lymphadenopathy may produce local symptoms (e.g. bronchial or SVC compression) or direct extension (e.g. to lung, pericardium, pleura or rib). Pleural effusions in 20%.
- Extranodal spread may also occur via bloodstream (e.g. to bone marrow (1–4%), lung or liver). Presence of disseminated extranodal disease is generally accompanied by generalised lymphadenopathy and splenic involvement; usually a late event.
- ~33% patients have ≥1 associated constitutional 'B' symptoms at presentation: weight loss >10% body weight during the previous 6 months, unexplained fever or drenching night sweats. 'B' symptoms correlate with disease extent, bulk and prognosis. Further systemic symptoms associated with HD (but not 'B' symptoms) are generalized pruritus and alcohol-induced lymph node pain.
- A defect in cellular immunity has been documented in patients with HL rendering them more susceptible to TB, fungal, protozoal and viral infections including *P carinii* and HZV.
- NLPHL more frequent in ♂ (2–3×); median age 35 years; typically localised at presentation; usually cervical or inguinal; infrequent 'B' symptoms; late relapses occur; increased risk of DLBCL; otherwise favourable prognosis; 10 year OS 80–90%.
- NSHL occurs typically in young adults (median age 26) and has a good prognosis if stage I/II.
- MCHL has a median age of 30 years and an intermediate prognosis.
- LDHL is more common in older adults; has a relatively poor prognosis.
- LRCHL ♂>♀; tendency to localised disease; favourable prognosis.

Investigation, diagnosis and staging

- Document 'B' symptoms in history.
- Document extent of nodal involvement by clinical examination.
- Confirm diagnosis by biopsy: best histology from lymph node excision biopsy; image guided needle biopsy or even laparotomy, mediastinoscopy or mediastinotomy may be necessary to obtain a tissue diagnosis.
- Clinical staging is now usual; routine staging laparotomy for 'pathological staging' abandoned; useful only if result may substantially reduce treatment.
- Clinical staging includes the initial biopsy site and all other abnormalities detected by non-invasive methods.

- Pathological staging requires biopsy confirmation of abnormal sites.
- FBC: may show normochromic normocytic anaemia, reactive leucocytosis, eosinophilia and/or a reactive mild thrombocytosis.
- ESR/plasma viscosity; U&E; LFTs; urate; LDH.
- CXR.
- CT chest, abdomen and pelvis to define occult nodal and extranodal involvement.
- Bone marrow trephine biopsy to exclude marrow involvement in patients with stage III/IV disease or B symptoms (not essential in stage IA/IIA disease); BM may show reactive features.
- Isotope bone scan, MRI or PET scan may be necessary.
- Biopsy of other suspicious sites may be necessary e.g. liver or bone.
- Attempt semen cryopreservation in young males with advanced disease (often unsuccessful in those with 'B' symptoms).

Ann Arbor staging classification (Cotswolds modification)

The Ann Arbor staging classification has strong prognostic value and is determined by the number of lymph node regions (not sites) involved and the presence or absence of 'B' symptoms. The Cotswolds modification reflects the use of modern imaging techniques, recognises clinical and pathological staging and clarifies differences in disease distribution and bulk.

Stage	**I**	involvement of a single lymph node region or structure
Stage	**II**	involvement of two or more lymph node regions on the same side of the diaphragm (number of anatomical sites indicated by a subscript, e.g. II_3).
Stage	**III**	involvement of lymph node regions or structures on both sides of the diaphragm
	III_1	± involvement of spleen, splenic hilar, coeliac or portal nodes;
	III_2	with involvement of para-aortic, iliac or mesenteric nodes
Stage	**IV**	involvement of one or more extranodal sites (e.g. BM, liver or other extranodal sites not contiguous with LN—*cf.* 'E' below).

A	absence of constitutional symptoms
B	fever, weight loss >10% in 6 months or drenching night sweats
	Additional subscripts applicable to any disease stage:
X	bulky disease (widening of mediastinum by >33% or mass >10cm)
E	involvement of a single extranodal site contiguous or proximal to known nodal site.
CS	clinical stage
PS	pathological stage

Clinical imaging criteria

- Lymph node involvement: >1cm on CT scan is considered abnormal.
- Spleen involvement: splenomegaly may be 'reactive'; filling defects on CT or USS confirm involvement.
- Liver involvement: hepatomegaly insufficient; filling defect on imaging and abnormal LFTs confirm involvement.
- Bulky disease: ≥10cm in largest dimension or mediastinal mass greater than one third the maximal intrathoracic diameter.

Initial therapy

- Aim of treatment is to provide each patient with the best probability of cure while minimising early and late treatment-related morbidity.
- Best strategy is determined by tumour-related and patient-related factors.
- Clinical trials remain necessary to evaluate therapeutic regimens in order to achieve this objective. BNLI/UKLG coordinate nationwide multicentre studies in UK.

Early stage HL

Prognostic factors: patients with stage I or II disease are generally divided into favourable and unfavourable prognostic groups using risk factors, e.g.

- Age >40.
- ESR >50mm/h or >30 in presence of 'B' symptoms.
- ≥4 separate sites of nodal involvement; mediastinal mass ratio > 0.35.
- Other risk factors identified in studies have been gender, histology, disease confined to upper cervical nodes, anaemia and low serum albumin.

Favourable prognosis: stage I or II HL without any risk factors

Aim: cure with minimal side effects.

- Treatment of choice is combined modality treatment, using attenuated duration chemotherapy, e.g. ABVD × 4 cycles + involved field radiotherapy (36–40Gy).
- Aims to eliminate local disease and treat occult disease with reduced toxicity using limited field and attenuated number of cycles of chemotherapy.
- Expected outcome: ~90% failure-free survival (FFS) and >95% OS at 5 years.

Alternative therapeutic options:

Subtotal lymphoid irradiation (36–40Gy) offers ~80% FFS and >90% OS. It has been argued that most patients relapsing after radiotherapy alone can be salvaged by chemotherapy (e.g. ABVD) thus sparing most patients the toxicity of combined modality therapy. However, long term toxicity from extended field radiotherapy is significant.

or

EBVP × 6 plus involved field radiotherapy (36–40Gy).

A very favourable subgroup (stage I, age <40, no 'B' symptoms, ESR <50, ♀ and MT ratio <0.35) may achieve 65–75% FFS and >90% OS at 10 years following extended field radiotherapy treatment alone.

Patients with non-bulky NLPHL presenting with unilateral high cervical or epitrochlear lymphadenopathy may be treated with involved field radiotherapy alone; at median follow up >7 years, more patients with NLPHL and LRCHL die of treatment-related toxicity than recurrent HL; may be best treated with limited dose, limited field radiotherapy alone; with similar aim of reduced toxicity anti-CD20 antibody treatment may prove useful in NLPHL.

Stage IA patients with subdiaphragmatic disease should receive chemotherapy ± involved field radiotherapy to avoid extended pelvic/abdominal fields that are myeloablative and sterilising in women; patients with NLPHL localised to inguinal or femoral region may receive regional irradiation only.

Unfavourable prognosis: stage I or II HL with any risk factors

Aim: cure with some acceptable side effects.

- Combined modality treatment essential, e.g. ABVD × 6 cycles + involved field radiotherapy (36–40Gy).
- Expected outcome: >85% DFS and ~90% OS at 5 years.
- Alternative therapeutic option: MOPP-ABV × 6 cycles + involved field radiotherapy (36–40Gy).

Advanced stage HL

Prognostic factors: a prognostic score has been devised by the International Prognostic Factors Project[1] for patients with advanced HL.

Seven factors were identified:

- Hb <10.5g/dL.
- ♂ gender.
- Stage IV.
- Age ≥45.
- WBC >16 × 10^9/L.
- Lymphopenia <0.6 × 10^9/L or <8% of differential.
- Albumin <40g/L.

Patients with no adverse factors had 5 year failure-free progression of 84%. Each additional factor reduces 5 year failure-free progression by ~7% until the group with 4–7 factors have ~40% failure-free progression at 5 years.

Combination chemotherapy

- Enter patient in a multicentre randomised clinical trial if possible.
- ABVD (📖*p596*) is the standard regimen for patients with advanced HL (stage III or IV) not enrolled in a clinical trial.
- In a randomised trial of 361 patients 6–8 cycles of ABVD was equivalent to 12 cycles of MOPP-ABVD alternating regimen (CR 82% *vs.* 83%; FFS at 5 years 61% *vs.* 65%) and superior to 6–8 cycles of MOPP (CR 67%; 5 year FFS 50%)[2].
- ABVD has a much lower risk of infertility than MOPP regimens and is not associated with increased risk of leukaemia but the anthracycline

component may exacerbate the cardiac and pulmonary complications of mediastinal irradiation.
- Often poorly tolerated by elderly patients due to cumulative doses of doxorubicin and bleomycin.
- Alternative: brief duration dose intensified regimens, e.g. Stanford V low cumulative doses of alkylators, doxorubicin and bleomycin over 12 weeks followed by radiotherapy to sites of bulk disease (≥5cm); FFS 89%, OS 96% at 6 years in a single institution study; multicentre randomised trials in progress; fertility preserved in a high proportion; very low risk of leukaemia.

Adjuvant radiotherapy

Involved field radiotherapy is frequently give to bulky mediastinal disease after completion of combination chemotherapy. This improves DFS but has no effect on OS. Meta-analysis suggest an overall 11% improvement in DFS and that the benefits are greatest for NSHL histology (least for MCHL and LDHL), for mediastinal bulk rather than other bulky sites and that no benefit is gained in stage IV disease[3]. Late toxicity is increased. The lack of difference in overall survival was attributed to a greater number of second malignancies and poorer response and survival after relapse among patients who received combined modality therapy.

Evaluation of response

- Evaluate by physical examination and repetition of abnormal investigations at initial staging.
- Often performed after 3–4 courses of chemotherapy to ensure adequate response and to determine total duration of treatment.
- Residual masses sometimes present at completion of therapy, notably in mediastinum: may be residual fibrotic tissue with no viable tumour.
- If residual mass evident on CT, gallium scintigraphy, MRI or PET scan may exclude active disease if negative and obviate need for invasive biopsy.

Cotswolds criteria:

CR: complete resolution of all radiological and laboratory evidence of active HL.

CRu: 'uncertain CR', identifies the presence of a residual mass that remains stable or regresses on follow-up.

Salvage therapy

- >50% of patients relapsing from primary radiotherapy of early stage HL may be cured by ABVD chemotherapy.
- Durable FFP and prolonged survival are not generally achieved by conventional chemotherapy for patients relapsing after initial chemotherapy.
- High-dose chemotherapy (BEAM or CBV) with autologous peripheral blood stem cell transplantation (SCT) has become the standard salvage approach for most patients relapsing after chemotherapy, producing high complete response rates (up to 80%), durable complete remissions in 40–65% and low morbidity and mortality in selected patients.

- HDT plus autologous SCT may be the best option for patients with refractory disease at initial therapy though patients with progressive disease on conventional therapy still have an unfavourable prognosis.
- Allogeneic SCT has been performed in a small number of patients.

Late complications of therapy

- Treatment-induced sterility is frequently seen in ♂ after treatment with MOPP and MOPP-like regimens regardless of age (90% azoospermic 1 year after ≥6 courses); the ABVD regimen produces significantly less infertility. Abnormal menstruation due to MOPP is more common in women over 30 (60–70%) and less common in those <20 (20–30%).

- Premature menopause is more common after MOPP in older ♀.
- ABVD + mantle radiotherapy causes higher incidence of post-irradiation paramediastinal fibrosis causing persistent effort dyspnoea.
- Patients cured of HL are at ↑ risk of a second malignancy with a relative risk of 6.4.
- Solid tumours (commonly breast, lung, melanoma, soft tissue sarcoma, stomach and thyroid) comprise >50% of second malignancies; proportion increases as follow-up lengthens; risk ~13% at 15 years and ~22% at 25 years; associated with radiotherapy and young age at time of treatment; 75% occur within radiation fields.
- Acute myeloblastic leukemia risk ~3% at 10 years after treatment; peak incidence between 5–9 years; risk ↓ 10 years after therapy; particularly associated with MOPP chemotherapy and age >40 and radiotherapy dose >30Gy to mediastinum; risk 10 years after ABVD <1%.
- NHL risk 7%; rises beyond 10 years and declines after 15 years; no clear association with type of therapy.
- Cardiac toxicity: myocardial infarction, radiation-induced pericarditis, valvular disease and congestive failure occur at an increased frequency in patients previously treated for HL; higher risk in patients <40 at treatment.
- Pulmonary toxicity: generally mild, usually asymptomatic changes in pulmonary function; associated with mediastinal irradiation and bleomycin containing chemotherapy (ABVD).
- Thyroid toxicity: 50% risk at 20 years after radiation to the neck and upper mediastinum; risk highest for ages 15–25; usually hypothyroidism, minority develop hyperthyroidism, Hashimoto's thyroiditis, nodules or thyroid cancer.
- Patients treated with HDT and autologous SCT have an increased incidence of myelodysplasia and AML and azoospermia in males and premature ovarian failure in females is usual.

1 Hasenclever, D. & Diehl, V. (1998) A prognostic score for advanced Hodgkin's disease. International Prognostic Factors Project on Advanced Hodgkin's Disease. *N Engl J Med*, **339**, 1506–1514 **2** Canellos, G.P. *et al.* (1992) Chemotherapy of advanced Hodgkin's disease with MOPP, ABVD, or MOPP alternating with ABVD. *N Engl J Med*, **327**, 1478–1484 **3** Loeffler, M. *et al.* (1998) Meta-analysis of chemotherapy versus combined modality treatment trials in Hodgkin's disease. International Database on Hodgkin's Disease Overview Study Group. *J Clin Oncol*, **16**, 818–829.

Lymphoma

Myelodysplasia

6

Myelodysplastic syndromes (MDS)

The myelodysplastic syndromes (MDS) are a group of biologically and clinically heterogeneous clonal disorders characterised by ineffective haematopoiesis and peripheral cytopenia due to increased apoptosis and by a variable tendency to evolve to acute myeloblastic leukaemia.

Incidence

Predominantly affects elderly but may occur at any age; median age 69; annual incidence 4/100,000 in general population; rising from 0.5/100,000 aged <50 years to 89/100,000 aged ≥80 years.

Risk factors

- Age.
- Prior cancer therapy: notably with radiotherapy, alkylating agents (chlorambucil, cyclophosphamide, melphalan; peak 4–10 years after therapy) or epipodophyllotoxins (etoposide, teniposide; peak within 5 years). *Note*: prolonged alkylator therapy used in rheumatology and other specialties.
- Environmental toxins: notably benzene and other organic solvents; related to intensity and duration of exposure; also smoking, petroleum products, fertilisers, semi-metal, stone dusts and cereal dusts.
- Genetic: rare familial syndromes; MDS increased in children with Schwachman–Diamond syndrome, Fanconi anaemia and neurofibromatosis type 1.

Pathophysiology

- Clonal haematopoietic stem cell disorder characterised by stepwise genetic progression possibly due to a combination of genetic predisposition and environmental exposures.
- Abnormalities in the marrow microenvironment described: e.g. aberrant cytokine production (increased inhibitory pro-apoptotic cytokines including TNF-α, IL-6, TGF-β, IFN-γ and Fas ligand) and altered stem cell adhesion.
- MDS marrow stem cells display lowered apoptotic threshold to TNF-α, IFN-γ & anti-Fas antibodies and less response to haemopoietic growth factors.
- Early indolent pro-apoptotic MDS transforms to aggressive proliferative MDS as genetic lesions accumulate (*ras*, *FLT3*, *FMS* and *p53* mutations associated with disease progression).
- Symptoms relate not only to the degree of cytopenia but to impaired function of granulocytes and platelets and may occur at near-normal or normal levels.

Myelodysplasia

Classification systems

French–American–British (FAB) system

- Morphology based classification widely adopted since 1982.
- Defines five subtypes.
- Requires dysplastic changes in ≥ 2 lineages.
- Useful for predicting prognosis and risk of evolution to acute leukaemia.

FAB classification

Refractory anaemia (RA): cytopenia of one peripheral blood (PB) lineage; normo- or hypercellular marrow with dysplasia ≥2 lineages; <1% PB blasts; <5% BM blasts. 25% of patients.

Refractory anaemia with ringed sideroblasts (RARS): defined as for RA plus ringed sideroblasts account for >15% nucleated erythroid cells; 15% of patients.

Refractory anaemia with excess blasts (RAEB): cytopenia of ≥2 PB lineages; dysplasia of all 3 BM lineages; <5% PB blasts; 5–20% BM blasts; 35% of patients.

Refractory anaemia with excess blasts in transformation (RAEB-t): cytopenia of ≥2 PB lineages; dysplasia of all 3 BM lineages; ≥5% PB blasts; 21–30% BM blasts or Auer rods in blasts; 15% of patients.

Chronic myelomonocytic leukaemia (CMML): PB monocytosis ($>1 \times 10^9$/L); <5% PB blasts; ≤20% BM blasts; 10% of patients[1].

World Health Organisation (WHO) system

- Proposed reclassification of MDS based on morphology, karyotype and clinical features; not yet universally accepted.
- Lower threshold for diagnosis of AML from 30%→20% blasts in PB or BM; eliminates FAB category 'RAEB-t'.
- Refined definitions for low grade MDS: RA and RARS.
- Addition of new category 'refractory cytopenia with multilineage dysplasia' (RCMD).
- Defines two subtypes of RAEB: RAEB-1 (5–9% BM blasts) and RAEB-2 (10–19% BM blasts) reflecting worse clinical outcomes with ≥10% blasts.
- Recognises the '5q– syndrome' as a distinct narrowly defined entity.
- Removes CMML to a newly created disease group: MDS/MPD.

WHO Classification System

Condition	PB findings	BM Findings
Refractory anaemia (RA)	anaemia >6 months no or rare blasts	erythroid dysplasia only <5% blasts <15% ringed sideroblasts
Refractory anaemia with ringed sideroblasts (RARS)	anaemia >6 months no blasts	erythroid dysplasia only ≥15% ringed sideroblasts <5% blasts
Refractory cytopenia with multilineage dysplasia (RCMD)	cytopenias (bi- or pan-) no or rare blasts no Auer rods <1 × 10^9/L monocytes	dysplasia in ≥10% cells in ≥2 myeloid cell lines <5%blasts no Auer rods <15% ringed sideroblasts
Refractory cytopenia with multilineage dysplasia and ringed sideroblasts (RCMD-RS)	cytopenias (bi- or pan-) no or rare blasts no Auer rods <1 × 10^9/L monocytes	dysplasia in ≥10% cells in ≥2 myeloid cell lines ≥15% ringed sideroblasts <5% blasts no Auer rods
Refractory anaemia with excess blasts (RAEB-1)	cytopenias <5% blasts no Auer rods <1 × 10^9/L monocytes	unilineage or multilineage dysplasia 5–9% blasts no Auer rods
Refractory anaemia with excess blasts (RAEB-2)	cytopenias 5–19% blasts Auer rods ± <1 × 10^9/L monocytes	unilineage or multilineage dysplasia 10–19% blasts Auer rods ±
Myelodysplastic syndrome, unclassified (MDS-U)	cytopenias no or rare blasts no Auer rods	unilineage dysplasia in granulocytes or megakaryocytes <5% blasts no Auer rods
MDS associated with isolated del(5q)	anaemia <5% blasts platelets normal or ↑	normal to increased megakaryocytes with hypolobated nuclei <5% blasts no Auer rods isolated del(5q)

Vardiman, J.W. *et al.* (2002) The World Health Organization (WHO) classification of the myeloid neoplasms. *Blood*, **100**, 2292–2302.

Comparison of FAB and WHO classifications

FAB	WHO
RA	RA (unilineage) 5q– syndrome RCMD
RARS	RARS (unilineage)
RAEB	RCMD-RS RAEB-1 RAEB-2
RAEB-t	AML
CMML	MDS/MPD – MDS-U

1 Bennett, J.M. *et al.* (1982) Proposals for the classification of the myelodysplastic syndromes. *Br J Haematol*, **51**, 189–199.

Myelodysplasia

Clinical features of MDS

- Presentation ranges from mild anaemia to profound pancytopenia.
- May be asymptomatic with mild anaemia identified on routine FBC.
- Macrocytic or normochromic anaemia usual (60–80%) ± neutropenia (50–60%) ± thrombocytopenia (40–60%).
- Isolated thrombocytopenia would be a most unusual presentation for MDS.
- Symptoms of underlying cytopenias and cellular dysfunction may develop:
  - Anaemia: fatigue, shortness of breath, exacerbation of cardiac symptoms.
  - Neutropenia and dysfunctional granulocytes: recurrent infection.
  - Thrombocytopenia and dysfunctional platelets: spontaneous bruising, purpura, bleeding gums.
- Constitutional symptoms including anorexia, weight loss, fevers and sweats usually feature of the more 'advanced' subgroups; may be due to cytokine release.
- Splenomegaly commonly occurs in CMML and may cause abdominal pain and easy satiety.

Investigation and diagnosis

- History: prior exposure to chemotherapy/radiation; FH of MDS/AML; recurrent infection or bleeding/bruising.
- Examination: pallor; infection; bruising; splenomegaly.
- FBC: macrocytic/normochromic anaemia ± neutropenia ± thrombocytopenia ± neutrophilia ± monocytosis ± thrombocytosis.
- Blood film: may demonstrate dimorphic red cells ± Pappenheimer bodies in RARS; basophilic stippling in RBCs; dysplastic granulocytes: pseudo-Pelger forms, hypersegmented neutrophils, hypogranular neutrophils, dysmorphic monocytes ± blasts; platelets may be large or hypogranular.
- U&E, LFTs, ECG and CXR: to assess co-morbidity.
- Serum ferritin, vitamin B_{12} and RBC folate: usually normal levels; ferritin may be elevated in RARS.
- Serum Epo level: indicates probability of therapeutic response to Epo.
- BM aspirate: demonstrates >10% dysplastic cells in ≥ 2 lineages (for FAB system): megaloblastoid erythropoiesis, nuclear-cytoplasmic asynchrony in myeloid or erythroid precursors, dysmorphic megakaryocytes or micro-megakaryocytes; normal or increased storage iron; ≥15% ringed sideroblasts in RARS; increased monocytes in CMML.
- BM trephine biopsy: allows assessment of cellularity—usually ↑ or normal; may demonstrate abnormal localisation of immature myeloid precursors centrally in the intertrabecular interstitium (ALIPs), megakaryocyte dysplasia, fibrosis or hypocellular MDS variant.
- BM cytogenetic analysis: may demonstrate clonal chromosome abnormality(s) confirming diagnosis and with prognostic value.
- Definitive diagnosis of early MDS (e.g. isolated cytopenia) may be difficult; regular review with repeat blood count and film assessment recommended; in all cases a measure of the pace of the disease over a 2–6 week period is of prognostic value.

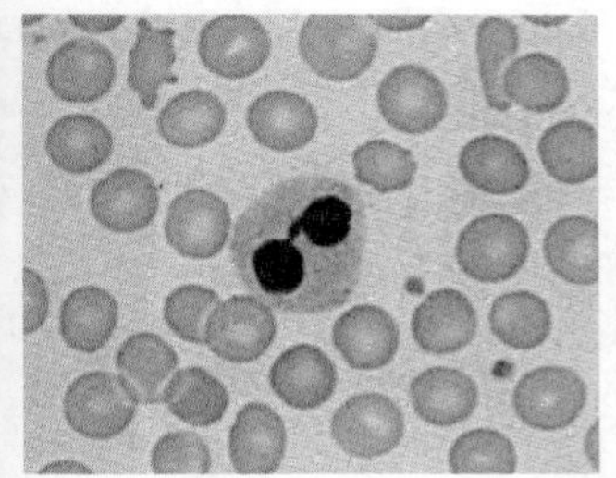

Blood film in MDS showing bilobed pseudo-Pelger neutrophil.

Cytogenetic analysis

- Abnormalities found in BM cytogenetic analysis of 40–70% of patients with *de novo* MDS and 80–90% of patients with secondary MDS.
- Single or complex abnormalities at diagnosis may evolve during course of disease.
- More complex abnormalities associated with more aggressive subtypes and higher % blasts and with secondary MDS.
- Most frequent abnormalities involve chromosomes 5, 7, 8, 11, 12 and 20; most typical are 8+, 7– or 7q–, 5– or 5q–.
- Isolated 5q–, 20q– and normal karyotype favourable; complex karyotypes (≥3 abnormalities), 7– or 7q– unfavourable.

Differential diagnosis

Exclude:

- Other causes of anaemia (haematinic deficiency, haemolysis, blood loss, renal failure).
- Other causes of neutropenia (drugs, viral infection).
- Other causes of thrombocytopenia (drugs, ITP).
- Other causes of bi-/pancytopenia (drugs, infection, aplastic anaemia).
- Other causes of monocytosis (infection, AML) or neutrophilia (infection, CML).
- Reactive causes of BM dysplasia: megaloblastic anaemia, HIV infection, alcoholism, recent cytotoxic therapy, severe intercurrent illness.
- Other causes of marrow hypoplasia in hypoplastic MDS: aplastic anaemia, PNH.

Prognostic factors in MDS

FAB classification	RA	RARS	RAEB	RAEB-t	CMML
Proportion of patients	25%	15%	12%	15%	10%
Median survival (months)	43	73	12	5	20
Transformation to AML	15%	5%	40%	50%	35%
Transformed at 1 year	5%	0	25%	55%	np
Transformed at 2 years	10%	0	35%	65%	np

np – data not provided

CMML median survival <5% blasts 53 months; 5–20% blasts 16 months.

Greenberg P.L. (2000) In: Hoffman R *et al.* eds *Hematology: Basic Principles & Practice*. 3rd ed. New York, NY: Churchill Livingstone 2000:1106–1129.

International Prognostic Scoring System (IPSS)

- Uses BM blast %, BM cytogenetics and number of cytopenias to compute a risk score and stratify patients into 4 distinct groups.
- Improved prognostic power for both survival and evolution into AML compared with earlier systems.
- Analysis excluded CMML with a WBC >12 × 10^9/L as this was considered myeloproliferative rather than MDS.
- IPSS score should be calculated during a stable clinical state not, for example, during florid infective initial presentation.
- May be used to assist management decisions.

	Score value				
Prognostic variable	**0**	**0.5**	**1.0**	**1.5**	**2.0**
BM blast %	<5	5–10	–	11–20	21–30
Karyotype	Good	Intermediate		Poor	
Cytopenias	0/1	2/3			

Karyotype: *Good*: normal, –Y, del(5q), del(20q); *Poor*: complex (≥3 abnormalities) or chromosome 7 anomalies; *Intermediate*: other abnormalities.
Cytopenias: Hb <10g/dL; neutrophils <1.8 × 10^9/L; platelets <100 × 10^9/L.

IPSS risk group	Combined score	Median survival	25% AML evolution
Low	0	5.7 yrs	9.4 yrs
Intermediate–1	0.5–1.0	3.5 yrs	3.3 yrs
Intermediate–2	1.5–2.0	1.2 yrs	1.1 yrs
High	>2.5	0.4 yrs	0.2 yrs

Greenberg, P. *et al.* (1997) International scoring system for evaluating prognosis in myelodysplastic syndromes. *Blood*, **89**, 2079–2088.

Myelodysplasia

Clinical variants of MDS

CMML: classified as MDS/MPD in the WHO classification; clinical outcome relates to BM blast % rather than PB monocyte count (📖p234).

5q– syndrome: clinically distinct form of MDS in WHO classification; characterised by more indolent clinical course, lower rate of evolution to AML, macrocytic anaemia, thrombocytosis and dysplastic megakaryocytes

Pure sideroblastic anaemia (PSA): defined as sideroblastic anaemia with dysplasia confined to erythropoietic cells (RARS in WHO classification); survival better (77% OS at 3yrs) than where dysplastic features are also present in myeloid or megakaryocytic lineages (RCMD-RS in WHO classification; 56% OS at 3yrs) and very low risk of AML, even in the long term.

Secondary MDS: incidence increasing due to successful chemotherapy and increased pollution; multiple chromosomal abnormalities in almost all patients; poorer prognosis than *de novo* MDS.

Hypoplastic MDS: <15% of cases of MDS have hypocellular BM on biopsy (<30% cellularity age <60; <20% aged ≥60); dysplastic megakaryocytes ± myeloid cells or excess blasts should be present; may be difficult to distinguish from aplastic anaemia in which pancytopenia usually more severe: cytogenetic findings typical of MDS may be necessary; no particular age range, FAB type and no difference in prognosis; may respond to immunosuppressive therapy.

Fibrotic MDS: up to 50% of cases have increased BM fibrosis but <15% have marked fibrosis; all FAB types; more common in secondary MDS; BM hypercellular with myelofibrosis; PB shows pancytopenia and dysplastic features and sometimes leucoerythroblastic picture; organomegaly unusual; rapid deterioration usual.

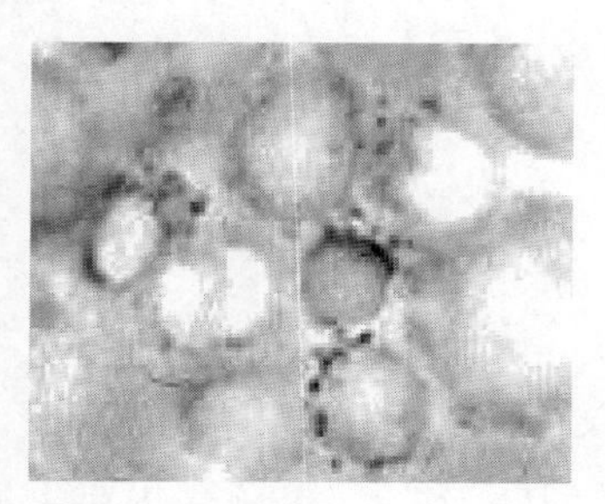

Bone marrow in RARS stained for iron: note iron granules round the nucleus of the erythroblast.

Myelodysplasia

Management of MDS

For patients with low risk indolent MDS, a watch and wait approach may be adopted prior to the introduction of therapy.

Supportive care

Supportive care is administered to most patients with MDS with the aim of reducing morbidity and maintaining quality of life. For many if not most patients this will be the mainstay of management.

Red cell transfusion should be administered for symptomatic anaemia; individual symptomatology rather than 'trigger' level should initiate red cell support.

Iron chelation therapy should be considered once a patient has received 25 units of RBCs if long term transfusion is likely e.g. pure sideroblastic anaemia or 5q– syndrome; Desferrioxamine 20–40mg/kg by 12h SC infusion 5–7 nights/week reduced to 25mg/kg when ferritin <2000mg/L; vitamin C 100–200mg/day PO may be added after 1 month; audiometric and ophthalmological assessments prior to therapy and annually; aim for serum ferritin <1000mg/L.

Platelet transfusion should be administered for patients with haemorrhagic problems and those with severe thrombocytopenia with the aim of maintaining a platelet count $>10 \times 10^9$/L.

Anti-infective therapy i.e. empirical broad spectrum antibiotics and/or antifungals should be administered promptly for neutropenic sepsis; no evidence to support routine use of prophylactic anti-infectives in neutropenic patients; prophylactic anti-infective agents may be useful in neutropenic patients with recurrent infection.

Low intensity therapy

Erythropoietin ± G-CSF treatment of symptomatic anaemia in MDS: maintenance of stable augmented Hb may provide better quality of life than the cyclical fluctuations of transfusion programmes; responses in 20–30% to Epo alone, 40–60% to Epo+G-CSF; synergistic effect most evident in RARS or patients with serum Epo levels <500U/L; check iron stores and replete if necessary.

- For patients with RA/RAEB with symptomatic anaemia, transfusion requirement <2 units/month and a basal Epo level of <200U/L consider trial of Epo (10,000 units daily for 6 weeks); in non-responders consider adding daily G-CSF (1mg/kg/day) SC or double dose Epo or both for further 6 weeks; no response after 2–3 months = treatment failure; in responders, reduce G-CSF to 3 × weekly and Epo in steps to lowest dose retaining response.
- For patients with RARS with symptomatic anaemia, transfusion requirement < 2 units/month and basal Epo levels <500 U/L combined therapy should be used from outset; consider Epo dose escalation if no response after 6 weeks; no response after 2–3 months = treatment failure; in responders titrate doses and frequency as tolerated.

G-CSF treatment of neutropenia: for patients with neutropenia and recurrent or antibiotic resistant infections but not recommended for chronic prophylaxis.

Immunosuppression: may be effective notably for patients with hypoplastic MDS but also for other patients with low risk MDS (IPSS≤ intermediate-1).

- ATG in clinical trials at a dose of 40mg/kg/d × 4d achieved transfusion independence in ~33% patients (median response >2 years); sustained neutrophil and platelet responses in up to 50%; response associated with significant survival benefit.
- Cyclosporin A has achieved transfusion independence in a high proportion of patients with RA in small clinical trials; improved neutrophil and platelet counts also.
- Younger age, shorter duration of transfusion dependence, HLA-DRB1* 15, hypoplastic BM and presence of a PNH clone associated with response to immunosuppression.

Non-intensive chemotherapy: may be tolerated by elderly patients with transformed or 'transforming' MDS; but transient reductions in blast counts may be at the price of increased cytopenia and transfusion dependence.

- Hydroxyurea is used to control monocytosis in CMML; titrate dose to achieve optimum control of myeloproliferation with minimum additional cytopenia; it is preferable to oral etoposide.
- Low dose melphalan (2mg/d) is under examination after small trials show a response rate of 40% in patients with RAEB or RAEB-t without severe side effects and prolonged survival in responders; best responses in hypoplastic MDS.
- 5-azacytidine: shows promise with 60% responses, decreased risk of AML transformation, improved QoL and improved survival in phase III trials.

High intensity therapy

Chemotherapy

- AML-type chemotherapy should be considered in patients <60 years with relatively high risk disease and good performance status (high risk IPSS/RAEB or RAEB-t); responses lower (40–50%) and treatment related morbidity and mortality higher than *de novo* AML; age >50 and karyotypic abnormalities associated with poor response.
- 5-aza-2-deoxycytidine achieved 64% responses in patients with high risk IPSS scores; myelosuppressive; requires hospitalisation; phase III trials under way.

High dose therapy

- Sibling allogeneic SCT offers the best prospect of prolonged survival and possible cure (35–40% 3 year DFS); few eligible but treatment of choice for patients aged <50 with ≥IPSS intermediate-1 and sibling donor; high treatment related mortality (>40%); relapse rate up to

40%; relapse risk relates to IPSS score—low risk <5%, high risk >25% as does DFS—IPSS low/intermediate-1 60%, intermediate-2 36% and high risk 28% at 5 years; favourable outcome associated with younger age, shorter disease duration, compatible graft, primary MDS, <10% blasts, good risk cytogenetics; lower intensity non-myeloablative regimens under trial for toxicity and response rate and may increase age range to 65 years.

- MUD allogeneic SCT associated with lower DFS (<30% at 2 years), higher treatment related mortality (>50%) but lower relapse rates (<15%); high mortality associated with patient age; this treatment should be discussed with patients ≤40 with ≥IPSS intermediate-1 who lack a sibling donor.
- Autologous SCT under trial for patients in CR after AML regimens; poor harvests; low TRM; high relapse rate.

A 'treatment algorithm' (BCSH Guideline: *Br J Haematol* (2003), 120, 187–200)

- *IPSS low:* high intensity therapy inappropriate; for symptomatic anaemia and RA with serum Epo <200U/L, RARS <500U/L consider trial of Epo±G-CSF; otherwise supportive care.
- *IPSS intermediate-1:* offer allograft to patients <50 years with sibling donor; consider patients aged 50–65 with good performance status and sibling donor for non-ablative conditioning and allograft within clinical trial; offer allograft within clinical trial (ablative or non-ablative conditioning) to patients ≤40 with MUD donor; *Note*: pre-transplant cytoreductive chemotherapy not recommended for IPSS intermediate-1; patients ≥65 or <65 without donors should be offered supportive care or Epo±G-CSF.
- *IPSS intermediate-2/high*: consider patients <65 for AML-type cytoreductive chemotherapy; those achieving CR or good PR after induction and consolidation chemotherapy should receive sibling or MUD allograft as detailed for IPSS intermediate-1 patients; those in CR or good PR without any donor but with good performance status and adequate harvest should receive autologous SCT within clinical trial.

Myelodysplasia

Myelodysplastic/myeloproliferative diseases (MDS/MPD)

This category was created in the World Health Organisation (WHO) classification of myeloid neoplasms for a group of disorders that have both dysplastic and proliferative features at diagnosis and are difficult to assign to either myelodysplastic or myeloproliferative groups.

WHO classification MDS/MPD diseases

- Chronic myelomonocytic leukaemia.
- Atypical chronic myeloid leukaemia.
- Juvenile myelomonocytic leukaemia.
- MDS/MPD unclassifiable.

Chronic myelomonocytic leukaemia (CMML)

Myeloproliferative element in CMML formerly recognised by subclassification into MDS-like or MPD-like on the basis of the WBC at presentation; MPD-like CMML associated with WBC >12 × 10^9/L, splenomegaly and constitutional symptoms; not a distinct condition as many patients who present with low WBC count and minimal splenomegaly ultimately progress to meet 'proliferative' criteria.

Clinical features

- Predominantly presents in >60 age group.
- Often asymptomatic and found on routine FBC.
- Weight loss, fatigue, night sweats may occur.
- Skin and gum infiltration may occur.
- Splenomegaly (50%) and hepatomegaly (up to 20%) usually only in cases with leucocytosis and symptoms.
- Serous effusions (pericardial, pleural, ascitic and synovial) associated with high PB monocytosis.

Investigation and diagnosis

- Investigation as for MDS.
- Variable leucocytosis; marked in 50%; neutrophilia in some patients.
- Monocyte count >1.0 × 10^9/L is diagnostic minimum.
- Variable anaemia; platelets usually normal or decreased.
- Marrow typically hypercellular; blasts and promyelocytes <20%.
- Karyotypic abnormalities associated with MDS found in most patients but no specific cytogenetic features apart from rarity of 5q–.
- Lysozyme raised in serum and urine.
- Hypokalaemia may be present.
- Reactive causes of monocytosis must be excluded (📖p144).

WHO diagnostic criteria for CMML

1. Persistent peripheral blood monocytosis >1.0 × 10^9/L.
2. No Philadelphia chromosome or *BCR-ABL* fusion gene.
3. <20% myeloblasts, monoblasts and promyelocytes in PB or BM.
4. Dysplasia in ≥1 myeloid lineages or if myelodysplasia absent but above criteria present, CMML may be diagnosed if:
   - An acquired clonal cytogenetic abnormality present in BM cells ***or***
   - Monocytosis persistent for ≥3 months and all other causes excluded.

Diagnose CMML-1 if <5% PB blasts and <10% BM blasts.

Diagnose CMML-2 = 5–19% PB blasts or 10–19% BM blasts or Auer rods present with <20% BM blasts.

Diagnose CMML-1 or CMML-2 with eosinophilia with above criteria + PB eosinophil count $>1.5 \times 10^9$/L.

Prognostic factors

BM blasts: median survival for CMML with <5% BM blasts 53 months versus 16 months for those with 5–20%.

Management

- Asymptomatic cases with near normal haematology apart from a monocytosis of $>1.0 \times 10^9$/L require no intervention and should simply be monitored. Therapy otherwise supportive.
- Patients with symptoms, organomegaly and/or ↑↑ WBC may respond to oral chemotherapy e.g. hydroxyurea (preferred) or etoposide.
- Rare young patients may be treated with myeloablative therapy and allogeneic SCT which offers only curative option.

Natural history

Prognosis for asymptomatic patients is favourable (several years). For those requiring therapy median survival is 6–12 months. Acute myelomonocytic leukaemia (AMML) develops in ~20%; poorly responsive to intensive chemotherapy.

Atypical chronic myeloid leukaemia (ACML)

- Heterogeneous group of patients with Philadelphia chromosome and *BCR-ABL* fusion gene negative CML.
- Other cytogenetic abnormalities frequent.
- Dysplastic myeloid series and often multilineage dysplasia; monocytosis frequent; no basophilia (*cf.* CML).
- Short median survival (11–18 months).

Juvenile myelomonocytic leukaemia (JML)

- Clonal disorder arising in pluripotent stem cell causing selective hypersensitivity to GM-CSF due to dysregulated signal transduction through *Ras* pathway.
- Affects infants and young children usually ≤5 years of age.
- Marked hepatosplenomegaly, neutrophilia and monocytosis, anaemia and thrombocytopenia.
- ↑ haemoglobin F.
- No Philadelphia chromosome or *BCR-ABL* fusion gene.
- Normal karyotype in >80%.
- No consistently effective therapy including allogeneic SCT (relapse rates up to 55%). 5 year survival after allograft 25–40%.

Myelodysplastic/myeloproliferative disease, unclassifiable

Category for patients with features of both MDS and MPD who do not meet the criteria for the three conditions above.

Myeloproliferative disorders 7

WHO classification of chronic myeloproliferative diseases

- Chronic myeloid leukaemia (Ph chromosome, t(9;22)(q34;q11), BCR-ABL-positive).
- Chronic neutrophilic leukaemia.
- Chronic eosinophilic leukaemia (and hypereosinophilic syndrome).
- Polycythaemia vera.
- Chronic idiopathic myelofibrosis (with extramedullary haematopoiesis).
- Essential thrombocythaemia.
- Chronic myeloproliferative disease, unclassifiable.

Chronic myeloid leukaemia

📖*p164.*

Chronic neutrophilic leukaemia (CNL)

- Very rare; <150 cases reported.
- Exclude underlying infection or neoplasia e.g. myeloma, before considering diagnosis of CNL.
- Neutrophilia without left shift, eosinophilia or basophilia.
- Modest splenomegaly common ± hepatomegaly.
- NAP usually ↑↑.
- Marrow hypercellular.
- BM cytogenetics usually normal.
- Most patients asymptomatic.
- Treatment often unnecessary.

Chronic eosinophilic leukaemia (CEL) and hypereosinophilic syndrome (HES)

- Must exclude infectious, inflammatory and neoplastic causes of eosinophilia including CML, AML with inv(16), other chronic myeloproliferative disorders, lymphoma (esp. Hodgkin's).
- Evidence of clonality = CEL; no evidence of clonality = HES.
- CEL is uncommon; marked increase in mature and immature eosinophils in PB and BM. Often >5% blasts in BM. Associated with tissue infiltration by immature eosinophils, anaemia and thrombocytopenia. No dysplastic features. No Philadelphia chromosome or *BCR-ABL* fusion gene. Short history of malaise, sweats, weight loss, skin rash and increased susceptibility to infection. Splenomegaly common. End-organ damage as per HES may occur. Proliferative element may be controlled by hydroxyurea. In symptomatic younger patients consider sibling allogeneic SCT.
- HES is characterised by PB eosinophilia $>1.5 \times 10^9$/L for >6 months and by end-organ damage, commonly endomyocardial fibrosis, skin lesions (angioedema, urticaria), thromboembolic disease , pulmonary lesions and CNS dysfunction. Associated with polyclonal increased in immunoglobulins including IgE. Splenomegaly 40%. Anaemia 50%; neutrophilia with left shift frequent; platelets may be normal, decreased or increased. BM hypercellular with 25–75% eosinophils with left shift. Eosinophilia may be controlled by prednisolone, hydroxyurea or IFN-α. Allogeneic SCT may be curative in younger patients.

Myeloproliferative disorders

Polycythaemia vera (PV)

Erythrocytosis is defined as increase in total red cell mass (RCM). It is suspected by finding a raised haematocrit (Hct) (packed cell volume, PCV). The term 'polycythaemia' is widely used synonymously but lacks precision and can lead to confusion. Polycythaemia vera (PV) is a neoplastic clonal disorder of the BM stem cell causing excessive proliferation of the erythroid, myeloid and megakaryocyte lineages and carrying a risk of thrombotic complications. Persistent elevation of Hct >0.48 in adult female and >0.51 in adult male is abnormal (*Note*: Hct can be raised with a normal RCM if plasma volume is reduced).

Classification of polycythaemia

See table opposite.

Clinical evaluation of a patient with suspected erythrocytosis

May be asymptomatic or may present with thrombosis or vague symptoms of headache, dizziness, tinnitus or visual upset. Take detailed history with attention to smoking habits, alcohol consumption and diuretic therapy. History of pruritus (especially after bathing) suggests PV (occurs in 50%). Burning sensation in fingers and toes (erythromelalgia) typical of PV. Physical examination may identify plethoric facies or abnormalities associated with a cause of secondary erythrocytosis such as gross obesity, hypertension, evidence of obstructive airways disease or cyanotic cardiac conditions. The presence of hepatomegaly or splenomegaly should be sought. An elevated Hct in the absence of identifiable factors in clinical assessment requires referral for specialist evaluation.

Investigation and diagnosis

- FBC: ↑↑ RCC and ↓ or ↔ MCV and MCH (may be evidence of iron deficiency).
- Neutrophils and platelets ↑ in PV (rare in other causes of erythrocytosis).
- NAP score: ↑ score usually present in PV (*but not diagnostic in isolation*).
- Red cell mass and plasma volume: patient red cells labelled with ^{51}Cr and re-injected; simultaneous plasma volume measurement using ^{131}I-labelled albumin. RCM ↑ >25% above mean predicted value is diagnostic of absolute erythrocytosis. Plasma volume also ↑ if marked splenomegaly present.

	PV	SE	RE
Red cell mass	↑	↑	↑ within NR or N
Plasma volume	N or ↑	N	↓ within NR or ↓

PV, polycythaemia vera; SE, secondary erythrocytosis; RE, relative erythrocytosis

- Arterial oxygen saturation: pulse oximetry most convenient to detect chronic hypoxia. SaO_2 <92% suggests causal relationship with absolute erythrocytosis. Sleep studies may be indicated by a history of snoring, waking unrefreshed and somnolence.
- Haematinic assays: serum ferritin: ↓ or ↔ (esp. PV) and occasionally overt iron deficiency. Serum vitamin B_{12}: levels commonly ↑ in PV due to ↑ transcobalamin reflecting associated granulocytosis. Folate deficiency may occur.

Myeloproliferative disorders

Classification of erythrocytosis

Primary erythrocytosis	*Congenital*	Truncation of erythropoietin receptor
	Acquired	Polycythaemia vera (PV) (*syn.* polycythaemia rubra vera (PRV); primary proliferative polycythaemia (PPP)).
Secondary erythrocytosis (SE) due to ↑ endogenous Epo production	*Congenital*	High oxygen-affinity haemoglobin Congenital low 2,3-DPG Autonomous high Epo production
	Acquired	
	Hypoxaemia	COAD Cyanotic congenital heart disease with right⟶left shunt Living at high altitude Chronic alveolar hypoventilation e.g. gross obesity Sleep apnoea syndromes
	Other causes of impaired tissue O_2 delivery	Smoking (↑ COHb)
	Renal disease	Polycystic kidneys Renal tumours Renal artery stenosis Post-renal transplantation
	Tumours	Cerebellar haemangioblastoma Uterine leiomyoma Hepatoma Bronchial carcinoma Adrenal tumours
	Liver disease	Cirrhosis Hepatitis Drugs Androgens
Idiopathic erythrocytosis (IE)		Persistent ↑ RCM, no cause found but no evidence of myeloproliferative disease or clear cause of secondary erythrocytosis.
Relative erythrocytosis (RE) Syn. apparent polycythaemia, spurious erythrocytosis, pseudopolycythaemia		Normal RCM and ↓ plasma volume Diuretic therapy or dehydration Gaisbock's syndrome (*see p248*) Smoking, alcohol, hypertension, obesity.

Investigation and diagnosis, cont.

- Serum U&E: to screen for renal impairment.
- Uric acid: often ↑ in MPD.
- Urinalysis: haematuria or proteinuria should prompt further renal investigations.
- LFTs: to screen for liver disease.
- Abdominal USS: for hepatosplenomegaly, renal or pelvic abnormalities.
- CXR: to screen for pulmonary disease (plus pulmonary function tests if indicated) and congenital cardiac abnormalities.
- Serum erythropoietin: assays not yet part of routine laboratory investigation in UK: serum Epo ↓ in PV and ↑ in SE; may also be low in RE and idiopathic erythrocytosis.
- BM examination: trephine may be diagnostic in PV. Typical features include hypercellularity and trilineage hyperplasia with abnormal megakaryocytes (clustering with giant forms and increased ploidy). Increased fibrosis may be present. Normal BM histology does *not* exclude PV but is more usual in SE.
- Cytogenetics: not routine; ~30% have abnormalities, typically 20q–. 8+, 9+ and 13q–.
- BFU-E culture: not routine; PV progenitors show increased sensitivity to growth factors and develop 'endogenous erythroid colonies' without added Epo.

Proposed diagnostic criteria for PV	
A1	Raised RCM (>25% above mean normal predicted value) or Hct ≥0.60 in ♂ or 0.56 in ♀
A2	Absence of cause of secondary erythrocytosis
A3	Palpable splenomegaly
A4	Clonality marker, i.e. acquired abnormal BM karyotype
B1	Thrombocytosis (platelet count >400 × 10^9/L)
B2	Neutrophil leucocytosis (neutrophils >10 × 10^9/L; >12.5 × 10^9/L in smokers)
B3	Splenomegaly demonstrated on isotope or ultrasound scan
B4	Characteristic BFU-E growth or reduced serum erythropoietin
A1 + A2 + A3 or A4 establishes PV	
A1 + A2 + two of B establishes PV	

Pearson, T.C. & Messinezy, M. (1996) The diagnostic criteria of polycythaemia rubra vera. *Leuk Lymphoma*, **22 Suppl 1**, 87–93.

Natural history of PV

Untreated PV carries a significant risk of thrombotic complications and a further long term risk of transformation into myelofibrosis or less commonly AML. There is also an ↑ risk of bleeding notably from peptic ulcers. The aim of treatment is to reduce the risk of thrombotic complications and to prevent progression to myelofibrosis or leukaemia. Current treatments improve the untreated median survival of 18 months to >15 years though some myelosuppressive treatments (notably chlorambucil and ^{32}P) have been associated with an increased risk of AML. Thrombotic complications notably MI, stroke and venous thromboembolism are the most common causes of death. Age and thrombotic history are the most important risk factors.

PV characteristically presents during the proliferative phase when control of erythrocytosis and prevention of thrombotic complications is often an urgent priority. This is often followed by a stable phase of variable (but often short) duration where near normal counts are maintained without therapy due to decreasing proliferative capacity due to early myelofibrosis. This is followed by an advanced or 'spent phase' which is due to extensive myelofibrosis and associated with progressive hepatosplenomegaly and pancytopenia. Incidence 10–15% after 10 years rising to >30% at 20 years; median survival <18 months. The incidence of AML is estimated at 2% in the absence of therapy but is over 14% after myelosuppressive therapy.

Management of PV

In younger patients (<40) who have a low risk of cerebrovascular or cardiovascular events the use of venesection in combination with low dose aspirin and non-leukaemogenic therapy such as anagrelide or IFN-α should be considered to reduce the risk of leukaemia.

Venesection: to ↓ blood volume to normal as rapidly as possible and prevent complications (target Hct <0.45). Removal of RBCs by venesection is the quickest way of reducing red cell mass. 450mL blood (± isovolaemic replacement with 0.9% saline) removed safely from younger adults every 2–3 days (↓ volume or frequency to twice weekly in older patients). If Hct very high (>0.60) venesection may be technically difficult due to extreme viscosity.

Maintenance therapy: venesection alone can be used to maintain the Hct at 0.42–0.45. Individual requirements are variable (e.g. 2 procedures per year to monthly venesection). However, early studies showed ↑ risk of thrombosis in first 3 years after treatment with venesection alone thus additional myelosuppressive treatment is required in most patients.

Hydroxyurea: an antimetabolite (ribonucleotide reductase inhibitor), is most commonly used therapy. Onset of myelosuppression with hydroxyurea is rapid, but overdosage quickly corrected by temporary withdrawal. Once Hct ↓, a daily dosage of 10–20mg/kg/d normally sufficient as maintenance therapy. Lower incidence of thrombosis by ensuring better Hct (<0.45) and platelet counts ($<400 \times 10^9$/L). Lower incidence of leukaemia than ^{32}P/alkylator therapy but still concerns.

Radioactive phosphorus (^{32}P) and busulfan: long established treatments for PV. Produce ↓ in RCM 6–12 weeks after administration (^{32}P 2.3 mCi/m^2 by IV injection every 12 weeks as necessary; busulfan by single oral dose 0.5–1mg/kg). Either agent may be repeated after 3–6 months if further myelosuppression is required. Both individually ↓ thrombosis and myelofibrosis but markedly ↑ the risk of AML. The use of ^{32}P and either busulfan or hydroxyurea in an individual is associated with a very high risk of AML. Neither is recommended for patients ≤65 years who should receive hydroxyurea. However, in patients >65 in whom compliance or regular monitoring of hydroxyurea dose may be a problem busulfan or ^{32}P can be considered as both offer intermittent therapy rather than long term maintenance.

Anagrelide: oral imidazoquinazoline with anti-cyclic AMP phosphodiesterase activity and profound effect on megakaryocyte maturation resulting in reduced platelet production. No evidence of mutagenic activity. Useful for control of thrombocytosis in PV but no effect on splenomegaly or other lineages. Side effects: headache (50%), forceful heartbeat, fluid retention, dizziness, arrhythmia (<10%) and CCF (2%). Use with caution in patients with known or suspected cardiac disease.

Aspirin: 75mg daily as antiplatelet therapy is common practice in myeloproliferative conditions. Higher doses are associated with haemorrhage. Large trial of low dose aspirin (40mg/d) in progress. Meantime reasonable to use 40mg/d aspirin in patients with history of MI or thrombotic CVA, erythromelalgia and other microvascular neurological and ocular disturbances. Avoid in those with a history of haemorrhage particularly in the GI tract.

Interferon-α therapy at a dose of 3–5MU three times weekly can control erythrocytosis and ↓ leucocytosis, thrombocytosis and splenomegaly in 60–75% of patients over 6–12 months. A useful observation is that it can diminish the severity of pruritus in 80% of patients. Tolerance is a problem but may be reduced by the use of pegylated-interferon.

Supportive treatment: maintain adequate fluid intake and avoid dehydration. Give allopurinol to minimise complications of hyperuricaemia. Acute gout is managed by standard therapies. Pruritus is a troublesome complication for some patients, unfortunately there is no satisfactory treatment. Sometimes abates when excess myeloproliferation controlled and Hct reduced but may persist despite adequate control of the Hct. Worth trying antihistamines, H_2-antagonists or interferon-α.

Surgical procedures relatively contraindicated in active PV: defer until Hct and platelets normalised for ≥2 months due to risk of thrombotic and haemorrhagic complications; if emergency surgery necessary perform venesection and cytapheresis.

Continued care and follow-up

Patients with PV and idiopathic erythrocytosis should have long-term haematological follow-up. Measure Hct at least 3 monthly. For patients on cytotoxic therapy with hydroxyurea the FBC should be checked every 8–12 weeks.

Treatment of advanced phase PV

Symptomatic management should be prioritised and the patient often requires blood product support. Splenectomy is often considered due to discomfort, recurrent infarction or hypersplenism but is often followed by massive hepatomegaly due to extramedullary haematopoiesis.

Myeloproliferative disorders

Secondary erythrocytosis

Causes of secondary erythrocytosis are listed in the table on page 241.

Effects of the increased red cell mass

- ↑ peripheral vascular resistance.
- ↓ cardiac output.
- ↓ systemic O_2 transport resulting in e.g. ↓ cerebral blood flow and oxygen and glucose delivery to the brain.
- Thromboembolic complications also occur. Thus 'compensatory' erythrocytosis is a pathological rather than physiological condition.

Symptoms and signs are non-specific and those of the underlying cause (particularly if cardiac or pulmonary) may predominate. Pruritus, splenomegaly or the presence of leucocytosis or thrombocytosis suggest the alternative diagnosis of PV.

Investigation as listed under PV, notably RCM and plasma volume, arterial oxygen saturation, renal and hepatic function, urinalysis, serum erythropoietin, renal ultrasound and if necessary abdominal CT.

The aim of therapy must be correction of the underlying cause where possible and reduction of the red cell mass. Venesection is the treatment of choice and if possible should be continued until a target Hct of <0.45 is achieved. In patients with cyanotic congenital heart disease, pulmonary disease or high O_2-affinity haemoglobin, the extent of venesection can be determined by symptomatic response or by using the serum Epo level as a measure of tissue hypoxia. Induction of iron deficiency by chronic venesection assists control of erythrocytosis. Myelosuppressive therapy is not indicated.

Myeloproliferative disorders

Relative erythrocytosis (RE)

Elevation of Hb and Hct with normal or minimally ↑ RBC mass and normal or ↓ plasma volume defines RE. Apparent/spurious polycythaemia, pseudopolycythaemia, stress erythrocytosis and Gaisbock's syndrome are synonymous terms for this disorder.

Aetiology

Unclear. Some cases may represent extreme ends of normal ranges for red cell and plasma volumes, but in most obesity, cigarette smoking and hypertension are present singly or in combination. Haemoconcentration from dehydration or diuretic therapy should be excluded.

Investigation

- FBC generally shows only modest ↑ Hct.
- Further investigations should be undertaken as appropriate for persistent erythrocytosis but, by definition, fail to reveal any other abnormality.
- RCM studies demonstrates normal RCM and ↓ plasma volume in ~33%; most have high normal RCM and low normal plasma volume.
- Important to exclude renal disease and arterial hypoxaemia.
- Bone marrow biopsy is not usually necessary but is normal when carried out.

Management

- Involves dealing with reversible associated features, i.e. weight reduction, cessation of smoking, control of ↑ BP and reduction in stress (where possible). Correction of these factors will result in spontaneous improvement.
- Venesection is not standard management; however, it is suggested that patients with Hct levels chronically >0.54 should be considered for venesection.

Natural history and treatment

- Not clear. Retrospective analysis appears to suggest an ↑ incidence of vaso-occlusive episodes that may relate to associated risk factors in the lifestyle of the patients under observation (rather than the ↑ PCV).
- Low dose aspirin (75mg/d) advisable for patients with overt thrombotic risks and no GI contraindication.
- No role for myelosuppressive therapy.
- Many patients improve with the simple measures specified. In ~33% the Hct returns to the normal range. In a further 33% the Hct oscillates between minimal elevation and the normal range. In the remaining 33% the Hct remains elevated and these patients should receive long term follow-up. In a minority absolute erythrocytosis may develop.

Idiopathic erythrocytosis (IE)

Heterogeneous group with absolute erythrocytosis (↑ RCM) but no clear cause of primary or secondary erythrocytosis.

- May be physiological variant.
- 5–10% show definite features of PV after several years follow up.
- Others develop clear evidence of SE, e.g. sleep apnoea.
- Long term follow-up is required in these patients.

Pearson, T.C. (1991) Apparent polycythaemia. *Blood Rev*, **5**, 205–213.

Essential (1°) thrombocythaemia (ET)

ET (*syn.* primary or idiopathic thrombocythaemia) is characterised by persistent thrombocytosis that is neither reactive (i.e. secondary to another condition; *p*XXX) nor due to another myeloproliferative or myelodysplastic disorder. It is a diagnosis of exclusion and may be biologically heterogeneous.

Incidence

True incidence unknown; slight excess in ♀; median age at diagnosis 60 years; frequently occurs <40 years; very rare <20 years.

Pathogenesis

Aetiology unknown. No association with radiation, drugs, chemicals or viral infection. Not all cases are clonal. Clonal and non-clonal cases may have different natural histories: thrombosis is less common in polyclonal ET as is the risk of leukaemic transformation. Platelets in ET are often functionally abnormal showing impaired aggregation *in vitro*. High platelet counts (>1000 × 10^9/L) are associated with an acquired von Willebrand syndrome; reduction in the platelet count corrects the abnormality and reduces haemorrhagic episodes.

Clinical features

- Diagnosis often follows routine FBC; up to 30% patients asymptomatic.
- Presentation may be due to 'vasomotor', thrombotic and/or haemorrhagic symptoms.
- Vasomotor symptoms occur in 40%: headache, light-headedness, syncope, atypical chest pain, visual upset, paraesthesiae, livedo reticularis and erythromelalgia (erythema and burning discomfort in hands or feet due to digital microvascular occlusion).
- Haemorrhagic symptoms occur in 25% (major <5%): easy bruising, mucosal or GI bleeding or unexplained or prolonged bleeding after trauma or surgery.
- Thrombosis occurs in ~20% (major <10%): arterial > venous, e.g. MI, CVA.
- Splenomegaly is found in <40% (less common and less marked than in other myeloproliferative disorders).
- Splenic atrophy may occur from repeated microvascular infarction.
- Recurrent abortions and fetal growth retardation due to multiple placental infarctions may occur in young women with ET.

Investigation and diagnosis

- FBC
  - Platelets persistently >600 × 10^9/L (may be as high as 5000 × 10^9/L).
  - Hb usually normal; may be ↓ with ↓ MCV due to chronic blood loss.
  - WBC usually normal; raised platelet distribution width (PDW).
  - Mean platelet volume (MPV) usually normal.
  - Automated FBC may give erroneous data in severe cases as giant platelets may be counted as RBCs.
- Blood film
  - Thrombocytosis, variable shapes and sizes (platelet anisocytosis), giant platelets and platelet clumps; megakaryocyte fragments; basophilia may be present; variable degree of RBC abnormality:

may be hypochromic and microcytic; may be changes of hyposplenism (*p44*).
- Bone marrow aspirate: not reliable for diagnosis; may show ↑ platelet clumps, atypical megakaryocytes including micromegakaryocytes and other maturation abnormalities.
- Bone marrow trephine biopsy: cellularity usually ↑; megakaryocytes ↑, with clustering, nuclear pleomorphism and atypical nuclear ploidy. Other elements may show abnormal distribution and maturation abnormalities. Reticulin normal or ↑ (25%); no fibrosis.
- Cytogenetics: abnormal in 5%; no recognised diagnostic abnormalities; occasionally 20q– or 21q–.
- Uric acid: ↑ in 25%.
- Pseudohyperkalaemia: in 25%.
- Acute phase proteins: CRP and fibrinogen, and ESR usually normal.
- Bleeding time: usually normal (↑ in ~20%)—rarely necessary; platelet aggregation studies not clinically helpful nor diagnostic.

Diagnostic criteria for ET
1. Persistent elevation of the platelet count $>600 \times 10^9$/L.
2. Absence of identifiable cause of reactive thrombocytosis.
3. Normal red cell mass or Hct <0.40.
4. Normal BM iron stores or normal serum ferritin or normal MCV.
5. Absence of Ph chromosome and *BCR-ABL* fusion gene.
6. Absence of significant BM fibrosis (<33% of biopsy in absence of splenomegaly and leucoerythroblastosis.
7. Absence of cytogenetic or morphological evidence of MDS.

Differential diagnosis
Before a diagnosis of ET is made, causes of reactive thrombocytosis (*p254*) must be excluded as must PV, CML, idiopathic myelofibrosis (IMF) and MDS with a predominant thrombocytosis which can mimic ET.

Prognostic factors in ET
- Thrombosis associated with previous thrombosis and age >60.
- Haemorrhage associated with extreme thrombocytosis ($>1000 \times 10^9$/L) and antiplatelet therapy.

Risk stratification in ET
Low risk
- Age < 60 *and*
- No history of thrombosis *and*
- Platelet count $< 1500 \times 10^9$/L *and*
- No cardiovascular risk factors (smoking, obesity, hypertension)

Intermediate risk
- Neither low risk nor high risk.

High risk
- Age ≥ 60 *or*
- Previous history of thrombosis.

Natural history

ET generally follows an indolent course and life expectancy is near normal. The risk of life-threatening complications or of leukaemic transformation is very low. However, the risk of AML is increased by cytotoxic therapy and such treatment should be used cautiously. The need for therapy must be individualised balancing risks of therapy against thrombotic risks (e.g. cigarette smoking, family history), FBC results, co-morbidity and age. Risk of AML 5–10%; risk of evolution to myelofibrosis ~5%.

Management

- Aim to ↓ risks and incidence of haemorrhagic and thrombotic complications by normalisation of platelet count (target <400 × 10^9/L); need to balance these risks with potential short and long term risks of therapy (e.g. aspirin) and cytotoxic therapy.
- Patients should be advised to make lifestyle changes (smoking, exercise, obesity) to reduce their risk of thrombosis and atherosclerosis.
- NSAIDs and standard dose aspirin should be avoided.

Low risk patients

- Incidence of thrombosis <2/100 patient years and haemorrhage ~1/100 patient years only; no added risk with pregnancy or surgery.
- Observation ± aspirin 75mg/d (if no contraindication) without cytotoxic therapy.

Intermediate risk patients

- Cytoreductive therapy (*see below*) for patients with marked thrombocytosis (>1500 × 10^9/L) who are at increased risk of thrombosis.
- Others in this group may be treated with low dose aspirin (if no contraindication) and observation.
- Smokers should be encouraged to stop smoking and obese patients to lose weight to reduce their risks of thrombosis.

High risk patients

- Control of thrombocytosis with hydroxyurea reduces the risk of thrombosis in these patients (<4% *vs.* 24% after 2 years in a randomised study).
- *Hydroxyurea*: treatment of choice for patients >60 years (0.5–1.5g/d maintenance after higher initial doses to bring platelets <400 × 10^9/L); used in symptomatic patients <60 intolerant of anagrelide and interferon-α; some patients may need combination therapy with anagrelide or interferon-α to achieve normalisation of the platelet count; side effects myelosuppression, oral ulceration, rash; contraindicated in pregnancy and breast feeding.
- *Anagrelide* (2–2.5mg/d) is preferred in younger patients <60 years (especially those of childbearing potential); interferes with megakaryocyte differentiation; side effects: headache, palpitations, fluid retention; contraindicated in pregnancy and patients with CCF or known cardiac disease.
- *Interferon-α*: (3–5mU 3–5 × weekly) can control thrombocytosis due to ET in younger patients intolerant of anagrelide; not associated with risk of AML; rarely used due to inconvenience of administration and poor tolerance.
- *^{32}P therapy* (2.3mCi/m^2 IV which may be repeated after 3–6 months) may be more appropriate in elderly patients (>75) or those unable to

comply with regular hydroxyurea therapy; side effects: myelosuppression, long term risk of AML.
- *Aspirin* 75mg/d recommended for patients with thrombotic event; increases risk of haemorrhage (safest when platelets <1000 × 10^9/L); relieves erythromelalgia quickly (2–4 days); extreme caution in patients with haemorrhagic complications or history of peptic ulceration; H_2-antagonist or proton pump inhibitors may be needed; markedly increased bleeding risk with higher aspirin doses. *Dipyridamole* is an alternative agent for those unable to tolerate aspirin.

ET in pregnancy
- First trimester abortion frequent in young women with ET (>40%).
- Low dose aspirin and interferon-α are treatments of choice because of the theoretically greater teratogenic risk of hydroxyurea.
- However, successful pregnancy reported following first trimester treatment with hydroxyurea.

Life-threatening haemorrhage in ET
- Stop anti-platelet agents.
- Identify site of bleeding.
- DDAVP/Factor VIII concentrate if evidence of acquired von Willebrand disease.
- Platelet transfusion if no evidence of acquired vWD.
- Plateletpheresis if persistent haemorrhage.
- Hydroxyurea 2–4g/day × 3–5d (takes 3–5d for effect).

Arterial thrombosis in ET
- Commence aspirin 75mg/d (rapid response in TIA and erythromelalgia).
- Hydroxyurea to normalise platelet count.
- Plateletpheresis if life threatening.

Surgery in ET
- Surgical procedures may require specific antithrombotic strategies e.g. heparin.
- Thrombotic risks lessened if platelet count normal.

Murphy, S. *et al.* (1997) Experience of the Polycythemia Vera Study Group with essential thrombocythemia: a final report on diagnostic criteria, survival, and leukemic transition by treatment. *Semin Hematol*, **34**, 29–39.

Reactive thrombocytosis

Platelet counts of >450 × 10^9/L occur as a reactive phenomenon and may be seen in:

- Infection.
- Following surgery, especially splenectomy.
- Malignancy e.g. underlying carcinoma.
- Trauma.
- Chronic inflammatory states e.g. collagen disorders.
- Blood loss and iron deficiency.
- Rebound in response to haematinics and/or chemotherapy.
- Any severely ill patient on ITU.

Raised platelet count in clonal haematological disorders occurs in CML, ET, PV, IMF and also in MDS (esp. 5q– syndrome).

In reactive thrombocytosis platelets are usually <1000 × 10^9/L but levels of 1500 × 10^9/L may occur. Platelet morphology usually normal but differentiation from ET relies on full clinical evaluation. No specific treatment is required for reactive thrombocytosis. Short term anticoagulant or antiplatelet therapy is advised for marked thrombocytosis in the immediate post-splenectomy period.

Myeloproliferative disorders

Idiopathic myelofibrosis (IMF)

Idiopathic myelofibrosis (*syn.* agnogenic myeloid metaplasia) is a myeloproliferative disorder characterised by marrow fibrosis, splenomegaly, extramedullary haematopoiesis and a leucoerythroblastic peripheral blood.

Incidence

Rare disorder; ~5 cases per million per annum; predominantly elderly patients (median 65 years).

Pathogenesis

- Clonal neoplastic proliferation arising from early haematopoietic stem cell.
- May evolve from PV (~9% of cases evolve into MF) or ET (~2% of cases evolve to MF); minority may follow previous chemotherapy or radiotherapy.
- Haemopoietic cells clonal, fibroblasts not clonal.
- Fibrosis is a cytokine-mediated reactive process (TGF-β, PDGF, IL-1, EGF, calmodulin and βFGF); can develop in response to chronic myeloproliferative disorders, myelodysplasia and secondary carcinoma.
- Exaggeration of normal BM reticulin pattern progresses to intense collagen fibrosis which disrupts and finally obliterates normal marrow architecture; ultimately osteosclerosis may develop.
- High levels of immature progenitors appear in PB.
- Extramedullary haemopoiesis develops in spleen and/or liver–occasionally other sites, e.g. lymph nodes, skin and serosal surfaces.

Clinical features and presentation

- ≤20% may be asymptomatic at diagnosis: mild abnormalities identified on routine FBC or splenomegaly at clinical examination.
- Most present with symptoms of progressive anaemia and hepatosplenomegaly associated with hypercatabolic features of fatigue, weight loss, night sweats and low grade fever.
- Abdominal discomfort (heavy sensation in left upper quadrant) and/or dyspepsia from pressure effects of splenic enlargement may prompt presentation.
- Symptoms and signs of marrow failure: lethargy, infections, bleeding.
- Splenomegaly is almost universal (>90%): moderate to massive (35%) enlargement; variable hepatomegaly (up to 70%); lymphadenopathy is uncommon (<10%).
- Gout in ~5%; portal hypertension, pleural effusion and ascites (due to portal hypertension or peritoneal seeding) also occur.

Investigation and diagnosis

- FBC: Hb usually ↓ or normal (<10g/dL in 60%); normochromic normocytic indices; WBC ↓, normal or ↑ (rarely $>100 \times 10^9$/L); platelets usually ↓ or normal; occasionally ↑.
- Blood film: leucoerythroblastic anaemia (nucleated red cells, myelocytes) with tear drop poikilocytes (96%) and polychromasia; giant platelets and megakaryocyte fragments.
- Bone marrow aspirate: usually unsuccessful ('dry tap').

- BM trephine biopsy: essential for diagnosis; characteristically shows patchy haemopoietic cellularity (often focally hypercellular) and variable reticulin fibrosis (often coarse and branching); ↑ numbers of large irregular megakaryocytes; distended marrow sinusoids with intravascular haematopoiesis.
- Coagulation screen: features of DIC in 15%; usually occult but causes problems at surgery (e.g. splenectomy); defective platelet aggregation common.
- Cytogenetics: abnormalities in up to 75%: 13q–, 20q– and 1q+ most frequent.
- Serum chemistry: bilirubin ↑ in 40%; alkaline phosphatase and ALT ↑ in 50%; urate ↑ in 60%.
- MRI: readily distinguishes fibrotic BM from cellular BM.

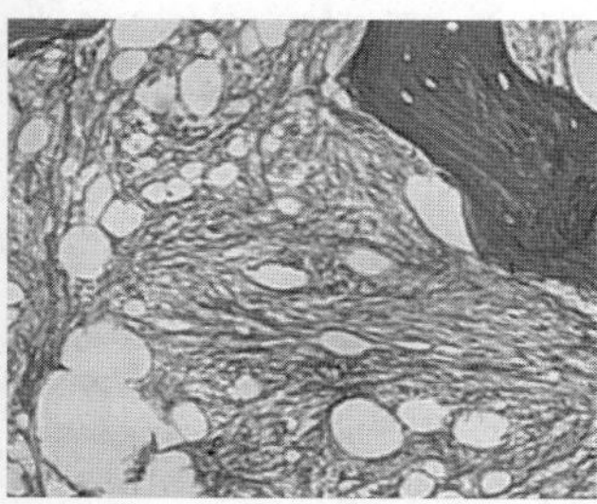

Bone marrow trephine in myelofibrosis: note streaming effect caused by intense fibrosis

Differential diagnosis

- Exclude other myeloproliferative disorders (CML, PV, ET) M7 AML (acute myelofibrosis), myelodysplasia, lymphoproliferative disorders (particularly hairy cell leukaemia), metastatic cancer (esp. breast, lung, prostate, stomach), tuberculosis, histoplasmosis and SLE, Gaucher's disease.
- IMF is –ve for Ph chromosome and *BCR-ABL* fusion gene.
- Metastatic cancer in marrow, especially breast, prostate and thyroid, can give similar FBC features but without splenomegaly; metastatic carcinoma cells are apparent on marrow biopsy and/or aspirate.
- Prefibrotic stage recognised: classical features may be minimal or absent and difficult to distinguish from PRV/ET; prominent neutrophil proliferation, decreased erythroid precursors and markedly abnormal megakaryocytes.

Prognostic factors

Short survival associated with:

- Hb <10 g/dL.
- WBC $<4 \times 10^9$/L or $>30 \times 10^9$/L.
- Constitutional symptoms.

- ≥1% blasts in PB or >10% blasts + promyelocytes + myelocytes in BM.

Management

- Myelofibrosis incurable except by allogeneic SCT; no other treatment alters disease course or prevents leukaemic transformation.
- Treatment palliative; aiming to improve anaemia, alleviate symptomatic organomegaly and hypercatabolic symptoms.
- Asymptomatic cases with minimal FBC abnormalities and splenic enlargement should simply be observed with regular follow-up.
- *Regular blood transfusion* for anaemic symptoms; transfuse on basis of symptoms not at a specific Hb level; iron chelation therapy with desferrioxamine should be considered after 25 units.
- *Corticosteroids*: ~33% of anaemic patients respond to combination therapy with an androgen (oxymethalone 50mg tds) and corticosteroid (prednisolone 1mg/kg/day).
- *Allopurinol* to treat or prevent hyperuricaemia.
- *Hydroxyurea*: often effective in reducing spleen size, leucocytosis, thrombocytosis, hypercatabolic symptoms.
- *Analgesia*: for acute splenic infarction; severe pain may respond to splenic irradiation.
- *Splenectomy* indicated for massive or symptomatic splenomegaly, excessive blood transfusion requirements, refractory thrombocytopenia, hypercatabolic symptoms unresponsive to hydroxyurea; evaluate coagulation system pre-operatively; 10% mortality; 40% morbidity.
- *Splenic irradiation* to reduce splenic size and discomfort in those unfit for splenectomy (3–6 month benefit).
- *Radiotherapy* also a useful treatment of extramedullary haemopoietic infiltrates at other sites e.g. pleural and peritoneal cavities.
- *Allogeneic SCT*: should be discussed with younger patients (e.g. ≤55) with ≥ 2 adverse risk factors (*see above*) and a sibling donor; median 5 year survival ~50%; actuarial probability of disease recurrence at 5 years ~30%.

Prognosis

- Median survival 4–5 years (range 1–30 years).
- Hypersplenism often develops as the spleen enlarges.
- Progressive cachexia occurs due to hypercatabolic state in advanced IMF.
- Death in symptomatic cases usually due to infection and haemorrhage.
- Around 5–10% transform to AML refractory to intensive chemotherapy.
- Asymptomatic cases usually die from unrelated causes.

Myeloproliferative disorders

Mast cell disease (mastocytosis)

Mastocytosis is a heterogeneous group of diseases characterised by abnormal proliferation of mast cells in one or more organ systems, including skin, bone marrow, liver, spleen and lymph nodes.

Epidemiology

Median age of systemic mastocytosis 50–60 years; range 5–88; median age of urticaria pigmentosa 2.5 months; after age 10 median age of urticaria pigmentosa 26 years.

Pathogenesis

Mast cells are derived from pluripotential haemopoietic dells and are the effector cells of the immediate allergic reaction via high affinity receptors for IgE. Most varients of systemic mast cell disease are clonal and a somatic mutation of *c-KIT*, the proto-oncogene that encodes the receptor for stem cell factor, is usually present. These mutations lead to constitutive activation of KIT which causes mast cell proliferation and prevents mast cell apoptosis. In paediatric mastocytosis KIT-activating mutations are rare. Clinical symptoms are due to the release of mast cell mediators (including histamine, tryptase, heparin, TNF-α, PGD2, cytokines and chemokines) which have both local and systemic effects, and to organ infiltration.

WHO classification of mast cell disease (mastocytosis)

- Cutaneous mastocytosis.
- Indolent systemic mastocytosis.
- Systemic mastocytosis with associated clonal, haematological non-mast cell lineage disease.
- Aggressive systemic mastocytosis.
- Mast cell leukaemia.
- Mast cell sarcoma.
- Extracutaneous mastocytoma.

Clinical features and presentation

- Patients usually present with symptoms of mediator release: urticaria, flushing, dermatographism, pruritus, angioedema; paroxysmal hyper- or hypotension; abdominal pain, dyspepsia, diarrhoea and malabsorption (80% of SM), multiple peptic ulcers, haemorrhage; wheezing, dyspnoea, rhinorrhoea; neuropsychiatric symptoms (headache, fatigue, irritability, cognitive disorganisation, nightmares); bone pain (25%).
- Most cases are seen in infants and children; involvement is generally limited to the skin; commonest forms are solitary cutaneous tumours (mastocytomas) or widespread cutaneous involvement with a few or many small lightly pigmented red-brown macules and papules (urticaria pigmentosa). Usually transient; begins in first year of life and disappears at puberty.
- Adult urticaria pigmentosa is associated with small heavily pigmented macular lesions; onset in young adults; often progressive with systemic organ involvement usually bone marrow (46%), lymph nodes (~25% at diagnosis), spleen (~50% at diagnosis), liver and GI tract.
- Familial mastocytosis causes cutaneous disease in infancy, persists into adult life and may progress to systemic involvement; rare.

Investigation and diagnosis

- Diagnosis of cutaneous mastocytosis (usually in children) based on typical clinical and histological skin lesions and absence of definitive signs of systemic involvement.
- Diagnosis of systemic mastocytosis (SM):
  - Bone marrow trephine biopsy: essential for diagnosis; multifocal lesions consisting of foci of spindle shaped mast cells with eosinophils and lymphocytes in a fibrotic stroma (90%); in advanced SM diffuse mast cell infiltration may occur.
  - Bone marrow aspirate: increased numbers of mast cells; clusters of confluent mast cells are a more specific finding (<30%); features of accompanying haematological disorder may be present, usually myelodysplastic or myeloproliferative disorder rarely lymphoproliferative.
  - Biopsy of other extracutaneous tissue: notably liver or lymph node; rarely necessary.
  - Serum mast cell tryptase and/or histamine:elevated in SM but not in isolated urticaria pigmentosa.
  - 24 hour urine for mediators (histamine metabolites, tryptase, PGD2 metabolites).
  - Bone scan/skeletal survey: bone lesions in 60%; generalised osteosclerosis, focal sclerosis or generalised osteopenia.
  - FBC and film: no characteristic features; circulating mast cells rare (2%) unless very advanced disease or mast cell leukaemia; mild to moderate anaemia in about 45%; eosinophilia up to 25%; thrombocytopenia about 20%; monocytosis about 15%; pancytopenia may develop due to BM infiltration or hypersplenism.
  - GI studies: as necessary.
  - EEG: if necessary.

Variants of SM

- Indolent SM: commonest form of SM; associated with maculopapular skin lesions (90%), slow involvement of target organs and good prognosis.
- Aggressive SM: characterised by impaired organ function due to infiltration of BM, liver, spleen, GI tract or skeletal system and predisposition to severe mediator release attacks with haemorrhagic complications.
- SM with associated haematological non-mast cell disease: <50% have urticaria pigmentosa; generally CML or CMML; classified according to FAB/WHO criteria; poorer survival.
- Mast cell leukaemia: defined by ≥20% MC in BM aspirate and ≥10% in PB; diffuse infiltration on trephine biopsy; no skin lesions, severe peptic ulcer disease, hepatosplenomegaly, anaemia, multiorgan failure and short survival.
- Mast cell sarcoma: a tumour consisting of atypical MC; locally destructive growth; no systemic involvement.

Differential diagnosis

Diagnosis often delayed due to protean clinical features. Exclude reactive mast cell hyperplasia, mast cell activation syndromes, myeloproliferative disorders with increased mast cells, carcinoid syndrome, phaeochromocytoma, myelofibrosis, liver disease and lymphoma.

Management

- No curative treatment; management consists of prevention of mediator effects and treatment of accompanying haematological disease where present.
- Avoid factors triggering acute mediator release: extremes of temperature, pressure, friction; aspirin, NSAIDs, opiates, alcohol, specific allergies.
- Treat acute mast cell mediator release.
- Anaphylaxis: epinephrine (adrenaline) 0.3mL of 1:1000 dilution (adult dose) every 10–15 minutes as needed.
- Refractory hypotension and shock: fluid resuscitation and epinephrine (adrenaline) IV bolus plus infusion of 1:10,000 dilution (up to 4–10mg/min); add inotropes if unresponsive.
- Commence H_1 plus H_2 receptor antagonists and steroids.
- Treat chronic mast cell mediator release: H_1 plus H_2 receptor antagonists: H_1 antihistamines: diphenhydramine (25–50mg PO 4–6 hourly; 10–50mg IM/IV), hydroxyzine (25mg PO tid or qid; 25–100 mg IM/IV) or loratadine (non-sedating; 10mg PO od); H_2 antihistamines: ranitidine (150mg PO bd; 50mg IV) or cimetidine (400–1600mg/day PO in divided doses; 300mg IV). Titrate doses for individual patient requirements; prednisolone 40–60 mg/day PO for malabsorption tailing; bisphosphonates and radiotherapy for bone pain; PUVA for urticaria pigmentosa; a small number of patients gain symptomatic relief from interferon-α or cyclosporin-A for refractory symptoms.
- Treat any associated haematological disorder: generally achieve short partial remission at best; splenectomy may help pancytopenic patients. SCT should be considered in appropriate patients.
- Attempt to control organ infiltration by mast cells: daunorubicin plus cytarabine and CVP have been reported to produce partial responses.

Prognosis

Most patients with SM have only slowly progressive disease and many survive several decades. 33% evolve into a haematological malignancy, frequently leukaemia. Mast cell leukaemia is resistant to intensive chemotherapy and has a survival of only a few months.

Escribano, L. *et al.* (2002) Mastocytosis: current concepts in diagnosis and treatment. *Ann Hematol*, **81**, 677–690; Valent, P. *et al.* (2001) Diagnostic criteria and classification of mastocytosis: a consensus proposal. *Leuk Res*, **25**, 603–625.

Myeloproliferative disorders

Paraproteinaemias

Paraproteinaemias

Heterogeneous group of disorders characterised by deranged proliferation of a single clone of plasma cells or B lymphocytes and usually associated with detectable monoclonal immunoglobulin (paraprotein or M-protein) in serum and/or urine.

Conditions associated with paraprotein production

Stable production

- Monoclonal gammopathy of undetermined significance (MGUS).
- Asymptomatic (smouldering) myeloma.

Progressive production

- Multiple myeloma (MM).
- Complete immunoglobulins: IgG, IgA, IgD, IgM, IgE.
- Free light chains (Bence Jones protein).
- 'Non-secretory'.
- Plasma cell leukaemia (PCL).
- Solitary plasmacytoma of bone (SPB).
- Extramedullary plasmacytoma (SEP).
- Waldenström's macroglobulinaemia (WM).
- Chronic lymphocytic leukaemia.
- Malignant lymphoma.
- Primary amyloidosis (AL).
- Heavy chain disease.

Paraproteinaemias

Monoclonal gammopathy of undetermined significance (MGUS)

MGUS describes the presence of a stable monoclonal paraprotein in serum or less commonly in urine in the absence of clinicopathological evidence of multiple myeloma (MM), Waldenström's macroglobulinaemia (WM), amyloidosis (AL) or other lymphoproliferative disorder.

Incidence
Median age 66 years. Incidence rises with age. Occurs in 1% population >50 years of age, 3% >70 years, 5% >80 years. More frequent in Afro-Caribbeans than Caucasians.

Pathophysiology
There is intraclonal variation in the Ig gene mutation and MGUS appears to arise from a pre-germinal centre cell whose progeny pass through the germinal centre and undergo mutation. Progression to MM may be due to outgrowth of a single clone. There is a continuing rate of progression to MM, WM, AL and other lymphoproliferative disorders. FISH demonstrates same MM cytogenetic abnormalities in MGUS often acquired over time. Expression microarrays show MGUS much closer to MM than to normal plasma cells. No specific trigger for progression yet identified.

Natural history
- >50% patients die of unrelated causes over a ~25 year follow-up period.
- 1% progress to MM, WM, AL or other lymphoproliferative disorder per annum.
- ~10% progress within 8 years; 26% after 25 years.
- 5% patients do not progress, some may show a ↑ in paraprotein levels.

Clinical features
- Typically asymptomatic and often incidental finding on investigation of ↑ ESR/PV or ↑ globulin on routine LFTs.
- No abnormal physical findings (end-organ damage) except unrelated.
- Lack of progression and absence of additional evidence of progressive plasma cell or B-cell lymphoproliferative malignancy.

Investigation and diagnosis
- Perform investigations listed for MM (📖*p273*).
- Serum protein electrophoresis with immunofixation and densitometry to detect, characterise and quantitate paraprotein levels: IgG 66%; IgA 20%; IgM 10%; biclonal 1%; light chain 1%; median ~15g/L.
- Urine electrophoresis: identifies only low levels of Bence Jones proteinuria (generally <1g/24h).
- Stable paraprotein and other parameters on prolonged observation.
- Immunoglobulin quantitation: by nephelometry; only 25% have immuneparesis of uninvolved Ig classes (*cf.* myeloma).
- Serum β_2-microglobulin levels normal (unless renal impairment).
- BM aspirate: <10% plasma cells in BM; median ~5%.

- BM cytogenetics: normal by conventional techniques but all abnormalities in MM described in MGUS by FISH; del(13), t(4;14), *ras* mutations, *p16* and *p53* inactivation less common.
- BM trephine biopsy: no evidence of diffuse plasma cell infiltration or osteoclast erosion of trabeculae.
- FBC: no anaemia or other cytopenia except due to unrelated causes.
- Serum chemistry: no hypercalcaemia or unexplained renal impairment.
- Skeletal radiology: no evidence of lytic lesions or pathological fracture; osteoporosis may co-exist from other causes e.g. post menopausal females.
- Other imaging: not routine; MRI of the spine; FDG-PET and ^{99m}Tc-MIBI scan are negative in MGUS.

Diagnostic criteria for MGUS

- Paraprotein <30g/dL.
- BM plasma cells <10%.
- No evidence of other B-cell lymphoproliferative disorder.
- No myeloma-related organ or tissue impairment (end-organ damage, see *Myeloma-related organ or tissue impairment below*).

Differential diagnosis

- Exclude conditions listed on p266 notably MM, WM and AL.
- Bone pain/damage, unexplained anaemia or impaired renal function suggests MM.
- Lymphadenopathy or splenomegaly with an IgM paraprotein suggests WM.

Risk factors for progression

- No specific features at initial presentation predict those who will progress but risk increased if:
- Paraprotein >15g/L.
- Paraprotein type: IgM>IgA>IgG;
- BM plasma cells >5%.
- Circulating plasma cells by immunofluorescence.
- Other possible risk factors under examination: immuneparesis; presence of urinary paraprotein; BM angiogenesis.

Management

- No treatment; long term follow-up with review of clinical and laboratory features required due to risk of progression.
- Clinical and laboratory (FBC, PV, renal function, serum Ca^{2+}, serum Igs, paraprotein quantitation and urine electrophoresis) re-evaluation at 3 months then 6 months then annually.
- Where diagnosis in doubt (e.g. elderly woman with paraprotein <30g/L and osteoporosis) review over 3–6 months usually differentiates MGUS from MM.
- Advise patients to seek early assessment if unexplained symptoms develop.

Kyle, R.A. (1997) Monoclonal gammopathy of undetermined significance and solitary plasmacytoma. Implications for progression to overt multiple myeloma. *Hematol Oncol Clin North Am*, **11**, 71–87; Kyle, R.A. *et al.* (2002) A long-term study of prognosis in monoclonal gammopathy of undetermined significance. *N Engl J Med*, **346**, 564–569.

Asymptomatic (smouldering) myeloma

Asymptomatic or smouldering myeloma identifies patients with a paraprotein over 30g/dL and/or more than 10% plasma cells in the bone marrow but in whom the natural history is that of MGUS rather than MM, i.e. no clinical evidence of progression or of complications associated with MM.

Prognosis

- Important to recognise because there is no survival advantage from chemotherapy before progressive or symptomatic disease develops.
- Clinical stability may persist for months or years and careful clinical follow-up is required.
- Survival is same as for newly diagnosed myeloma from the time chemotherapy is started.

Clinical and laboratory features

- Absence of symptoms or physical signs attributable to myeloma.
- Performance status >50%.
- Perform investigations listed for MM (📖*p273*).
- FBC: pre-transfusion haemoglobin >10g/dL.
- Serum chemistry: post-rehydration creatinine <130μmol/L; normal serum Ca^{2+}.
- β2-microglobulin: normal or minimally raised.
- BM aspirate: plasmacytosis >10% but normally <25%.
- BM cytogenetics: FISH identifies the abnormalities associated with MM; some patients have detectable chromosomal abnormalities by standard karyotype analysis.
- Skeletal radiology: should be normal.
- Other imaging: not yet routine; CT, MRI of spine FDG-PET and ^{99m}Tc-MIBI scan identify bone lesions in ~25% of patients with normal conventional radiology.
- BM plasma cell labelling index: (when measured) <1%.
- Stable paraprotein and other parameters on prolonged observation.

Diagnostic criteria for asymptomatic (smouldering) myeloma

- Paraprotein ≥30g/dL and/or
- BM clonal plasma cells ≥ 10%.
- No evidence of other B-cell lymphoproliferative disorder.
- No myeloma-related organ or tissue impairment (end-organ damage, see *Myeloma-related organ or tissue impairment below*).

Risk factors for early progression of asymptomatic MM

Shorter time to progression associated with:

- Abnormal MRI (median <2 years *vs.* ~7 years).
- Serum paraprotein >30g/L.
- β2-microglobulin >2.5mg/L.
- BM plasmacytosis >25%.
- Suppression of uninvolved IgM to ≤3g/L.
- IgA protein type.
- Urinary Bence Jones proteinuria >50mg/day.

These risk factors have no impact on survival after progression. Other risk factors for progression are high plasma cell labelling index; circulating plasma cells and karyotype abnormalities on conventional cytogenetics.

Management

- Chemotherapy is not indicated for these patients until there is evidence of clinical progression.
- Review of clinical and laboratory features as for MGUS; more frequent review may be appropriate for patients with risk factors for progression.
- Median survival following chemotherapy is 3–5 years, i.e. identical to that of *de novo* symptomatic myeloma.

Weber D. *et al.* (2003) Risk factors for early progression of asymptomatic multiple myeloma. *Hematol J.* **4**(Suppl. 1): S31–S32.

Multiple myeloma (MM)

MM (*syn.* myelomatosis) is a clonal B-cell malignancy characterised by proliferation of plasma cells that accumulate mainly within bone marrow and usually secrete paraprotein. MM is associated with lytic bone lesions or diffuse osteoporosis and normal Ig production is impaired by immuneparesis (hypogammaglobulinaemia). <1% cases are non-secretory.

Epidemiology

MM accounts for 1% of all malignancies; 10% of haematological malignancies. Incidence ~4 per 100,000 per annum, 2500 new cases/year in UK. Median age 65 years; <3% <40 years. Incidence in Afro-Caribbeans 2 × Caucasians; lowest in Asians. Most present *de novo* but minority arise from MGUS. Association with radiation, benzene and pesticide exposure and farm working.

Pathophysiology

MM arises from a post germinal centre B cell (probably in LN or spleen) that has undergone antigen selection, VDJ recombination, somatic hypermutation of V regions and switch-recombination of IgH genes. Aberrant class-switch recombination may contribute to neoplastic transformation (IgH translocations common in MM). BM microenvironment critical to clonal expansion. Secretion of IL-6, IL-1, TNF-α and RANK-ligand stimulate MM proliferation and osteoclast proliferation and activation (causes bone destruction plus hypercalcaemia). BM infiltration causes anaemia. Immuneparesis of normal Ig production predisposes to infection. Physicochemical properties of paraprotein determine amyloid deposition, renal damage and hyperviscosity (IgA and IgG_4).

Clinical features and presentation

- Spectrum from asymptomatic paraproteinaemia detected on routine testing (~20%) to rapidly progressive illness with extensive, destructive bony disease.
- Most present with bone (usually back) pain (~75%) or pathological fracture; kyphosis and loss of height may occur from vertebral compression fractures.
- Weakness and fatigue (>50%), recurrent infection (10%) and thirst, polyuria, nocturia or oedema due to renal impairment (~10%) also common.
- Acute hypercalcaemia, symptomatic hyperviscosity (mental slowing, visual upset, purpura, haemorrhage), neuropathy, spinal cord compression, amyloidosis and coagulopathy less frequent at presentation.

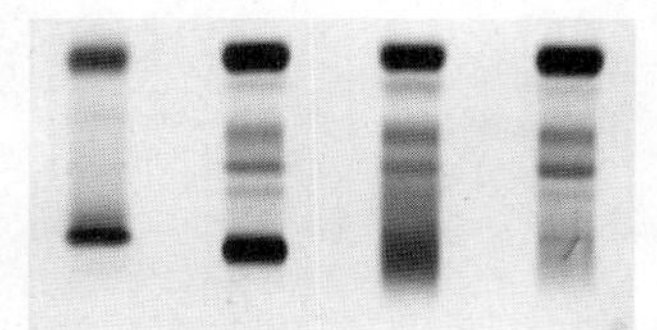

Electrophoresis: from L ⟶ R, urine BJP, serum M band (myeloma); polyclonal Igs; normal.

Investigation of patients with suspected myeloma	
Screening tests	
FBC and film	Normochromic normocytic anaemia in 60%; film may show rouleaux
ESR or PV	↑ in 90% ; not in LC or NS MM
Urea & creatinine	May identify renal impairment (~25%)
Uric acid	May be ↑
Serum albumin, calcium, phosphate, alk phos:	may reveal low albumin or hypercalcaemia (~20%) with normal alk phos
Serum immunoglobulins	To detect immuneparesis
Serum protein electrophoresis	To detect serum paraprotein (80%)
Routine urinalysis	To detect proteinuria (~70%)
Urine electrophoresis with immunofixation:	To detect Bence Jones proteinuria: 22% have BJP only and no serum M-band: LC myeloma)
X-ray sites of bone pain	May reveal pathological fracture(s) or lytic lesion(s)
Diagnostic tests	
BM aspirate	Demonstrates plasma cell infiltration—may be only way to diagnose non-secretory (NS) myeloma
Radiological skeletal survey	Identifies lytic lesions, fractures and osteoporosis (80%; 5–10% osteoporosis only; 20% normal)
Paraprotein immunofixation and densitometry	Characterises and quantifies paraprotein; IgG ~55%; IgA ~22% IgD ~2%; IgM 0.5%; IgE <0.01%; LC ~22%; *Note*: serum & urine EPS –ve in NS ~1%
Tests to establish tumour burden and prognosis	
Serum β2-microglobulin	Measure of tumour load
Serum C-reactive protein	Surrogate measure of IL-6 which correlates with tumour aggression
Serum LDH	Measure of tumour aggression
Serum albumin	Hypoalbuminaemia correlates with poor prognosis
BM cytogenetics	Clear prognostic value (*see below*)
BM trephine biopsy with immunohistochemistry	Shows light chain restriction, extent of infiltration and haematopoietic reserve
Tests which may be useful in some patients	
Creatinine clearance	With 24h protein—to assess renal damage
MRI	Not routine but useful in patients with cord compression or solitary plasmacytoma; abnormal in ~25% of patients with normal skeletal survey
CT	Not routine but useful for detailed evaluation of localised sites of disease
Biopsy for amyloid + SAP scan	Where amyloid suspected (📖 p288)
Serum free light chain assay	Provides treatment response parameter in LC myeloma, amyloidosis and most cases of 'non-secretory' MM
FDG-PET scan	Under evaluation; abnormal in ~25% with normal skeletal survey; persistent positive post-therapy may predict early relapse; identifies focal recurrent disease and focal extramedullary disease
^{99m}Tc-MIBI scan	Under evaluation; may identify extensive BM involvement

Diagnostic criteria for multiple myeloma
Paraprotein in serum and/or urine (*Note*: no minimum level).
BM clonal plasma cells (*Note*: no minimum level; 5% have <5% plasma cells) or plasmacytoma.
Myeloma-related organ or tissue impairment (end-organ damage)

Myeloma-related organ or tissue impairment (end-organ damage)

- Elevated calcium levels: serum calcium >0.25mmol/L above upper limit of normal or corrected serum calcium >2.75mmol/L or >11mg/dL.
- Renal insufficiency: (creatinine >173µmol/L or >2mg/dL).
- Anaemia: Hb 2g/dL below normal range or Hb <10g/dL.
- Bone lesions: lytic lesions or osteoporosis with compression fractures recognised by conventional radiology.
- Others: symptoms of hyperviscosity; amyloidosis; recurrent bacterial infection.

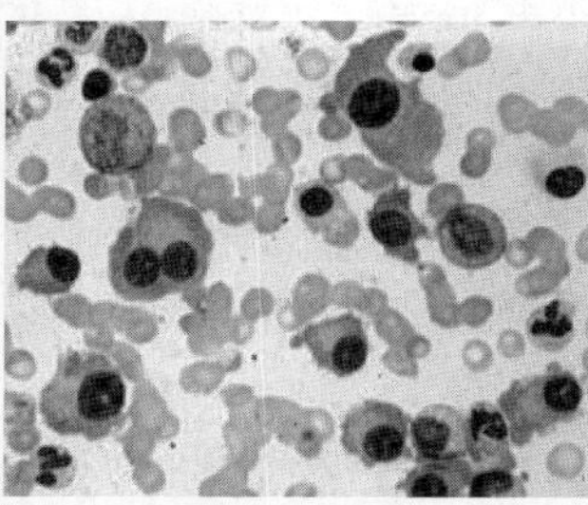

Bone marrow aspirate in myeloma showing numerous plasma cells (note binucleate cell, centre left).

Cytogenetics

- Using conventional techniques abnormal karyotypes found in 30–50%; heterogeneous pattern and complex abnormalities are common.
- FISH techniques demonstrate aneuploidy in nearly all patients:
  - Monosomies in vast majority (8, 13, 14, 16, 22).
  - Abnormalities involving 14q32 (Ig heavy chain locus) in 60–75% (esp. non-hyperdiploid karyotypes): t(11;14), t(4;14), t(14;16) and non-recurrent.
  - Hyperdiploidy in 50–60% (trisomy 3, 5, 7, 9, 11, 15, 19).
  - del(13) in 50%.
  - del(17p;13.1): loss of *p53* tumour suppressor gene also occurs in MM.
- Prognostic value
  - Poor prognosis: t(4;14), t(14;16), del(17p), del(13), hypodiploidy.
  - Favourable prognosis: others including t(11;14).

Differential diagnosis

- Suspect MM in a patient >50 with bone pain, lethargy, anaemia, recurrent infection, renal impairment, hypercalcaemia or neuropathy or in whom rouleaux or an ↑ ESR or PV is detected.

- Exclude MGUS and other conditions associated with a paraprotein (📖p266), notably solitary plasmacytoma, primary amyloidosis and lymphoproliferative disorders.

Prognostic factors: adverse prognostic factors at diagnosis
- Age >65.
- Performance status 3 or 4.
- High paraprotein levels (IgG >70g/L; IgA >50g/L; BJP >12g/24h).
- Low haemoglobin (<10g/dL).
- Hypercalcaemia.
- Advanced lytic bone lesions.
- Abnormal renal function (creatinine >180μmol/L).
- Low serum albumin (<30g/L).
- High β2-microglobulin (≥6mg/mL).
- High C-reactive protein (≥6mg/mL).
- High serum LDH.
- High % BM plasma cells (>33%).
- Plasmablast morphology.
- Adverse cytogenetics (*see above*).
- Circulating plasma cells in PB.
- High serum IL-6 (measured in only a few centres).
- High plasma cell labelling index (measured in only a few centres).

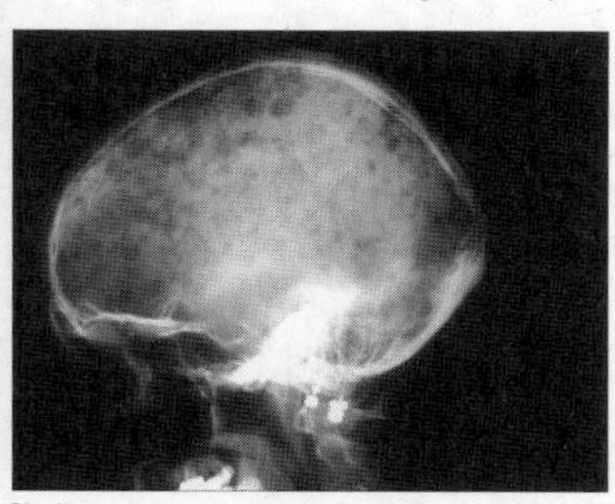

Skull x-ray in myeloma showing multiple lytic lesions.

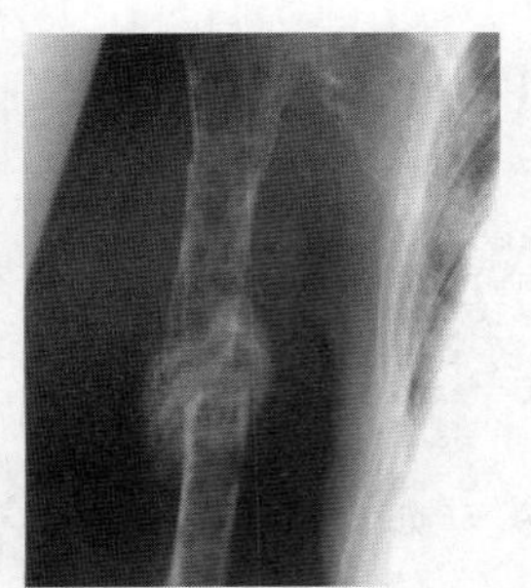

Myeloma: humerus shows marked osteoporosis, lytic lesions and healing pathological fracture.

Staging systems

Durie–Salmon staging system in wide use since 1975 attempts to assess tumour bulk but may not provide as good prognostic discrimination as newer systems:

Patients staged as I, II or III & A or B; stage represents tumour burden			
	Stage I	**Stage II**	**Stage III**
Tumour cell mass	*Low* all of the following:	*Medium* not fitting Stage I or III	*High* one or more of the following:
Monoclonal IgG (g/L)	<50		>70
Monoclonal IgA (g/L)	<30		>50
BJP excretion (g/24h)	<4		>12
Hb (g/dL)	>10		<8.5
Serum Ca^{2+} (mmol/L)	<2.6		>2.6
Lytic lesions	none or one		advanced
Stage A: serum creatinine	<175µmol/L		
Stage B: serum creatinine	>175µmol/L		

Durie, B.G. & Salmon, S.E. (1975) A clinical staging system for multiple myeloma. Correlation of measured myeloma cell mass with presenting clinical features, response to treatment, and survival. *Cancer*, **36**, 842–854.

Serum β2-microglobulin ($β_2$-M) is most powerful prognostic factor (measure of tumour bulk) and can be used with serum C-reactive protein (CRP) a surrogate measure for serum IL-6 (measure of tumour aggression) to assess prognosis:

Low risk	*both* β_2-M <6mg/L & CRP <6mg/L	median survival 54 mo
Intermed. risk	*either* β_2-M or CRP ≥6mg/L	median survival 27 mo
High risk	*both* β_2-M ≥6mg/L & CRP ≥6mg/L	median survival 6 mo

Bataille, R. *et al.* (1992) C-reactive protein and beta-2 microglobulin produce a simple and powerful myeloma staging system. *Blood*, **80**, 733–737.

International Prognostic Index (IPI) has been devised using serum β_2-M and serum albumin (ALB):

Stage 1	β_2-M <3.5mg/L; ALB ≥35g/L	median survival 62 mo
Stage 2	β_2-M <3.5mg/L; ALB <35g/L or β_2-M 3.5–5.5mg/L	median survival 41 mo
Stage 3	β_2-M >5.5mg/L	median survival 29 mo

Greipp, PR. *et al.* (2003) Development of an international prognostic index (IPI) for myeloma: report of the international myeloma working group. *Hematol J*, **4**, (Suppll) 542–44.

Good and poor risk groups in IPI

- Age is only additional factor that significantly impacts outcome:
  - Survival >5 years associated with age <60 years (very low risk if stage 1).
  - Survival <2 years associated with age >60years, platelets <130 × 10^9/L or ↑ serum LDH.
- Cytogenetics affect outcome but do not add to impact of age, β_2-M and ALB.

Management (UKMF Guidelines, Br J Haematol **115**, 522–540)

Initial considerations and general aspects

- *Pain control*: titrate simple analgesia and opiates (MST + prn Oramorph) ± NSAIDs (monitor renal function) ± local radiotherapy (8–20Gy) ± spinal support corset for severe back pain.
- *Correction of renal impairment*: rehydration with high fluid input (3–4L/day) and rapid treatment of hypercalcaemia, infection and hyperuricaemia may improve renal function; caution with nephrotoxic drugs including NSAIDs; ?role of plasmapheresis in established renal failure; peritoneal or haemodialysis if required (<5%); VAD-type regimen treatment of choice after response to rehydration or established CRF; follow with PBSC harvest (mobilised by G-CSF alone) and HDM (140mg/m^2) and SCT in younger patients; after response EFS and OS same as other patients.
- *Hypercalcaemia*: rehydration (3–6L/day IV); loop diuretics; IV bisphosphonate; (pamidronate 30–90mg IV or zoledronate 4mg IV; ↓ dose in renal impairment); chemotherapy.
- *Bone disease*: local radiotherapy for localised pain (8-20Gy); fixation of fractures/potential fractures; long term bisphosphonate prophylaxis.

- *Infection*: vigorous antibiotic therapy; annual influenza immunisation.
- *Anaemia*: blood transfusion for symptomatic anaemia; Epo for Hb persistently ≤10g/dL (10,000IU tiw or 30,000IU once weekly ~70% response rate with ≥2g/dL rise in Hb).
- *Hyperviscosity syndrome*: plasmapheresis (3L exchange) followed by prompt chemotherapy.
- *Cord compression*: MRI scan to define lesion; oral dexamethasone stat; urgent local radiotherapy.

Melphalan and prednisolone (M&P)

- 4 day courses of M&P (M 6–9mg/m^2/day PO; P 40–100mg/day PO) at 4–6 week intervals achieve ≥50% reduction of paraprotein in 50–60% patients; monitor response by serum/urine paraprotein level (serum free light chains in most non-secretors); response often slow; continue treatment to maximum response (9–12 months); CR uncommon.
- Patients with ≥50% response may achieve plateau phase (stable paraprotein without further treatment; median duration 12–18 months); maintenance chemotherapy in plateau ineffective and toxic; monitor paraprotein 6–8 weekly to detect progression; further responses to M&P after durable plateau; melphalan resistance ultimately develops in all patients.
- Median survival ~36 months; well tolerated; remains appropriate first line treatment for elderly patients treated outside a clinical trial; side effects myelosuppression and steroid toxicity (add PPI or H_2 antagonist).

Combination chemotherapy

- ABCM (📖*p620*),VMCP/VBAP and VBMCP showed improved objective responses in 3 large studies; CR still <10%; but no survival benefit over M&P on meta-analysis; ?superior results in younger patients with poor risk disease; side effects myelosuppression and infection; more toxicity in elderly patients.
- VAD infusional regimen (📖*p624*) produces improved overall responses (60–80%) and CRs (10–25%); maximum response rapidly achieved (~12 weeks); responses not durable without consolidation by melphalan-containing regimen; non-toxic to stem cells thus good initial therapy in patients destined for PBSC harvest, HDT and autograft; useful regimen in patients with renal failure; VAMP gives similar results; no convincing advantage for C-VAMP (📖*p622*); side effects myelosuppression, infection (esp. indwelling IV catheter), alopecia, neuropathy, proximal myopathy (add PPI or H_2 antagonist).

Approach to treatment of myeloma in non-trial patients	
Age ≥65 years	M&P to plateau Repeated on progression if durable response to initial therapy Thal-Dex or low dose CTX for short response/ refractory disease
Age <65 or very fit ≥65	VAD × 4–6; PBSC mobilisation; HDM; repeat on progression if durable response; Thal-Dex for short response/refractory disease

Thal-Dex, thalidomide + dexamethasone; CTX, cyclophosphamide.

Other agents

- Bisphosphonates inhibit osteoclast activation; patients on long term therapy experience less bone pain and fewer new bone lesions and fractures; there is evidence of improved quality of life and possible prolongation of survival; as yet no evidence for superiority of either daily oral clodronate or monthly IV pamidronate/zoledronate.
- Interferon-α administered as maintenance therapy during plateau phase at a dose of 3mu/m^2 SC tiw improves response duration on a meta-analysis (median 6 months) and has a small effect on survival; side effects reduce patient compliance and cost–utility profile is unfavourable.
- Cyclophosphamide (300–500mg PO/IV once weekly; 'C-weekly') may be used as a single agent for patients intolerant of melphalan due to persistent cytopenia and is capable of achieving durable plateau phase.

Radiotherapy

- Important modality of treatment in myeloma at all stages of disease; local radiotherapy (8–20Gy) often rapidly effective treatment for bone pain associated with pathological fracture.
- Multiple widespread lesions may be palliated with hemibody irradiation: 10Gy for the lower hemibody or 6Gy for the upper hemibody; side effect myelosuppression; sequential hemibody irradiation may be performed after an interval of 6 weeks.

High dose therapy and stem cell transplantation

- Autologous SCT after high dose melphalan (HDM; 200mg/m^2) achieves high CR rates (25–80%) after initial therapy with a VAD-type regimen and PBSC harvest; median duration of response 2–3 years; treatment of choice for patients <65 years; best responders have best survival, median >5 years; improved progression free survival (32 *vs.* 20 mo) and overall survival (54 *vs.* 42mo) in large randomised study[1]; side effects: myelosuppression, infection, delayed regeneration; not curative.
- Addition of TBI to melphalan 140mg/m^2 with autologous SCT adds toxicity but no benefit; no convincing benefit for 'double/tandem' autografts though may be of value for those converted to CR after second procedure; no benefit from stem cell purification procedures.
- Intermediate dose melphalan (60–80mg/m^2) + G-CSF offers an alternative consolidation treatment for patients with failed PBSC mobilisation.
- Allogeneic SCT: applicable to fit patients ≤50 years; transplant-related mortality with standard conditioning regimens (📖*p310*) is high (~33%) due to infection and GvHD; 35–45% long term survival (>5 years); ~33% chance of durable remission and possible cure; ~33% chance of survival with recurrence; evidence of graft *vs.* myeloma effect; non-myeloablative regimens (📖*p310*) reduce toxicity, increase age limit but reduce response rate; allogeneic SCT should be discussed with all patients <55 with a suitable sibling donor.

Treatment of primary refractory disease

- Patients with MM who progress or fail to respond (<25% reduction in paraprotein) to initial therapy with melphalan may respond to single agent dexamethasone (20–40mg/d × 4 days weekly × 3 weeks), VAD-type regimens thalidomide and dexamethasone or combination chemotherapy; failure to respond to VAD is an indication for thalidomide based therapy followed by HDM and autologous SCT where possible.

Disease progression

- Patients who achieve a durable response (>12 months) to initial therapy may respond to further treatment with the same regimen (response rate 25–50%).
- Patients who relapse early after initial therapy with M&P or fail to respond at relapse may respond to single agent dexamethasone (20–40mg/day × 4 days weekly × 3 weeks/month initially) or thalidomide (50–200mg/day) or these drugs in combination (response rate up to 70%) to which may be added cyclophosphamide (300–500mg/week) or clarithromycin (↑ responses).
- Thalidomide (50–400mg/day) as a single agent achieves up to 30% responses in chemotherapy-resistant myeloma; addition of dexamethasone (20–40mg/day × 4 days/month) ↑ response rates (up to 70%); side effects constipation, tremor, headache, oedema, somnolence; thromboembolism risk esp. in combination with anthracyclines (full dose warfarin or LMW heparin prophylaxis advised).
- Patients who relapse after prolonged response to HDM (>18 months) with a PBSC harvest sufficient for 2 procedures or with a further successful harvest may benefit from second HDM ± re-induction with VAD.
- There is evidence of a graft-versus-myeloma effect and DLI has re-induced responses in patients with recurrence after allogeneic SCT.
- The immunomodulatory drug Revimid and the proteosome inhibitor Velcade are both active in refractory and resistant myeloma; studies to define the role of these agents are in progress.
- Cyclophosphamide (50–100mg/day PO) is well tolerated palliative therapy for patients with advanced refractory disease or cytopenia who are intolerant of thalidomide or dexamethasone.

1 Child, J.A. *et al.* (2003) High-dose chemotherapy with hematopoietic stem-cell rescue for multiple myeloma. *N Engl J Med*, **348**, 1875–1883.

Variant forms of myeloma

Non-secretory myeloma

- ~1% of MM cases; no detectable serum or urine paraprotein by immunofixation; (*Note*: serum free light chain ratio abnormal in 70%); clonal plasma cells ≥5% in BM or plasmacytoma on biopsy; myeloma-related end-organ damage.
- Treat as above; response rates comparable to secretory MM; response more difficult to assess in absence of paraprotein; serum free light chain assay provides alternative to surrogate markers (β_2-M, CRP) and BM assessment.

IgD myeloma

- ~1% of cases of MM; younger mean age; high rate of Bence Jones proteinuria and associated higher frequency of acute and chronic renal failure; tendency to present with other poor prognostic features (high β_2-M; low Hb).
- Treat aggressively when possible.

IgM myeloma

- Very rare; <0.5% of MM; 1% of all IgM gammopathies; plasma cell infiltrate in BM associated with osteolytic lesions as opposed to lymphoplasmacytoid infiltrate characteristic of WM; response and survival equivalent to MM.

IgE myeloma

- Rarest form of MM; younger age; high incidence of plasma cell leukaemia.
- ?shorter survival.

Plasma cell leukaemia

- Defined as PB plasma cells >2 × 10^9/L or 20% of differential count; may occur *de novo* at presentation or in the terminal stages of otherwise typical MM.
- Aggressive disease associated with BM failure and organomegaly; poor response to conventional dose therapy; few survive >6 months; better responses to HDM.

Cryoglobulinaemia

- Rare complication of paraprotein precipitation at low temperature;
- Leg ulcers, Raynaud's phenomenon, renal impairment, gangrene, CNS and GI symptoms; biopsy usually shows vasculitis.
- Treat myeloma and avoid cold.

POEMS syndrome

- Polyneuropathy, Osteosclerosis, Endocrinopathy, M-protein, Skin changes.
- Association of plasmacytoma with chronic inflammatory demyelinating polyneuropathy causing predominantly motor disability.

- Confirm diagnosis by demonstrating monoclonal plasma cells in osteosclerotic bone lesion (plasmacytoma).
- BM usually <5% plasma cells; low level paraprotein; hypercalcaemia and renal impairment rare.
- Other features: lymphadenopathy, organomegaly, diabetes mellitus, male gynaecomastia and impotence, female amenorrhoea, hypertrichosis and hyperpigmentation.
- Treat solitary bone lesions with aggressive radiotherapy (45Gy) ± surgery.

Solitary plasmacytoma of bone (SPB):

Diagnostic criteria

- Generally no paraprotein in serum or urine though small band may be present.
- Single area of bone destruction due to clonal plasma cells.
- BM not consistent with MM.
- Otherwise normal skeletal survey (and MRI of spine and pelvis).
- No myeloma-related organ or tissue impairment (end-organ damage).
- Represents ~5% plasma cell neoplasia: ♂:♀ ratio 2:1; median age 55.
- Lesion usually in axial skeleton; 66% in spine.
- Generally presents with bony pain; may cause cord/root compression.
- Diagnosis requires biopsy or FNA, exclusion of MM (p273) and exclusion of other bone lesions with MRI (FDG-PET/^{99Tc}-MIBI under examination).
- Serum or urine paraprotein detected in 24–72%; generally low level.
- Adverse prognostic factors for progression to MM include persistence of paraprotein >1 year after radiotherapy, immuneparesis and lesion >5cm.
- Negative MRI of spine is good prognostic feature.
- Treat with fractionated radical radiotherapy 40Gy (50Gy for lesions >5cm); local control 80–95%; curative in 50% if solitary lesion; DFS ~40% at 5 years.
- Treat non-responders with chemotherapy as for myeloma (p278).
- Regular follow-up to monitor paraprotein; disappears in 25–50% (often slowly over several years).
- ~75% progress to MM; treat as *de novo* MM (p278); high response rate.
- Some patients develop multiple solitary recurrences; treat each with local radiotherapy.
- Median survival ~10 years.

Extramedullary plasmacytoma (SEP)

Diagnostic criteria

- Generally no paraprotein in serum or urine though small band may be present.
- Extramedullary tumour of clonal plasma cells.
- BM not consistent with MM.
- Normal skeletal survey (and MRI of spine and pelvis).
- No myeloma-related organ or tissue impairment (end-organ damage).
- Rare; may occur anywhere but 90% in head and neck; most in upper airways.
- Diagnosis requires biopsy or FNA of the lesion; exclusion of MM and other lesions.
- <25% have serum or urine paraprotein.

- Treat with radical radiotherapy (40Gy; 50Gy if lesion >5cm) including cervical lymph nodes when involved; radical surgery only for SEP outside head and neck.
- Most cured; <5% local recurrence; relapse <30%; MM, SBP or soft tissue involvement: chemotherapy for refractory or relapsed disease (p278).
- >70% survival at 10 years.

Criteria for the classification of monoclonal gammopathies, multiple myeloma and related disorders: a report of the International Myeloma Working Group (2003) *Br J Haematol*, **121**, 749–757; BCSH UKMF Guidelines Diagnosis and management of solitary plasmacytoma of bone (SBP) and solitary extramedullary plasmacytoma (SEP). www.bcshguidelines.com

Waldenström's macroglobulinaemia (WM)

WM is an uncommon indolent chronic B-cell lymphoproliferative disorder characterised by bone marrow infiltration by lymphoplasmacytic cells and an IgM paraproteinaemia. It is classified as a lymphoplasmacytic lymphoma in the REAL and WHO classifications (p195).

Epidemiology

- Incidence <0.5 per 100,000 per annum; mean age 65; rare <40; M:F ~2:1.
- Cause unknown; several familial clusters described; 23% of patients have 1st degree relative with B-cell disorder.

Pathophysiology

WM appears to arise from IgM+ memory B lymphocytes (suggested by the immunophenotype and Ig somatic hypermutation without intraclonal variation); slowly progressive; symptoms may be due to infiltration of BM (BM failure) spleen (splenomegaly) or liver (hepatomegaly) or to hyperviscosity due increased serum levels of pentavalent monoclonal IgM (when IgM >30g/L). Autoimmune disorders may also develop due to the paraprotein: neuropathy, cold agglutinin disease

Clinical features and presentation

- Occasional diagnosis following routine ESR/PV/FBC/blood film.
- Usually insidious onset of weakness and fatigue.
- Often present with symptoms of anaemia, epistaxis, recurrent infection, dyspnoea, CCF and weight loss.
- Usually no bone pain and no evidence of destructive bone disease.
- Symptoms of hyperviscosity (headache, dizziness, visual upset, bleeding, ataxia, CCF and somnolence, stupor and coma) 15–20%.
- Peripheral neuropathy—usually sensory or sensorimotor (~20%): distal, symmetrical, slowly progressive, usually lower extremities.
- Hepatomegaly (~25%); splenomegaly and lymphadenopathy less frequent.
- Fundoscopy reveals distended sausage-shaped veins, retinal haemorrhage ± papilloedema.
- Cryoglobulinaemia (<5%) may cause Raynaud's syndrome, arthralgia, purpura, peripheral neuropathy, liver dysfunction and renal failure.
- Haemorrhagic symptoms (e.g. epistaxis or easy bruising) may develop as a result of abnormalities of platelet function or coagulation due to the paraprotein.
- Amyloidosis may occur (<5%) causing cardiac, renal, hepatic or pulmonary dysfunction or macroglossia.

Investigation and diagnosis

- FBC and film: normochromic normocytic anaemia 80% (often spuriously low due to increased plasma volume); rarely lymphocytosis or pancytopenia; blood film shows rouleaux or agglutination (cold agglutinins ~5%); may contain circulating lymphoplasmacytic cells.
- ESR/plasma viscosity: ↑ in almost all patients (~70% PV >1.8cP), often markedly (ESR commonly >100mm/h); risk of hyperviscosity symptoms

when PV >4cP (5–10% at diagnosis); most have symptoms when PV >6cP; PV often correlates well for symptoms in an individual though not between patients.
- Biochemistry: renal impairment unusual; LFTs may be abnormal in advanced disease or cryoglobulinaemia; uric acid may be ↑.
- Serum immunoglobulins: ↑ IgM; may be mild immuneparesis of IgG (60%) and IgA (20%).
- Serum protein electrophoresis, immunofixation and densitometry: confirms and quantifies IgM paraprotein.
- Urine electrophoresis: scanty Bence Jones protein present in ~50%.
- β2-microglobulin: ↑ in 33%.
- C-reactive protein: ↑ in ~66%.
- BM aspirate: often hypocellular; may show infiltration by lymphoplasmacytic cells of variable degrees of differentiation; mast cells may be increased.
- BM trephine biopsy—essential—usually hypercellular; demonstrates intertrabecular infiltrate (diffuse, interstitial or nodular) of lymphoplasmacytic cells (*Note*: paratrabecular infiltrate suggests follicular NHL); immunochemistry demonstrates light chain restriction.
- BM immunophenotyping: useful in differentiating WM from other B-cell disorders; characteristically pan B-cell marker (CD19, CD20, CD22, CD79) positive (*cf.* myeloma plasma cells); light chain restricted surface IgM; CD10 negative (*cf.* FL), CD23 negative (*cf.* CLL); 5–20% express CD5 (must differentiate from CLL and MCL); CD103 and CD138 rarely positive.
- Cytogenetics: no disease defining abnormality described; many normal; presence of IgH translocations (14q) suggests myeloma.

Proposed diagnostic criteria
- IgM monoclonal gammopathy of any concentration.
- BM infiltration by small lymphocytes, plasmacytoid cells and plasma cells.
- Intertrabecular pattern of BM infiltration.
- Immunophenotype: surface IgM+, CD5±, CD10–, CD19+, CD20+, CD22+, CD23–, CD25+, CD27+, FMC7+, CD103–, CD138–.
- WM may be divided into symptomatic WM and asymptomatic (smouldering) WM (~25%) by the presence or absence of symptoms attributable to either the IgM paraprotein (e.g. hyperviscosity or neuropathy) or tumour infiltration (BM failure or symptomatic organomegaly).

Differential diagnosis
- IgM MGUS: IgM monoclonal protein <30g/L; Hb >12g/dL; no BM infiltrate; no organomegaly or lymphadenopathy; no end-organ symptoms.
- IgM-related disorders: IgM monoclonal protein; no overt evidence of lymphoma; symptomatic cryoglobulinaemia, peripheral neuropathy, cold agglutinin disease or amyloidosis.

(Owen, R.G. *et al.* (2003) Clinicopathological definition of Waldenström's macroglobulinaemia. *Semin Oncol* **30**:110–115)

- Other B-cell lymphoproliferative disorders: IgM monoclonal protein can be demonstrated in most B-cell lymphoproliferative disorders e.g. CLL, NHL; generally very low levels; no lymphoplasmacytic BM infiltration; hyperviscosity rare; features of other lymphoproliferative disorder e.g. phenotype.
- IgM myeloma: very rare; BM contains plasma cells (cytoplasmic IgM+, CD20–, CD138+) not lymphoplasmacytic cells; myeloma associated cytogenetic abnormalities (esp. 14q translocations) and lytic bone lesions frequent.

Prognostic factors

Predictors of early progression in asymptomatic WM:

- Hb <11.5g/dL.
- β2-microglobulin ≥3.0mg/L.
- IgM >30g/L.

Predictors of shorter survival in WM:

- Age ≥60.
- Hb <10g/dL.
- High β2-microglobulin.
- Other less consistently identified factors: cytopenias: WBC $<4.0 \times 10^9$/L; neutrophils $<1.8 \times 10^9$/L; platelets $<150 \times 10^9$/L; ↓ serum albumin; ♂ sex; constitutional symptoms; plasmacytic and polymorphous morphology in BM.

Management

- Therapeutic principles as for CLL and FL; no indication for therapy in asymptomatic WM; regular review (3–6 monthly) of clinical and laboratory features required: consistently monitor paraprotein by densitometry (more reliable than IgM nephelometry).
- Initiation of therapy should not be based simply on IgM level alone as this does not correlate directly with clinical manifestations of WM but for:
  - Constitutional symptoms: recurrent fever, night sweats, fatigue due to anaemia, weight loss.
  - Progressive symptomatic lymphadenopathy or splenomegaly.
  - Hb ≤10g/dL and/or platelets $<100 \times 10^9$/L due to BM infiltration.
  - Hyperviscosity syndrome, symptomatic peripheral neuropathy, systemic amyloidosis, symptomatic cryoglobulinaemia, renal failure.
  - *Note*: avoid red cell transfusion simply to correct low Hb (plasma volume ↑ causing spuriously low Hb; low Hb protects against clinical effects of hyperviscosity).
- Plasmapheresis may be necessary as urgent initial therapy for patients with symptoms of hyperviscosity; 3L exchange efficiently reduces plasma viscosity (80% of large IgM molecule is intravascular); may rarely be required regularly in treatment of neuropathic or chemo-intolerant patients; in an emergency venesection and exchange transfusion will ↓ plasma viscosity.
- Chlorambucil at a dose of 6–10mg/d for 7–14 days ± prednisolone in a 28d cycle is widely used initial therapy; continue to maximum response; up to 75% achieve ≥50% reduction in paraprotein; duration of response 2–4 years; <10% achieve CR; reinstitute treatment when paraprotein approaches previously symptomatic levels; often effective on several occasions; resistance ultimately develops; side effects; myelosuppression; cyclophosphamide may achieve comparable results.

- Purine analogues: fludarabine (40mg/m^2 PO × 5d or 25mg/m^2 IV × 5d repeated monthly for 4–6 cycles) has a response rate of 40–80% in untreated patients and achieves ~33% response rate even after chlorambucil resistance; response duration 30–40 months; similar results with cladribine (0.1mg/kg continuous infusion × 7d); both agents achieve more rapid responses than chlorambucil; side effects: myelosuppression; profound immunosuppression (*see p558*); need *P carinii* prophylaxis and irradiated blood products; addition of cyclophosphamide to a purine analogue increases response rates.
- Rituximab: monoclonal anti-CD20 antibody administered on 4 occasions achieves 60% responses ≥25% ↓ in WM and useful in patients with marked cytopenia; abrupt elevation in serum paraprotein and PV may occur after rituximab therapy and patients should be closely monitored; may be of benefit for symptomatic neuropathy; administration of 4 further doses over 12 months extends the response from ~9 months to up to 3 years; under examination in clinical trials in combination with purine analogue therapy.
- High dose therapy and autologous or allogeneic SCT: has been undertaken in a small number of younger patients; high response rates (~80%; up to 40% CR) are achieved but relapse rate is high after autograft and treatment related mortality of ~40% occurs after allograft; the latter does offer survivors the prospect of long-term disease control; HDT should be performed in a trial context where possible and patients in whom this treatment is planned should have limited prior exposure to alkylator and purine analogue therapy.
- Treatment of relapse: if a response of >1year has been achieved most patients will respond to the same therapy; refractory patients or those relapsing shortly after prior therapy may respond to an alternative listed above; ~33% of patients with refractory WM respond to thalidomide (50–200mg) in combination with dexamethasone (20–40mg once weekly) and/or clarithromycin (250–500mg bd).

Prognosis

- Median time to progression of asymptomatic WM ~7 years.
- Median survival of patients with WM ~5 years; patients who achieve CR with chlorambucil have median survival of ~11 years.
- Up to 20% die of unrelated causes and 33% from infection; others from disease progression, transformation and bleeding.
- Indolent course may be interrupted by transformation into aggressive high grade NHL which is often poorly responsive to treatment; poor tolerance of aggressive treatment due to poor marrow reserve.

Gertz, M.A. *et al.* (2003) Treatment recommendations in Waldenstrom's macroglobulinemia: consensus panel recommendations from the Second International Workshop on Waldenstrom's Macroglobulinemia. *Semin Oncol*, **30**, 121–126; Kyle, R.A. *et al.* (2003) Prognostic markers and criteria to initiate therapy in Waldenstrom's macroglobulinemia: consensus panel recommendations from the Second International Workshop on Waldenstrom's Macroglobulinemia. *Semin Oncol*, **30**, 116–120; Weber, D. *et al.* (2003) Uniform response criteria in Waldenstrom's macroglobulinemia: consensus panel recommendations from the Second International Workshop on Waldenstrom's Macroglobulinemia. *Semin Oncol*, **30**, 127–131.

Heavy chain disease (HCD)

Uncommon lymphoplasmacytic cell proliferative disorder characterised by production of incomplete immunoglobulins comprising heavy chains without light chains. Alpha (α) HCD is most frequent, γ and μ HCD also described but rare.

α-HCD

- Usually occurs in residents or immigrants from Mediterranean or Middle East; associated with low socio-economic group, poor hygiene, recurrent infectious diarrhoea and chronic parasitic infection.
- Commonly presents with diarrhoea, steatorrhoea, weight loss, abdominal pain and vomiting; α-HCD protein detectable in serum of most patients, concentration often low; mild to moderate anaemia; low serum albumin; hypokalaemia and hypocalcaemia (tetany); infiltrative lesions in duodenum and jejunum in most patients; histology ranges from lymphoplasmacytic infiltration of mucosa (Stage A) to immunoblastic lymphoma invading entire intestinal wall.

- Progressive course without treatment; treat Stage A initially with oral metronidazole and tetracycline for 6 months; treat non-responders and Stage B or C with CHOP-type regimen.

AL (primary systemic) amyloidosis

AL (primary systemic) amyloidosis is a clonal plasma cell disorder in which systemic disease results from organ dysfunction due to extracellular deposition of fibrillar protein. It can also complicate most clonal B-cell lymphoplasmacytic disorders, notably myeloma, Waldenström's macroglobulinaemia, MGUS and lymphoma.

Incidence

Estimated incidence 0.5–1 per 100,000 per annum; ♂:♀ ratio 2:1; most cases aged 50–70; <10% <50 years; ~1% <40 years; 15% of patients with MM develop amyloid (lower % of MGUS and WM).

Pathophysiology

In AL amyloidosis the fibrillar deposits are composed of the variable regions of immunoglobulin light chains (VL) in association with glycosaminoglycans and amyloid P component derived from the normal plasma protein serum amyloid P (SAP) component. More commonly λ light chains. Unique amino acid insertions may render the proteins amyloidogenic. Without treatment deposits progressively accumulate in viscera notably kidneys, heart, liver and peripheral nervous system causing increasingly severe dysfunction. Under favourable circumstances, further amyloid deposition can be prevented, deposits can regress and improvement in organ dysfunction can occur.

Clinical features and presentation

- Renal involvement is the predominant feature in 33% with nephrotic syndrome (oedema, fatigue and lethargy) ± renal impairment (usually mild).

- Cardiac symptoms predominate in 20–30%: CCF due to restrictive cardiomyopathy notably with right sided features (↑ JVP, peripheral oedema and hepatomegaly).
- Peripheral neuropathy occurs in 20%; 10–15% present with isolated neuropathic symptoms; typically painful sensory polyneuropathy; carpal tunnel syndrome in 40%; autonomic neuropathy may cause postural hypotension, impotence and disturbed GI motility.
- GI involvement may be focal or diffuse: malabsorption, perforation, haemorrhage and obstruction may occur; hepatomegaly 25%; macroglossia 10%.
- Haemorrhage occurs at some time in up to 33% of patients; usually non-thrombocytopenic purpura, often periorbital causing characteristic 'raccoon eyes' appearance.
- Vocal cord infiltration may cause dysphonia; large joint arthropathy; adrenal and thyroid infiltration may cause endocrine dysfunction; cutaneous plaques and nodules usually on face or upper trunk; pulmonary infiltration rarely symptomatic.

Investigation and diagnosis

- High index of suspicion required; consider in patient with nephrotic syndrome, cardiomyopathy, peripheral neuropathy, hepatomegaly or autonomic neuropathy.
- Confirm diagnosis by histological examination of biopsy of affected organ or subcutaneous fat aspirate, rectal biopsy or labial salivary gland biopsy stained with Congo Red for red-green birefringence under polarised light; confirm AL amyloidosis by immunochemistry for κ or λ light chains (50% are negative).
- Assess severity of organ involvement:
  - FBC: ↓ Hb suggests probable myeloma.
  - Serum chemistry: to assess renal and hepatic function.
  - β2-microglobulin: prognostic indicator in MM (*see p276*).
  - Coagulation screen; may be a coagulopathy due to absorption of factor X and sometimes FIX by the amyloid.
  - Serum protein electrophoresis, immunofixation and densitometry: to detect, type and quantitate any paraprotein present (~70%; usually only modest quantity).
  - Serum immunoglobulins: to identify immuneparesis (suggests MM).
  - Serum free light chain assay: useful in patients with no detectable paraprotein in serum or urine (10–15%).
  - Creatinine clearance and 24h quantitative proteinuria: to assess renal dysfunction.
  - Urine electrophoresis: to detect, type and quantify paraprotein (85%; 90% have albuminuria).
  - BM aspirate and trephine biopsy: usually only mild ↑ in % plasma cells; overt MM in 20%.
  - Skeletal survey: if MM suspected.

- ECG and echocardiography: low voltage ECG; echo shows concentrically thickened ventricles, normal to small cavities and a normal or mild reduction in ejection fraction.
- SAP (serum amyloid protein) scan: radiolabelled serum amyloid P component allows detection and quantification of amyloid deposits and assessment of extent of organ involvement by scintigraphy. (In UK contact National Amyloidosis Centre at UCLMS Royal Free Hospital, London Campus).

Differential diagnosis

Exclude MM (*as above*), reactive (AA) amyloidosis (history of chronic inflammatory disorder) and familial amyloidosis (family history).

Prognostic factors

Poor prognostic features:

- CCF.
- Multisystem involvement.
- Renal failure.
- Jaundice.
- High total body amyloid load on SAP scan.

Management

Aims: suppress underlying plasma cell neoplasia and paraprotein production to reduce further deposition of amyloid and permit regression resulting in improvement in organ dysfunction.

Supportive care

- Nephrotic syndrome: loop diuretic + salt ± fluid restriction.
- Renal failure: peritoneal or haemodialysis if required; rigorous control of hypertension.
- CCF: diuretic + ACE inhibitors if tolerated; digoxin hypersensitivity common; calcium channel blockers and β-blockers contraindicated; cardiac transplantation should be considered in appropriate patients.

Chemotherapy

- Melphalan ± prednisolone: slow response rate; consider for patients not eligible for HDT; prolongs median survival in a randomised trial *vs.* colchicine (but survival only 12–18 months).
- VAD: induces a more rapid response than M&P; suitable initial therapy in those patients eligible for HDT; caution with vincristine in neuropathic patients and adriamycin in those with CCF; dexamethasone alone may produce responses.
- High dose melphalan and autologous PBSCT: improves organ function in up to 60% of survivors; up to 40% procedure related mortality; *Note*: stem cell mobilisation associated with mortality and morbidity due to cardiac complications (avoid cyclophosphamide), oedema and splenic rupture (low doses of G-CSF recommended); better tolerance of HDT if ≤2 organ systems involved; younger patients with good performance status and good renal and cardiac function do best; cardiac involvement or elevated creatinine poor prognostic factor; reduce melphalan dose to 100–140mg/m^2 in high risk patients; GI haemorrhage a frequent complication; HDT should be undertaken in trial context.
- Allogeneic SCT: few patients have been treated; complete resolution has been reported.

Follow-up
Response to therapy should be monitored by quantitation of the serum or urine paraprotein (or serum free light chains); SAP scintigraphy; ECG, echocardiography and assessment of other organ dysfunction should be reviewed every 6 months.

Prognosis
- Median survival 1–2 years; 4–6 months if CCF at diagnosis.
- Most common cause cardiac: progressive congestive cardiomyopathy or sudden death due to VF or asystole.
- Others succumb to uraemia or other complications.

Other causes of amyloid
Acquired
- AA amyloid: reactive systemic amyloidosis associated with chronic inflammatory diseases e.g. rheumatoid arthritis, TB; due to AA fibrils derived from serum amyloid A protein (SAA).
- Senile systemic amyloidosis due to transthyretin deposition.
- Endocrine amyloidosis, associated with APUDomas.
- Haemodialysis associated amyloidosis, localised to osteoarticular tissues or systemic due to β2-microglobulin deposition.
- Non-familial Alzheimer's disease, Down syndrome due to β-protein.
- Sporadic Creutzfeldt–Jakob disease, kuru due to prion protein deposition.
- Type II diabetes mellitus due to islet amyloid polypeptide.

Hereditary
- Numerous syndromes with characteristic patterns of peripheral or cranial neurological involvement or visceral or cardiac involvement due to a variety of proteins.
- Familial Alzheimer's disease due to a β-protein.
- Familial Mediterranean fever due to AA derived from SAA.

BCSH/UKMF Guideline. Guidelines on the dignosis and management of AL amyloidosis.
http://www.bcshguidelines.com

Transplantation

9

Stem cell transplantation

Stem cell transplantation (SCT) achieves reconstitution of haematopoiesis by the transfer of pluripotent haemopoietic stem cells. In allogeneic SCT stem cells are obtained from a donor e.g. a matched sibling or normal volunteer (matched unrelated donor; MUD), in syngeneic SCT the donor is a monozygotic (identical) twin. For autologous SCT the patient acts as his/her own source of stem cells. Placental cord blood has become a useful source of stem cells for paediatric transplants.

The aim of SCT is

1. To permit haemopoietic reconstitution after potentially curative but myeloablative doses of chemotherapy or chemoradiotherapy (high dose therapy; HDT) in the treatment of malignant disease.

or

2. To replace congenital or acquired life threatening abnormal BM or immune function with a normal haematopoietic and immune system.

Stem cells may be obtained from bone marrow (BMT) by multiple aspirations under general anaesthesia (BM harvest) or obtained from peripheral blood after 'mobilisation' by G-CSF (± chemotherapy in the case of autologous SCT) and collection by apheresis (peripheral blood stem cell transplants; PBSCT). Whether used fresh from donor harvest or thawed after cryopreservation, stem cells are re-infused IV. PBSCT carries the advantages of avoiding general anaesthesia for the donor and more rapid engraftment (~7 days) but may be associated with a higher incidence of chronic graft versus host disease (cGvHD). In the autologous setting not all previously treated patients will mobilise adequate numbers of stem cells.

Stem cell collection for autologous SCT with curative intent in diseases involving the bone marrow should be undertaken after a complete response has been achieved by initial therapy. In some settings e.g. myeloma where HDT is being used with the aim of disease control rather than with curative intent, BM involvement up to 30% is often accepted.

Comparison of autologous and allogeneic SCT

Autologous	Allogeneic
Wide age range, generally ≤65	Age range generally ≤55
No need for donor search if BM clear	Sibs have ~1 in 4 chance of match
Not feasible if BM involved	May be used in patients with BM disease
Risk of tumour cell re-infusion	No tumour contamination of graft
Not all patients can be mobilised	Donor search may impose delay
No GvHD	GvHD mortality and morbidity
No immunosuppression	Graft-versus-leukaemia (GvL) effect
Low early treatment related mortality (2-5%)	Higher early treatment related mortality from GvHD and infection (20-40%)
Risk of long term MDS from BM injury	Less risk of late MDS

Transplantation

Patient receives high dose chemo–(±radio)therapy (conditioning) which ablates the BM and immune system. After conditioning is completed, BM or PBSC are infused IV. After a period of profound myelosuppression (7–25d), engraftment occurs with production of WBCs, platelets and RBCs. Immunosuppression is required after allogeneic transplantation to prevent GvHD and graft rejection.

Early complications of the transplant procedure

Chemoradiotherapy

- Nausea/vomiting.
- Reversible alopecia.
- Fatigue.
- Dry skin.
- Mucositis.
- VOD* (p328).

Infection

- Bacterial (Gram –ve and +ve).
- Viral—HZV.
- CMV (particularly pneumonitis)*.
- Fungal—*Candida*, *Aspergillus**, *Mucor**.
- Atypical organisms—*Pneumocystis* (PCP)*, *Toxoplasma**, *Mycoplasma**, *Legionella**.

*Low risk in autologous SCT; significant to high risk in allogeneic SCT

Graft-versus-host disease (GvHD)

May occur in recipients of allogeneic SCT due to tissue incompatibility between donor and recipient undetected by standard tissue-typing tests. Acute and chronic forms occur. Higher incidence of severe GvHD following unrelated donor SCT and mismatched (haploidentical) grafts.

Late complications of transplantation

- Infertility (both sexes).
- Hypothyroidism.
- Secondary malignancy.
- Late sepsis due to hyposplenism.
- Cataracts (where TBI used).
- Psychological disturbance.

Follow up and post-transplant surveillance

Life-long supervision required. The particular risks and monitoring required depend on the type of graft and whether TBI was used. Suitable conditioning regimens are outlined on p310.

Allogeneic stem cell transplantation

Patient selection

- Recipients should be in good physical condition, and ≤55 years old.
- Donor and recipient should be fully or closely HLA-matched to reduce the risk of life threatening GvHD or graft rejection.
- Greatest chance of full HLA match is with siblings (small chance of full match with cousins); each sib has ~1:4 chance of full HLA-match.
- Matched-volunteer unrelated donor (MUD) may be sought from donor registries e.g. in UK The National Blood Authority and Anthony Nolan panels.
- Haploidentical sibling may considered as a donor for patients in whom no matched sibling or volunteer donor is available (~40%) and the increased risks of the procedure are acceptable (e.g. poor risk adult AML, Ph-positive adult ALL).

Indications for allogeneic SCT

- Adult AML (poor risk first CR or any second CR)[1].
- Adult ALL (poor risk first CR or any second CR)[2].
- Severe aplastic anaemia.
- Chronic myeloid leukaemia.
- Myelodysplasia.
- Multiple myeloma (stage II/III).
- Primary immunodeficiency syndromes.
- Thalassaemia major.
- Sickle cell disease.
- Inborn errors of metabolism.
- Relapsed aggressive histology NHL.
- Relapsed Hodgkin's lymphoma.

1. Good risk adult AML should not receive SCT in first remission as outcomes are good for most patients with standard treatment (p156)
2. Most children with ALL will be cured by standard chemotherapy alone—transplantation is reserved for those who relapse. (p475)

Outline of allogeneic SCT procedure

- Patient receives standard conditioning therapy with high dose chemoradiotherapy (e.g. cyclophosphamide (CTX) 120mg/kg + 14Gy fractionated total body irradiation (TBI)) or chemotherapy (e.g. cyclophosphamide 120mg/kg + busulfan 16mg/kg).
- Non-myeloablative conditioning regimens use moderate doses of chemotherapy and immunosuppression to achieve engraftment and have a lower transplant-related mortality and morbidity; utilised to increase age range for allogeneic SCT and permit the use of adoptive immunotherapy with donor lymphocyte infusion (DLI) for residual disease post-transplant.
- In patients receiving MUD or haploidentical SCT, Campath-1H (humanised anti-CD52 monoclonal antibody) is often administered daily for 5d prior to conditioning as an immunosuppressant to ↓ the risk of graft rejection.
- For patients with aplastic anaemia less intensive conditioning is used (200mg/kg CTX combined with anti-thymocyte globulin) and because

of sensitivity to alkylating agents in Fanconi's anaemia still less intensive conditioning is used.
- One day after completing conditioning treatment, BM or PBSC are harvested from donor and infused IV through a central line.
- In MUD and haploidentical SCT the graft is usually depleted of T lymphocytes prior to infusion to reduce the risk of severe GvHD.
- After 7–21d of severe myelosuppression, haematopoietic engraftment occurs.
- Reverse barrier nursing in a filtered air environment, prophylactic anti-infectives (ciprofloxacin, itraconazole, acyclovir) reduce the risk of infective complications.
- Immunosuppression is required to prevent GvHD and graft rejection; generally methotrexate (in the early engraftment phase) + cyclosporin A (for 6 months).

Mechanism of cure: evidence for graft versus leukaemia (GvL) effect

1. Reduced risk of relapse in patients with acute and chronic GvHD.
2. Increased risk of relapse after syngeneic SCT (no GvHD).
3. Increased risk of relapse after T-lymphocyte-depleted SCT.
4. Delayed clearance of minimal residual disease detected post-SCT.
5. Induction of remission by donor lymphocyte infusion (DLI) after relapse post-SCT.

Early complications of allogeneic SCT

- Overall transplant related mortality for matched sibling allografts is 15–30%, for volunteer unrelated donors may reach 45%.
- Infection: severe myelosuppression together with immune dysfunction from delayed reconstitution or GvHD predisposes to a wide variety of potentially fatal infections with bacterial (Gram +ve and –ve), viral, fungal and atypical organisms. Both HSV and HZV infections are common—may present with fulminant extensive lesions. Main causes of infective death post-transplant are: CMV pneumonitis and invasive fungal infections with moulds e.g. *Aspergillus*.
- Graft versus host disease (GvHD): Acute GvHD occurs ≤100d of transplant and chronic >100d. (p324–327)
- Other complications:
  - Endocrine infertility (both sexes), early menopause and occasionally hypothyroidism.
  - Cataract (TBI induced) >12 months post-transplant.
  - 2° malignancies (esp. skin).
  - EBV associated lymphoma.
  - Mild psychological disturbances common (serious psychoses rare).

Follow-up treatment and post-transplant surveillance

Immunosuppression requires careful monitoring to avoid toxicity. Unlike solid organ transplant recipients, lifelong immunosuppression not required and cyclosporin is usually discontinued at about 6 months post-transplant. Prophylaxis against pneumococcal sepsis secondary to hyposplenism, HZV reactivation and PCP infections required. Despite these complications, most patients return to an active, working life without the need for continuing medication.

Future developments

Molecular HLA gene loci mapping: improved DNA characterisation of HLA gene loci should permit greater applicability and success of transplants from volunteer unrelated donors.

Umbilical cord blood transplants: umbilical cord blood donation post-delivery shown to be safe for mother and child. Cord blood stem cells are immunologically immature and may be more permissive of HLA donor/recipient mismatches with less risk of GvHD. Successful grafts in children; cell dose insufficient for adult grafts.

Transplantation

Autologous stem cell transplantation

Patient selection

Patients should good physical condition; age range for some procedures can be extended up to ~70. BM should be uninvolved or in CR at the time of harvest/mobilisation unless disease control rather than cure is the primary intent *cf.* myeloma.

Accepted indications

- Relapsed aggressive and very aggressive NHL.
- Relapsed Hodgkin's lymphoma.
- Adult AML (poor risk first CR without allogeneic option or second CR without allogeneic option).
- Adult ALL (poor risk first CR without allogeneic option or second CR without allogeneic option).
- Multiple myeloma (stage II/III).
- AL amyloid.

Possible indications

- Sclerosing mediastinal B-cell NHL in 1st CR.
- Patients with aggressive or very aggressive NHL with 2 of: stage III/IV, high LDH, ECOG performance status 3 or 4, bulk disease (mass >10cm).
- Indolent NHL (aged ≤60) relapsing after 2nd line therapy if still responsive to therapy.
- Relapsed germ cell tumours.
- Ewing's sarcoma.
- Neuroblastoma.
- Soft tissue sarcoma.
- Autoimmune disease (multiple sclerosis, systemic sclerosis, rheumatoid arthritis, juvenile chronic arthritis, SLE).

Outline of autologous SCT procedure

- Haematopoietic stem cells harvested in CR are processed, frozen and stored in liquid N_2.
- SCT may take place within days of harvest or several years later after treatment for recurrent disease.
- Different conditioning chosen for underlying indication e.g. cyclophosphamide plus busulphan for AML or BEAM (p612) for NHL or HL.
- After completion of conditioning (generally plus 24 hours to allow clearance of chemotherapeutic agents), the stem cell product is thawed rapidly and infused IV. Bags are thawed by transfer directly from liquid N_2 into water at 37–43°C. Product is infused IV rapidly through indwelling central line.
- There is period of myelosuppression (7–25d) followed by WBC, platelet and RBC engraftment.

Early complications of the transplant procedure

- Overall transplant related mortality is 5–10%.
- Morbidity from conditioning regimens e.g. nausea from chemoradiotherapy and mucositis from the widespread mucosal damage to GIT:

oral ulceration, buccal desquamation, oesophagitis, gastritis, abdominal pain and diarrhoea may all be features.
- Spectrum of infective organisms seen is similar to allografts but severity and mortality are ↓.

Late complications of autologous SCT

- Single commonest long-term complication is relapse of underlying disease.
- Other late complications similar to allografts, but less frequent and less severe.

Follow-up treatment and post-transplant surveillance

- Regular haematological follow-up is mandatory and psychological support from the transplant team, family and friends is important for readjustment to normal life.
- Prophylaxis against specific infections required including *Pneumococcus*, HZV and PCP. Most patients return to an active, working life without continuing medication.

Investigations for BMT/PBSCT

Haematology

- FBC, reticulocytes, ESR.
- Serum B_{12} and red cell folate, ferritin.
- Blood group, antibody screen and DAT.
- Coagulation screen, PT, APTT, fibrinogen.
- BM aspirate for morphology (cytogenetics if relevant); BM trephine biopsy.

Biochemistry

- U&Es, LFTs.
- Ca^{2+}, phosphate, random glucose.
- LDH.
- TFTs.
- Serum and urine Igs.
- EDTA clearance.

Virology

- Hepatitis BsAg.

- Hepatitis C antibody.
- HIV I and II antibody (counselling and consent required).
- CMV IgG and IgM.
- EBV, HSV and VZV IgG.
- Parvovirus B19 titre (allografts only).
- Toxoplasma titre (allografts only).

Immunology

- Autoantibody screen.
- HLA type—(if not known) in case HLA matched platelets are subsequently required.
- HLA and platelet antibody screen (if previously poor increments to platelet transfusions).
- CRP.

Bacteriology

- Baseline blood cultures (peripheral blood and Hickman line).
- Routine admission swabs: throat, central line site.
- MSU, stool cultures.

Cardiology

- ECG.
- Echocardiogram, to include measurement of systolic ejection fraction.

Respiratory

- Lung function tests.

Radiology

- CXR.
- Sinus x-rays.

Cytogenetics

- Blood for donor/recipient polymorphisms (allografts only).

Other

- Consider semen storage.
- Dental opinion if caries/gum disease.
- Psychiatric opinion if previous history.

Bone marrow harvesting

Pre-operative preparations

Important to give advanced notice so that theatre time can be booked if necessary and the virological screening results obtained.

Within 30 days before the harvest procedure, arrange the following virological investigations

1. Hepatitis B surface antigen.
2. Hepatitis C antibody.
3. HIV 1 and 2.
4. VDRL.
5. Spare serum stored.

Admit patient day before harvest. Clerk patient and arrange:

- U&E.
- FBC.
- X match 2–3 units blood (CMV –ve). If harvest is on normal donor—offer autologous blood collection to donor. If declined, arrange for genotyped, CMV negative and irradiated X-matched blood to be available for the donor. A CXR and ECG may also be arranged, if felt clinically appropriate.

Harvest procedure

1. Give heparin 50units/kg IV at anaesthetic induction.
2. Prepare harvest bag: adding ACD with a dilution factor of 1:10 for the prospective marrow volume; i.e. 100mL of ACD if expected harvest is ~1L.
3. Heparinise aspirate needles/syringes (0.9% saline containing at least 100U heparin/mL).
4. Begin with posterior superior iliac crests, limiting the number of skin entry points, the aspirate needle should be manoeuvred to collect as much marrow as possible with 5–10mL maximum from each penetration of the bone. Each aspirate should be deposited in a sterile harvest bag and syringe rinsed in the heparinised saline prior to re-use. Gently agitate bag at intervals.
5. Midway through harvest (or 500mL) a bag sample should be sent for FBC to determine the adequacy of the harvest. The final total WBC count should be at least 2×10^8 cells/kg of the recipient for autografts and 3×10^8 cells/kg for allografts.

The volume of marrow required may be calculated as follows:

Total volume required for autograft
= 2.0 x recipient weight (kg) ÷ (bag WBC x 10)
e.g. recip. 100kg and bag WBC 20 $\times 10^9$/L then vol. required = (2.0 x100) ÷ (20 x10) = 1.0L

Volume still needed to be harvested = total volume – volume already taken at time of count + ~10%

Notes

1. The extra 10% compensates for reduced harvesting efficiency and the ACD.
2. The formula works at whatever volume you choose to do the first WBC but is a more accurate prediction at ~500mL.
3. If need to harvest >1L, remember to add additional ACD in the same 1 in 10 ratio.
4. For allograft calculations, substitute 3.0 for 2.0 in the formula.

If yield not adequate from the posterior iliac crests, other sites may be considered (e.g. anterior superior iliac crests and sternum). Review puncture sites the following morning for signs of local infection or continuing bleeding. For normal donors, offer out-patient follow-up appointment as additional safeguard and provide access to counselling services.

Peripheral blood stem cell mobilisation and harvesting

Properties of stem cells

- Stem cells are defined as the most primitive haemopoietic precursor cell.
- Unique property is capability of both infinite self-renewal and differentiation to form all mature cells of the haemopoietic and immune systems.
- In the resting state almost all stem cells reside in the bone marrow although a tiny minority circulate in peripheral blood.
- Stem cells in marrow can migrate into the blood after treatment with chemotherapy and/or haemopoietic growth factors.
- Once circulating, they can easily be harvested using a cell separator machine.
- Stem cell levels in peripheral blood can be assessed by CD34 immunophenotype analysis.
- More than one day of apheresis may be necessary to achieve required yield.
- The yield can be assessed for engraftment potential.

Protocols

Mobilisation and harvesting protocols differ between diseases. The following illustrate the principal types of schedule:

1. Mobilisation after standard chemotherapy

- No specific additional stimulus given.
- Harvest times determined by WBC and platelet recovery, and CD34 count.
- Yields variable. Improved by addition of G-CSF.

Suitable for

- NHL post DHAP chemotherapy.
- AML post ADE/DAT chemotherapy.
- ALL post high dose methotrexate.

2. *Mobilisation with chemotherapy and haemopoietic growth factors*

The commonest schedule and the best evaluated. Harvest timing and yields more predictable.

Typical protocol for NHL

Day 0 cyclophosphamide 1.5g/m^2 IVI with Mesna.
Day +4 to day + 10 G-CSF 5μg/kg/d SC continued until last day of harvesting.
Harvest ~day +10 when CD34 >10 × 10^6/L and/or WBC >10 × 10^9/L

Typical protocol for myeloma

Day 0 cyclophosphamide 4g/m^2 IVI with Mesna.
Day +1 to day +10 to14, G-CSF 5–10μg/kg/d SC.
Harvest day +10 to14 when CD34 > 10 × 10^6/L and/or WBC >10 × 10^9/L

Mobilisation with haemopoietic growth factor alone

Suitable for normal volunteers e.g. allograft donors.

G-CSF 5–10μg/kg/d SC for 4–5d.
Harvest days 4–5.

Yield evaluation

Common parameters are mononuclear cell counts (MNC); CD34 numbers and haemopoietic colony forming unit assays e.g. CFU-GM. All are a quantitative or functional assessment of engraftment potential expressed per kg of recipient weight.

Typical target yields

Daily apheresis and daily G-CSF continue until the collection exceeds:

(i) 4×10^8/kg mononuclear cells or
(ii) 10×10^4/kg CFU-GM or
(iii) 3×10^6/kg CD34+ cells

Microbiological screening for stem cell cryopreservation

Infective agents, particularly viruses, can be transmitted through stem cell preparations as through blood products and may cause significant morbidity and mortality in the recipient. It has been demonstrated that transmission of hepatitis B virus has occurred following common storage in a liquid nitrogen tank which contained one patient's hepatitis BsAg +ve bone marrow.

The following tests should be performed on all patients in whom it is planned to cryopreserve stem cells

- Hepatitis B surface antigen.
- Hepatitis B surface antibody.
- Hepatitis B core antigen.
- Hepatitis B core antibody.
- Hepatitis C antibody.
- HIV 1 and 2 antibodies.
- HIV 1 and 2 antigen.
- HTLV1 antibody.
- VDRL.
- Additional serum for storage for retrospective analysis.

These results must be available to transplant laboratories before cryopreservation. Since many of these patients will be receiving blood products as part of their on-going treatment, they must be performed within 30 days of cryopreservation to prevent false –ve antibody tests due to the interval between exposure and seroconversion. In practice these constraints dictate that samples should be taken between 7 and 30 days prior to cryopreservation.

Patient samples shown to be –ve for all the above infectious agents should have stem cells stored in a dedicated liquid nitrogen freezer conventionally in the liquid phase.

Patient samples shown to be +ve for any of the above agents should ***be double bagged and stored in a separate liquid nitrogen freezer in the vapour phase*** (to reduce transmissibility). Data on all stem cell product samples must be registered in a secure environment on a computerised database with a logical inventory and retrieval system. No material should be imported to the freezers unless a complete negative virological audit storage trail can be demonstrated.

Transplantation

Stem cell transplant conditioning regimens

Conditioning is the treatment the patient undergoes immediately prior to a stem cell transplant. The purpose is to reduce the burden of residual disease; in allogeneic transplant recipients, it also acts as an immunosuppressant to prevent rejection of the graft. There are many different protocols using chemotherapy alone or in combination with total body irradiation (TBI). Unrelated transplants require immunosuppression with ALG or anti-T-cell monoclonal antibodies or total lymphoid Irradiation (TLI).

Examples are

AML–allo and autografts

- Cyclophosphamide 120mg/kg + 13.2Gy fractionated TBI

or Cyclophosphamide 120mg/kg + busulfan 16 mg/kg.

ALL–Allo and autografts

- Cyclophosphamide 120mg/kg + 13.2Gy fractionated TBI

or Etoposide 60mg/kg + 14.4Gy fractionated TBI.

Non-myeloablative allografts

- Campath-1H 100mg + fludarabine 150mg/m^2 + melphalan 140mg/m^2.

NHL–autografts

- BEAM (BCNU, etoposide, ara-C and melphalan; p612).

Myeloma–autografts

- High dose melphalan 200mg/m^2.

Transplantation

Infusion of cryopreserved stem cells

Equipment

1. Dewar containing stem cells in liquid N_2.
2. Water bath heated to 37°C–40°C.
3. Tongs.
4. Protective gloves.
5. Patient's notes.
6. Trolley with: syringes, needles, ampoules of 0.9% saline, blood giving sets, sterile dressing towels, chlorhexidine spray, bags of 500mL N/Saline, sterile gloves.

Ensure the patient has had procedure and any possible side effects explained.

Method

1. Write up the stem cell infusion on the blood product infusion chart.
2. 30 mins before re-infusion, ensure water bath is filled and heated to 37°C–40°C and give (chlorpheniramine) 10mg IV and paracetamol 1g PO.
3. When ready to return the stem cells take the dewar and equipment trolley to the patient's bedside.
4. Check the patient's vital signs.
5. Set up a standard blood giving set with microaggregate filter. Never use additional filters. Prime with 500mL 0.9% saline, connect to the patient and ensure good flow before starting to thaw any cells.
6. Check the water bath is 37°C–40°C and using the protective gloves and large tongs remove a bag of cells from liquid nitrogen dewar and place on the trolley. Carefully remove from the outer sleeve and place in water bath and allow one minute. DMSO cryopreservative is very toxic to cells once thawed so it is important to go straight from rapid thaw to infusion.
7. Remove bag of cells from water bath using the tongs, spray with chlorhexidine and allow to dry. Check patient identification number and DOB with the patient and if correct then connect to the giving set.
8. Cells should be returned as quickly as possible. Each bag contains approximately 100–150mL. Providing the flow is good, start thawing the next bag. Only thaw the next bag if you are able to finish the previous bag within the next minute. Check the patient's details on every bag.
9. Check the patient's observations at 15 minute intervals.
10. If the patient complains of abdominal pain, nausea or feeling faint, slow down the IVI for a short time. If symptoms persist or patient develops chest tightness or wheezing—stop the infusion. O_2 ± nebulised salbutamol may be required. Anaphylaxis rarely occurs.
11. At the end of re-infusion ensure no more bags of stem cells in the dewar and clear away all equipment.
12. Write the infusion details in the patient's notes in red ink.

Special considerations

► If the bag splits/leaks do not re-infuse—contents will not be sterile. Very rarely, a bag could start to expand rapidly upon thawing if all air not removed from the bag before freezing. A sterile needle may be used to pierce the bag if release of pressure appears essential.

►► Acute anaphylaxis is very rare but epinephrine (adrenaline) (1mL of 1:1000) should be available in the patient's room for SC or IM administration.

Infusion of fresh non-cryopreserved stem cells

Explain procedure and side effects to patient. In general, bone marrow will be in a larger volume than an apheresis product.

Procedure

1. A medical staff member must be available to start the infusion and stay with the patient for the first 30 minutes.
2. Prime blood giving set without an in-line filter with 500mL 0.9% saline and connect to the patient—check there is a good flow.
3. Check BP, pulse and chest auscultation before the infusion.
4. Give paracetamol 1g PO and chlorpheniramine 10mg IV at beginning of infusion.
5. Give stem cells as slowly as possible for the first 15 minutes, then increase the rate to 100mL in 60 minutes. If after 2h the patient is tolerating infusion without problems, increase to 200mL/h until completion.
6. Watch for fluid overload—give diuretic if necessary.
7. Nursing staff should monitor BP and pulse every 15–30 mins.
8. Write infusion details in the patient's notes in red ink.

Complications of stem cell infusion

- Microemboli occasionally cause dyspnoea and cyanosis. O_2 should be available. Slow down or stop the stem cell infusion if dyspnoea.
- Pyrexia, rash and rigors can occur—treat with hydrocortisone 100mg IV and chlorpheniramine 10mg IV.
- Hypertension may occur (especially if patient fluid overloaded). Usually responds to diuretic.

►► Acute anaphylaxis is very rare but adrenalin (1mL of 1:1000) should be available in the patient's room for SC or IM administration.

Daily ward management

Each day check patient for

- Fever.
- Nausea and vomiting.
- Diarrhoea.
- Bleeding.
- Rashes.
- Fatigue.
- Dyspnoea.
- Pain.
- Weight loss.
- Jaundice.
- Mucositis.
- Skin surveillance needed to observe for signs of acute and chronic GvHD, HSV, HZV and drug related problems.
- Hickman line infections are common post-transplant. If any signs of infection and fever, line cultures and exit site swab should be taken. Remove line as soon as infusional support no longer needed.

Transplantation

Blood product support for stem cell transplantation

All cellular blood products, i.e. red cells and platelets, must be irradiated.

Irradiation

- All cellular blood products given to allogeneic and autologous SCT patients must be irradiated to prevent transfusion associated GvHD due to transfused T lymphocytes.
- Transfusion associated GvHD is usually fatal particularly in allografts.
- Fatality can sometimes be avoided by immediate administration of anti-lymphocyte globulin or Campath antibody.
- Irradiation protocol is standard 2500cGy.
- Commence blood product irradiation two weeks prior to allogeneic SCT until one year post-SCT or off all immunosuppression whichever is later.
- Commence blood product irradiation two weeks prior to autologous SCT until six months post-SCT.
- Cell-free blood products e.g. FFP, cryoprecipitate or albumin do not need to be irradiated.
- Marrow or blood stem cell transplant itself is never irradiated.

CMV status of blood products

- CMV is not destroyed by irradiation.
- All transplant recipients should ideally receive CMV –ve red cells and platelet transfusions regardless of their own CMV status if sufficient CMV –ve blood products available. This is because of good evidence that transfused CMV carried in donor white cells may cause disease post-transplant regardless of the CMV status of the patient. CMV –ve recipients must always have –ve products.
- Should CMV negative platelets not be available at any time, it is acceptable to use unscreened leucodepleted red cells or platelets. This is because CMV is carried predominantly in leucocytes.
- For allograft recipients, additional preventive measures are taken against CMV reactivation (see p334).

Indications for RBC and platelet transfusions

Identical to those for patients undergoing intensive chemotherapy (see, pp546–650).

Management of ABO incompatibility

ABO incompatibility between donor and recipient does not affect the long-term success of the transplant nor the incidence of graft failure or GvHD. However, major ABO incompatibility transfusion reactions will occur unless specific steps are taken to manipulate the graft where donor and recipient are ABO mismatched. Furthermore, additional care must be given post-transplant in providing appropriate ABO matched products.

ABO mismatched definitions

1. Major ABO mismatch. This is where the recipient has anti-A or anti-B antibody to donor ABO antigens e.g. group O recipients with group A donor.

2. Minor ABO mismatch. This is where the donor has antibodies to recipient ABO antigens e.g. group A recipient with group O donor.

Management of major ABO mismatch

Manipulation of donor marrow/stem cells: red cells are removed in the transplant laboratory by starch sedimentation or Ficoll centrifugation, prior to infusion of the graft.

Choice of red cell and platelet supportive transfusions

- Transfuse packed group O red cells only for all major mismatch donor–recipient pairs.
- The choice of platelet group is less critical and may be affected by availability. First, second and third choice groups for platelet transfusions are shown in the table below.

Management of minor ABO mismatch

Manipulation of donor stem cells: prior to infusion, the product will have been plasma reduced in the transplant laboratory by centrifugation to remove antibody that could be passively transferred. Delayed immune haemolysis, which may be severe and intravascular, can occur after minor ABO mismatch due to active production of antibody by engrafting donor lymphocytes. Maximum haemolysis occurs 9–16 days post-transplant.

Choice of red cell and platelet transfusions

- Always transfuse packed O red cells, i.e. the same as in major ABO mismatch.
- Platelet transfusions first, second and third choice group is shown in the table below.

Choice of ABO group of blood/platelets in ABO mismatch BMT

			Platelets		
Donor	Recipient	Red cells	1st choice	2nd choice	3rd choice
Major ABO mismatch					
A	O	O	A	B	O
B	O	O	B	A	O
AB	O	O	A	B	O
A	B	O	B	A*	O*
B	A	O	A	B*	O*
AB	A	O	A	B*	O*
AB	B	O	B	A*	O*
Minor ABO mismatch					
O	A	O	A	B*	O*
O	B	O	B	A*	O*
O	AB	O	A*	B*	O*
A	AB	O	A*	B*	O*
B	AB	O	B*	A*	O*

(*Risk of haemolysis but do not withhold)

Rhesus (D) mismatch

Anti-D is not a naturally occurring antibody but may be induced by sensitisation with D +ve cells through pregnancy or previous incompatible transfusion. Important to screen both recipient and donor serum for the presence of anti-D.

- When either donor or recipient serum contains anti-D, rhesus D –ve blood products should always be given post-transplant. *Note*: in the situation where a rhesus D +ve recipient receives a graft from a donor whose serum contains anti-D, immune haemolysis may occur despite plasma reduction of the donor marrow due to active production of donor lymphocyte derived anti-D. Cannot be prevented but is rarely severe.
- Provided neither donor nor recipient have anti-D in the serum, specific pre-transplant manipulation of the product is only required in the situation of rhesus D +ve donor going into rhesus D –ve recipient where red cell depletion is required pre-transplant.
- It will occasionally be necessary to give rhesus D +ve platelet support when rhesus D –ve is preferable simply due to lack of abundant availability of rhesus –ve platelet products.
- If rhesus D +ve platelets have to be given, give anti-D 250iu SC immediately post-transfusion.

Transplantation

GvHD prophylaxis

In vitro T-cell depletion of graft or *in vivo* T-cell depletion with Campath-1H or anti-lymphocyte globulin (ALG) are successful in reducing both the incidence and severity of GvHD in graft recipients. The former is associated with an increased risk of relapse. Both are used in MUD and haploidentical grafts where the risk of severe GvHD is increased. The 'Seattle protocol' is most commonly used post graft infusion: consists of a combination of stat pulses of IV methotrexate (MTX) with bd infusions of cyclosporin:

Methotrexate MTX (IV bolus) 15mg/m^2 on day +1, then 10mg/m^2 days +3, +6 and +11. Folinic acid rescue 15mg/m^2 IV tds may be given 24 hours after each MTX injection for 24 hours (rescue protocol designed to reduce mucositis).

Dosage reductions

- If renal/hepatic impairment ↓ MTX dose as follows:

Creatinine (μmol/L)	MTX dose (%)
<145	100
146–165	50
166–180	25
>180	omit dose

Bilirubin (μmol/L)	MTX dose (%)
<35	100
36–50	50
51–85	25
>85	omit dose

Side effects although reduced by folinic acid rescue mucositis may remain severe and require IV diamorphine.

Cyclosporin administration

Powerful immunosuppressant with profound effects on T-cell suppressor function. Available for IV and oral use.

Intravenous regimen—commence on day –1 at 1.5mg/kg IV bd as IVI in 100mL 0.9% saline/2h. If flushing, nausea or pronounced tremor, slow infusion rate 4–6h/dose. Following loading, on day +3 onwards, adjust cyclosporin dosage based on plasma cyclosporin A level together with renal and hepatic function.

Oral regimen—switch intravenous→oral when patient can tolerate oral medication and is eating (usually day +10 to +20). Dosage on conversion is ~1.5–2.0 × IV dose (still bd).

Monitoring cyclosporin levels

- Cyclosporin is toxic and renal impairment is the most frequent dose limiting toxicity.
- Cyclosporin A levels should be monitored at least twice weekly.
- Never take blood for cyclosporin A levels from the central catheter through which cyclosporin has been given as cyclosporin adheres to

plastic and falsely high levels will be obtained. One lumen should be marked for cyclosporin administration and another lumen marked for blood levels testing.
- 12h pre-dose trough whole blood levels are measured.

Instruct patient to delay the morning dose of cyclosporin until after the blood level has been taken. The optimum blood cyclosporin level is not known. Target range: 100–300ng/mL. Aim towards the top of the therapeutic range in the early post-transplant period and lower part of the range at other times. In practice, the dose is often limited by a rise in serum creatinine. If serum creatinine >130μmol/L—adjust dose. Do not give cyclosporin if serum creatinine >180μmol/L.

Dosage adjustment—cyclosporin has a very long $t_{1/2}$ so dosage adjustment similar to warfarin adjustment.

1. To ↓ cyclosporin level omit 1–2 doses and make a 25–50% reduction in ongoing maintenance dose, recheck levels at 48h.
2. To ↑ levels, give 1 additional dose, increase maintenance dose by 25–50%, recheck level in 48h.
3. Monitor renal function and LFTs daily. Check serum calcium and magnesium twice weekly.

Cyclosporin toxicity

- Nephrotoxicity (*see above*). Worse with concurrent use of aminoglycosides, vancomycin and amphotericin.
- Hypertension—often associated with fluid retention and potentiated by steroids. Treat initially with diuretic to baseline weight and then nifedipine if persists. Sub-lingual nifedipine useful where emergency reduction of blood pressure is required.
- Neurological syndromes, esp. grand mal seizures (usually if untreated hypertension/fluid retention).
- Anorexia, nausea, vomiting, tremor (almost always occurs—if severe suggests overdosage).
- Hirsutism and gum hypertrophy with prolonged usage.
- Hepatotoxicity—less common than nephrotoxicity. Usually intrahepatic cholestatic picture on LFTs. Potentiated by concurrent drug administration e.g. macrolide antibiotics, norethisterone and the azole antifungals.
- Hypomagnesaemia commonly occurs. Potentiated by combination with amphotericin. Give 20mmol IVI if levels <0.5μmol/L or if symptoms develop.

Note: only one orally absorbed preparation of magnesium. For hypomagnesaemia persisting on cyclosporin post-discharge, consider magnesium glycerophosphate tablets qds.

Cyclosporin drug interactions

There are substantial and important drug interactions with cyclosporin:

Drugs that ↑ cyclosporin A levels	*Drugs that ↓ cyclosporin levels*
Azole antifungals	Rifampicin ⟶ major effect
Digoxin	Phenytoin ⟶ major effect
Macrolide antibiotics, especially erythromycin	Sulphonamides
Imipenem/meropenem	Carbamazepine
Calcium channel blockers	
Oral contraceptives	

Drugs WORSENING cyclosporin nephrotoxicity
- Aminoglycosides.
- Amphotericin B.
- Ciprofloxacin.
- Cotrimoxazole.
- ACE inhibitors.

Note: This is not an exhaustive list. Check cyclosporin levels 48h after any drug addition or cessation.

Tacrolimus
- Calcineurin inhibitor that prevents early T-cell activation; mechanism of action, pharmacology, drug interactions and toxicity similar to cyclosporin.
- Superior to cyclosporin in three randomised trials when used in combination with methotrexate as GvHD prophylaxis.
- Dosage: 0.03mg/kg/day by continuous IV infusion from day –2; taper 20% every 2 weeks from day 180; monitor blood level and toxicities and modify dose accordingly; used with standard dose MTX or mini-MTX (5mg/m^2 IV days +1, +3, +6 and +11).

Transplantation

Acute GvHD

Risk factors for acute GvHD include: older recipients, older donors, male recipient of female SCT (↑ risk with previous donor pregnancies), matched unrelated donors, haploidentical sibling donor. Defined as GvHD occurring within first 100d post-transplant (usually starts between day 7 and 28 post-transplant). Ranges from mild self-limiting condition to extensive disease (may be fatal). Characterised by fever, rash, abnormal LFTs, diarrhoea, suppression of engraftment and viral reactivation, particularly CMV.

Classified according to the Seattle system by a staging for each organ involved (skin, liver, gut) and overall clinical grading based on the organ staging.

Skin—involved in >90% cases. May be mild and unremarkable maculopapular rash (esp. palms of hands and soles of feet, but can affect any part of the body). In more severe cases, erythroderma and extensive desquamation and exfoliation can occur.

Liver—typical pattern of LFT abnormalities is intrahepatic cholestasis with ↑ bilirubin and alkaline phosphatase (relative sparing of transaminases). Note: this picture often does not discriminate between other causes of post-transplant liver dysfunction (e.g. drugs, infection – particularly CMV and fungal).

Gut—may occasionally be only organ involved, with nausea, vomiting, diarrhoea. Stool appearance may be highly abnormal with mincemeat or redcurrant jelly stools or green coloration.

Diagnosis

- Perform skin biopsy—but do not delay treatment if strong clinical suspicion.
- Rectal biopsy may be helpful (to distinguish infective from pseudomembranous colitis) but beware risk of bleeding and bacteraemia—perform only if it will alter management.
- Where GI symptoms are predominantly upper GI, gastroscopy with oesophageal, gastric and duodenal biopsies may be helpful (e.g. to distinguish between CMV and fungal oesophagitis and gastritis). Liver biopsy is hazardous and should only be performed where other convincing diagnostic guides are not available. It should be performed only by the transjugular route by an experienced operator and covered appropriately with blood products.

Consensus criteria for grading acute GvHD

Stage	Skin	Liver	Gut
1	Rash <25% body	Bilirubin 35–50μmol/L	Diarrhoea >0.5L/d or persistent nausea
2	Rash 25–50% body	Bilirubin 51–100μmol/L	Diarrhoea 1–1.5L/d
3	Rash >50% body	Bilirubin 101–250μmol/L	Diarrhoea >1.5L/d
4	Generalised erythroderma with bullae	Bilirubin >250μmol/L	Severe abdominal pain ± ileus

Overall clinical grading for the patient

Grade					
I	Stage 1–2		None		None
II	Stage 3	or	Stage 1	or	Stage 1
III	–		Stage 2–3	or	Stage 2-4
IV	Stage 4	or	Stage 4	or	Stage 4

Treatment

General measures—good nutrition and weight maintenance important. TPN may be necessary. IV antibiotics and antifungals often necessary in the absence of neutropenia and signs of infection may be masked by steroids. Continue cyclosporin during acute GvHD ensuring levels are not toxic.

Specific treatment should always be discussed with an experienced haemato-oncologist. Now known that mild GvHD confers a GvL effect (see p297) in the patient and mild forms of skin GvHD may require no treatment.

Overall grade

I–II Begin with prednisolone 1–2mg/kg/d PO. If response, taper dose slowly. If no response, consider progressing to high dose methyl prednisolone.

II–IV Give high dose methylprednisolone 20mg/kg/over 1h bd IV for 48h, then ↓ dose by 50% every 48h.

Side effects of methylprednisolone

- Gastritis/peptic ulceration—use proton pump inhibitors rather than H_2 blockers.
- Hyperglycaemia, particularly when TPN in use. May require insulin infusion.
- Hypertension may be potentiated by cyclosporin and by fluid retention—treat with diuretics and nifedipine.
- Insomnia and psychosis.

Failure of response to high dose methylprednisolone

Discuss with senior colleague. Outlook poor. Various empirical possibilities include tacrolimus, infusion of Campath or ALG.

Chronic GvHD

Occurs between 100–300d post-allogeneic transplant. There may not have been preceding acute GvHD, and acute GvHD may have resolved prior to onset of chronic GvHD. Conventionally subdivided into limited or extensive chronic GvHD. Major clinical features are debility, weight loss with malabsorption, sclerodermatous reaction due to excessive collagen deposition, severe immunosuppression and features of autoimmune disease.

Limited chronic GvHD: clinical features

- Localised skin involvement <50% total surface.
- Hepatic dysfunction—portal lesions but lacking necrosis, aggressive hepatitis or cirrhosis.
- Other localised involvement of eyes, salivary glands and mouth.

Extensive chronic GvHD—clinical features

- Generalised skin involvement >50% of surface—may include sclerodermatous changes and ulceration.
- Abnormal liver function—histology shows centrilobular changes, chronic aggressive hepatitis, bridging necrosis or cirrhosis.
- Liver dysfunction ± localised skin GvHD with involvement of eyes, salivary glands or oral mucosa on labial biopsy.
- Involvement of any other major organ system.

Criteria for classification of chronic GvHD

Classification	Criteria
Subclinical	Histological evidence on screening biopsies without clinical signs or symptoms.
Limited	Localised skin or single organ involvement not requiring systemic therapy.
Extensive low risk	Platelet count $>100 \times 10^9$/L and extensive skin disease or other organ involvement requiring systemic therapy.
Extensive high risk	Platelet count $<100 \times 10^9$/L and extensive skin disease or other organ involvement requiring systemic therapy.

Prognostic factors

Thrombocytopenia is an adverse prognostic factor for survival from diagnosis of chronic GvHD. Other factors associated with poor outcome are progressive onset, lichenoid skin rash, elevated bilirubin, poor performance status, alternative donor and sex mismatched donor.

Treatment

Discuss with a senior member of transplant team.

General measures

1. Adequate nutrition, vitamin/calorie supplements may be required and severe cases may require TPN.
2. Pneumococcal prophylaxis must be continued lifelong.

3. Consider restarting conventional prophylactic antifungal and antibacterial agents.
4. CMV surveillance is critical (reactivation is more common).
5. *P carinii* prophylaxis must be commenced with cotrimoxazole or nebulised Pentamidine and continued for 6 months after immunosuppressive therapy.
6. Psychological support may be required to adjust to chronic disability.

Specific treatment

1. Commonest protocol used is the Seattle regimen of prednisolone and cyclosporin A on alternate days; typically: begin daily prednisolone 1mg/kg/day with cyclosporin A 10mg/kg/day divided bd.
2. If disease stable or improved after 2 weeks taper prednisolone by 25% per week to target dose of 1mg/kg every other day.
3. After successful completion of steroid taper, reduce cyclosporin A by 25% per week to alternate day dosage of 10mg/kg/day divided bd.
4. If resolved completely at 9 months, slowly wean patient from both medications with dose reductions every 2 weeks.
5. Incomplete responses should be re-evaluated after 3 months more therapy; if fail to respond or progress then salvage therapy required.
6. If no response or progression add in azathioprine 1.5mg/kg/d initially (monitor FBC, renal and liver function).
7. Severe refractory cases may respond to thalidomide, tacrolimus, hydroxychloroquine or mycophenolate mofetil (all of which may at least have a steroid sparing effect) or experimental measures such as extracorporeal PUVA therapy or anti-lymphocyte globulin.

Veno-occlusive disease

Presents clinically early post-transplant (usually within the first 14d). Pathophysiology poorly understood. Risk factors for severe VOD include: intensive conditioning regimens, pre-transplant hepatitis and second transplants. VOD is characterised by a triad of hepatomegaly, jaundice and ascites (resulting in rapid post-transplant weight gain) as a result of this. Commoner in allografts than autografts.

Diagnosis is largely clinical but may be supported by typical findings on Doppler ultrasound study of hepatic arterial and venous flows, or by elevated plasminogen activator inhibitor (PAI 1) levels. However, the only definitive diagnostic investigation is transjugular liver biopsy, the risks of which must be weighed against the importance of the information obtained.

There is no treatment currently universally accepted as effective prophylaxis.

Strategies include

- Heparin 100u/kg/d by continuous IVI.
- LMWH SC od or a prostaglandin E1 (PGE1) infusion.

No universally accepted effective treatment. The key is supportive therapy with management of fluid overload with spironolactone and frusemide while maintaining intravascular volume with albumin or plasma substitute. In severe VOD, infusion of TPA or PGE1 may be considered.

If thrombolysis required

- Ensure no active bleeding is occurring and keep platelets $>20 \times 10^9$/L.
- Give tissue-type plasminogen activator (Altaplase™).
  - 10mg IV into central line over 30 minutes
  - Then 40mg as IVI over next 60 minutes
    i.e. total dose of 50mg over 90 minutes
    (↓ doses proportionally for patients weighing <than 60kg).
- Give daily for 3 days minimum and assess against VOD parameters.

Transplantation

Invasive fungal infections and antifungal therapy

Invasive fungal infections are an important cause of morbidity and mortality after allogeneic SCT with a frequency of 10–25% and mortality of >70%.

Pathogenesis

- Majority of infections are due to *Candida* species and *Aspergillus* species though infections due to other opportunistic fungi increasing (*Trichosporon* spp., *Fusarium* spp., *Bipolaris* spp. and *Zygomycetes* amongst others.
- Invasive *Candida* infections classified as candidaemia or acute disseminated candidiasis and arise from invasion of bloodstream from infected mucosal surfaces or via central venous catheters; decreasing incidence due to introduction of fluconazole prophylaxis though increased non-albicans spp. (esp. *glabrata* and *krusei*).
- Invasive *Aspergillus* infections affect paranasal sinuses and lungs and arise from airborne exposure; increasing incidence, particularly late after transplantation.

- Risk factors: prolonged and profound neutropenia; use of corticosteroids.

Prophylaxis

- Prophylaxis: high efficiency (>90%) particulate air (HEPA) filtration or positive pressure ventilation; prophylaxis with fluconazole (400mg/day does not cover *Aspergillus* spp., *C glabrata* or *C krusei*) or itraconazole (200–400mg/day; poor absorption from capsules; extremely unpalatable liquid preparation).

Amphotericin

- If a febrile neutropenic transplant patient is unresponsive to second line antibiotics after 48–96h and/or there is a suspicion of possible fungal infection (unwell; chest symptoms; peripheral nodules, halo sign or cavitation on CT chest, evidence of candidaemia), then standard formulation of amphotericin (Fungisone™) should be started.
- Give test dose of 1mg IV over 30 mins with observation of the patient for abreaction for 30 mins followed by 1mg/kg daily.
- Daily urea and electrolytes are recommended and amiloride 5mg (increasing to 10mg if required) should be prescribed to counteract the frequently accompanying hypokalaemia. Oral K^+ supplements often required. Serum Mg^{2+} and LFTs should be checked twice weekly.
- All doses of amphotericin should be preceded by a 0.9% saline preload. 500mL 0.9% saline should be infused as fast as tolerated (usually over 1h)—reduces nephrotoxicity and side effects. Paracetamol 1g PO should be given 30 minutes prior to infusion together with chlorpheniramine 10mg IV. Pethidine 25–30mg IV stat may be given if a troublesome reaction occurs.

Liposomal amphotericin

Suggested indications for prescribing a liposomal or other lipid formulation of amphotericin.

1. Refractory fever >72h on standard amphotericin at 1mg/kg.

2. A rise in the creatinine to >50% baseline levels with standard amphotericin despite optimal hydration.
3. Deteriorating LFTs.
4. Evidence of severe disseminated fungal infection–ie multiple lesions on CXR or CT scan, or any two sites of sinuses, lung, liver, spleen or brain.
5. Patients receiving cyclosporin after an allograft. These patients should receive lipid formulation product if baseline creatinine is >130μmol/L. Otherwise, the indication for lipid formulation product is as in 1–4 above.

Lipid formulation amphotericin products

2 lipid formulations of amphotericin in extensive use—both expensive. No comparative trial of the 2 products but efficacy data appear similar. An appropriate protocol is suggested:

Commence either liposomal amphotericin (AmBisome™) at 1–5mg/kg/day or amphotericin B lipid complex (Abelcet™) at 2.5mg/kg (in practice round up or down to standard vial size to avoid wastage and minimize cost). Follow data sheet instructions carefully, observing for anaphylaxis. The dosage should be increased to a maximum of 5mg/kg Abelcet™ or 3–5mg/kg AmBisome™ in patients who have either a confirmed mycological diagnosis or a fever which does not respond within 72h on the lower dose.

Paracetamol and chlorpheniramine pre-medication cover is advised for Abelcet™ (may also be required for AmBisome™). 0.9% saline preload is not normally required unless renal or liver function deteriorate during treatment. Renal function should be checked on alternate days for the duration of the treatment. Serum Mg^{2+} and LFTs should be checked weekly.

Total duration of treatment difficult to asses. General principles are that therapy should continue for at least 2 weeks and until neutrophil recovery and no signs of progression radiologically.

Voriconazole

A second-generation triazole that has been shown to be superior to amphotericin in antifungal efficiency and survival in an international randomised trial and likely to become treatment of choice for invasive aspergillosis due to more favourable toxicity profile. Dose 6mg/kg IV bd day 1 then 4mg/kg IV bd maintenance converting to oral 200mg bd (may commence orally with 400mg bd loading dose on day 1). No dose adjustment required for renal or acute hepatic impairment but monitor renal and hepatic function. Side effects: visual disturbances, rash, elevated LFTs and with IV administration, flushing, fever, tachycardia and dyspnoea.

Caspofungin

An echinocandin which targets the fungal cell wall and is active against *Candida* and *Aspergillus* spp. Higher response rate demonstrated in comparison to amphotericin in treatment of invasive candidiasis. Loading dose of slow IV infusion of 70mg on day 1 followed by maintenance dose of 50mg/day (lower maintenance in moderate liver insufficiency). It may also be used for treatment of invasive aspergillosis refractory to amphotericin preparations. Caution with concomitant cyclosporin: monitor LFTs; adjust tacrolimus dose. Side effects: phlebitis, fever, headache, rash, abdominal pain, nausea, diarrhoea.

Note

As with all protocols check local policies since these may differ to those outlined in this handbook.

Transplantation

CMV prophylaxis and treatment

All transplant recipients who are CMV sero-negative should receive CMV –ve blood products. If supplies are available, this is recommended also for CMV sero-positive recipients. Limits risk of CMV blood product transmission regardless of donor/recipient serological status.

CMV surveillance

- All allograft patients and CMV sero-positive autograft recipients should receive CMV surveillance.
- The minimum surveillance required is the DEAFF (detection of early antigen fluorescent foci) test. Should detect CMV antigen in culture by immunofluorescence within 48 hours and virus culture continues for 1–2 weeks. Urine and throat washings are not sent routinely for CMV detection.
- 5 ml EDTA blood should be sent weekly on the above cohort of transplant patients from admission until day 100. Screening of allograft recipients should continue until 1 year post-transplant although the frequency of testing may be reduced in the absence of appropriate symptoms.

- More sensitive tests now available to detect CMV antigen or genome by PCR technology in buffy coat of EDTA peripheral blood will soon replace DEAFF as standard tests.

CMV prophylaxis

Indicated in allograft patients when either donor or recipient are CMV sero-positive. Not recommended when both donor and recipient are sero-negative, nor for autograft recipients, even if sero-positive.

Suggested protocol

1. Acyclovir 800mg tds IV from day –5 to discharge, then 800mg tds PO for 3 months *plus*
2. IVIg 200mg/kg IV day –1, day +13 and then every 3 weeks until day +100.

Note: The graft suppression of this dose of acyclovir may sometimes be dose limiting.

Treatment of CMV infection

A +ve CMV identification in buffy coat by either surveillance method should be treated even if the patient is asymptomatic:

- Gancyclovir: 5 mg/kg IV bd for 14 days minimum then continue maintenance dose 5mg/kg/day IV daily (6mg/kg/day 5 days weekly as outpatient).
- Stop acyclovir when gancyclovir commenced.
- Side effects: myelosuppressive, may be abrogated by G-CSF, nephrotoxic.
- Renal function must be monitored and dose reductions implemented according to the BNF.
- Abnormal LFTs may occur.
- Fever, rashes and headaches.
- Alternative—foscarnet 90 mg/kg IV bd for 14d minimum.
- Administer through a central line as IVI over 2 hours (may be given as a peripheral IVI but should be given concurrently with a fast running

litre of 0.9% saline). Side effects–nephrotoxic and hepatotoxic (follow BNF dosage adjustments).

Treatment plan

On a first episode of CMV antigenaemia, start with gancyclovir. Failure to become CMV antigen –ve by the end of the 2 week course would lead to immediate progression to foscarnet.

CMV-related disease

May cause pneumonitis, oesophagitis, gastritis, hepatitis, retinitis and myelosuppression. Where CMV antigenaemia accompanied by symptoms/signs of CMV disease high titre anti-CMV Ig 200mg/kg/day IV should be administered on days 1, 3, 5 and 7 of antiviral therapy with gancyclovir or foscarnet. Broncho-alveolar lavage (BAL) should be performed to establish the presence of CMV locally in the lung.

Post-transplant vaccination programme

General

The subject of re-vaccination post-transplant remains a contentious topic. The general principles are that live vaccination is forbidden, probably for the lifetime of the patient. Secondly, antibody and T-cell responses to vaccination in the first year following transplantation are sub-optimal. In allogeneic transplants, immune reconstitution continues beyond 1 and up to 2 years post-transplant. These general considerations have been used to suggest the following policy.

Allogeneic transplants

No immunisations should be given in the presence of acute or chronic GvHD. In the absence of this, proceed as follows:

At 12 months post-transplant

- Diphtheria and tetanus toxoid primary course (3 doses).
- Primary course of inactivated polio vaccine (3 doses).
- Pneumovax II (repeated every 6 years).
- *Haemophilus influenzae* B.
- Meningococcal A and C.
- Influenza vaccine (and annually thereafter).

The vaccinations should be staggered with only diphtheria and tetanus being administered concurrently. It would be reasonable to leave a gap of 2 weeks between each vaccination. Not only may this enhance antibody responses but it will easily identify the cause if there are any reactions.

At 2 years post-transplant

- Measles if the patient is at high risk but patient free of GvHD and off immunosuppressive therapy.
- Rubella if the patient is a female of child-bearing age who has a low titre but patient free of GvHD and off immunosuppressive therapy.

Autologous SCT for lymphoma or myeloma—1 year post-transplant

- Tetanus booster.
- Inactivated polio vaccine booster.
- Pneumovax II (repeated every 6 years).
- *Haemophilus influenzae* B.
- Meningococcal A and C.
- Influenza vaccine (repeated annually).

Foreign travel

All transplant recipients should take medical advice from their transplant team before travelling abroad.

- Typhoid, cholera, hepatitis A/B and meningococcal vaccines are safe.
- Yellow fever and Japanese B encephalitis are not safe.
- Remember malaria prophylaxis.

Avoid live vaccines. e.g.:

- Yellow fever

- BCG.
- Oral polio.
- Oral typhoid.

Post-transplant complications
- Bacterial and fungal infections.
- Pneumonitis.
- CMV reactivation.
- Veno-occlusive disease (VOD)—*see p328*.

Allografts only
- Acute GvHD (see p324).
- Chronic GvHD (see p326).

Longer term effects
- Endocrine: hypothyroidism may occur post-transplant. Check TFTs at 3 monthly intervals→1 year.
- Respiratory: check lung function tests at 6 months and 1 year if TBI has been given.
- Skin: advise about sun protection (following TBI avoid the sun). If exposure is unavoidable, total sun block factor 15 or higher is essential for at least 1 year.
- Fertility: most patients will be infertile after transplant (almost invariably if TBI given). Since this cannot be absolutely guaranteed, contraceptive precautions should be taken until the confirmatory tests have been performed.
- Males: check sperm counts at 3 and 6 months post-transplant. Zero motile sperm on both samples confirms infertility.
- Females: check FSH, LH and oestradiol at 3 months. FSH and LH levels should be high and oestradiol levels low if no ovulation is occurring.
- Menopause–women may have an early menopause due to the treatment and may experience symptoms such as hot flushes, dry skin, dryness of the vagina and loss of libido. Most women should have hormone replacement therapy (Prempak C 1.25 initially starting as soon as early menopause is confirmed) and counselled about HRT problems.
- Cataracts—patients who have had TBI are at risk of developing cataracts. Refer for ophthalmological assessment at 1 year post BMT.
- Immunisations at 12–24 months post-transplant (*see p336*).

Treatment of relapse post-allogeneic SCT

Recurrence of leukaemia, myeloma or lymphoma after an allogeneic SCT may be treated by donor lymphocyte infusion (DLI), a second transplant (in those patients with a durable first response who are fit enough to withstand the rigours of a second allograft) or conventional dose or palliative treatment.

DLI

- May be used in CML, AML and ALL, NHL, HL and myeloma.
- DLI can promote full donor chimerism in patients with mixed chimerism or residual tumour after reduced intensity non-myeloablative conditioning.
- Patient should discontinue cyclosporin and steroid therapy at least 2 weeks before DLI and chemotherapy at least 24h before DLI.
- Donor lymphocytes are collected by leucapheresis; a typical collection of 150mL contains ~50×10^8 T lymphocytes.
- Escalating doses are generally used to limit GvHD e.g. first dose 10^7 donor lymphocytes followed 12 weeks later if no response by 5×10^7 cells, then if no response 12 weeks later 10^8 cells then $>10^8$ cells 12 weeks later if no response; lower initial doses and increments are utilised in MUD SCT.
- Where possible e.g. CML, AML molecular monitoring may be undertaken and DLI may be utilised for molecular relapse with molecular monitoring of response.
- The main adverse effect of DLI is acute or chronic GvHD especially if administered early after SCT. The incidence of these complications has been reduced by the adoption of an escalating dose regimen but increased with MUD SCT.

Transplantation

Discharge and follow-up

Criteria for discharge

Blood counts should ideally be: Hb >10.0g/dL (but may require transfusion), neutrophils $>1.0 \times 10^9$/L, platelets $>25 \times 10^9$/L, and patients should be able to maintain a fluid intake of 2–3L/d, tolerating diet and oral medications particularly in allografts on cyclosporin. Should be apyrexial and no longer losing weight.

Counsel patients

1. Possible need for blood/platelets.
2. Adherence to neutropenic diet.
3. Check temperature bd and report immediately if febrile.
4. Fatigue post-transplant in irradiated patients due to the late TBI effect usually 6–10 weeks post transplant.
5. Risk of HZV (explain the early symptoms).
6. To continue with mouth care.
7. To report any new symptoms.

Blood tests—initially twice weekly

- FBC, reticulocytes and blood film.
- Biochemistry including LFTs.
- CyA levels pre-dose (EDTA sample)—allografts only.

Initially once a week

- Magnesium.
- CRP.
- Coagulation screen.
- CMV screening test e.g DEAFF—allografts and seropositive autograft recipients only.
- Stool culture—allografts only unless relevant symptoms.

Drugs

1. Cyclosporin capsules—allografts only.
2. Acyclovir prophylaxis against HZV 400mg qds PO for minimum of 3 months in non-TBI patients and 6 months in TBI autografts and all allografts. Allografts may be on 800mg tds if acyclovir chosen for CMV prophylaxis. Consider low dose 200mg bd maintenance until 1–2 years post-transplant.
3. Penicillin V 250mg bd PO should be given to all patients. Erythromycin 250mg od PO if penicillin allergic.
4. Ciprofloxacin 250mg bd PO if neutrophils $<1.0 \times 10^9$/L.
5. Cotrimoxazole 480mg bd PO Monday, Wednesday, Friday for 1 year minimum and until CD4 count >500. Cotrimoxazole should be started when neutrophils $>1.5 \times 10^9$/L and platelets $>60 \times 10^9$/L. Until then, use nebulised pentamidine 300mg every 3 weeks.
6. Itraconazole—allografts only.
7. Nystatin mouth care.
8. Folic acid 5mg bd until full engraftment.
9. Sanatogen Gold™ multivitamins 1/d may be advisable while gaining weight.
10. Antiemetics PRN.

Transplantation

Haemostasis and thrombosis 10

Coagulation disorders—a clinical approach

Haemophilia is the name given to an increased bleeding tendency. It can be heritable or acquired. The commonest heritable bleeding disorder is mild von Willebrand disease, affecting 1 per few hundred of the population. This heritable disorder is not typically referred to as haemophilia but in the broadest sense of the definition it is a form of haemophilia. 'Classical haemophilia', also termed 'haemophilia A', is due to factor VIII deficiency and affects only 1 per 10,000 male births. It is therefore encountered infrequently in non-haematological practice. The most common acquired form of haemophilia is that due to oral anticoagulant therapy as 1 per 100 of the population of many countries are now taking long-term warfarin or similar anticoagulants.

Conversely, thrombophilia is used to describe an increased tendency to thrombosis. This can also be heritable or acquired. Heritable thrombophilic defects are often insufficient on their own to cause thrombosis and an additional acquired factor, such as surgery, is often the trigger for an acute thrombotic event.

Bleeding disorders

Causes of bleeding—surgery, trauma, non-accidental injury, coagulation disorders (including anticoagulant drugs), platelet dysfunction (including aspirin and other anti-platelet drugs), vascular disorders.

Clinical features—is there a lifelong bleeding history, has the patient been previously challenged, is this an isolated symptom? Type of bleeding problem that led to presentation e.g. mucocutaneous, easy bruising, spontaneous, post-traumatic. Duration and time of onset. Menstrual history is important. Absence of obstetric bleeding may be misleading as haemostatic capacity increases significantly in pregnancy.

Systemic enquiry—do symptoms suggest a systemic disorder, bone marrow failure, infection, liver disease, renal disease?

Past medical history—previous episode, previous known disorder e.g. ITP. Exposure to trauma, surgery, dental extraction, or pregnancies.

Family history—similar bleeding tendency in other family members? Pattern of inheritance (autosomal dominant, sex-linked).

Drugs—thrombocytopenia (📖 *p384*), platelet dysfunction (📖 *p378*); not always obvious—aspirin, warfarin. Drug reaction—allergic purpura.

Physical examination

Signs of systemic disease—anaemia, lymphadenopathy ± hepatosplenomegaly?

Assess bleeding site—check palate and fundi. Check size e.g petechiae (pinhead); purpura (larger =1cm); bruises (ecchymoses) =1cm—measure them.

Joints—swelling or other signs of chronic arthritis, joint destruction or muscle contractures from previous bleeds?

Vascular lesions—purpura e.g. allergic, Henoch–Schönlein (*p376*), senile, steroid-related, hypergammaglobulinaemic, HHT—capillary dilatations (blanches on pressure), vasculitic lesions, autoimmune disorders, hypersensitivity reactions.

Investigation

- FBC (especially platelet count), film, biochemistry (especially creatinine and LFTs), ESR, coagulation tests (PT and APTT).
- Special tests will be dictated by history. The bleeding time is not a reliable test and is rarely indicated. von Willebrand's disease (vWD) often missed because PT and APTT and platelet count are normal. If history suggestive of vWD then plasma level of von Willebrand factor must be measured.
- Family studies should be considered to identify other family members at risk of bleeding.

Summary

Pre-operative history is most important aspect of identifying clinically significant bleeding risk. If abnormal bleeding does occur exclude surgical bleeding and take blood for testing before blood transfusion compounds the problem. Decide whether platelet or coagulation defect or both? Is it hereditary or acquired?

Treatment

Establish diagnosis and treat as appropriate.

Classification of bleeding disorders	📖
Inherited	
von Willebrand's disease (vWD)	p348
Haemophilia A and B	p352
Other congenital deficiencies	p356
Acquired	
Anticoagulant therapy	
Heparin	p588
Warfarin	p590
Thrombolysis	p516
Vitamin K deficiency	p360
Liver disease	p364
DIC	p512
Acquired inhibitors	p366
Massive blood transfusion	p524

Coagulation disorders—laboratory approach

Establish whether bleeding is of recent origin (suggests acquired) or long-standing (congenital), spontaneous or induced by trauma/surgery, mucocutaneous (?platelet defect) or generalised (?coagulation defect or ?drug induced).

Laboratory tests

- FBC with platelet count, coagulation tests (PT, APTT, fibrinogen).
- Fill blood sample tube to the mark to ensure correct anticoagulant concentration.
- Repeat test if result abnormal before investigating further.
- Check patient not on anticoagulants.

Further investigation

Abnormal platelet count

- Both high and low counts may cause bleeding.
- If isolated low platelets 📖 *p384*; if platelets high 📖 *p382*.
- If platelets low and coagulation screen abnormal—could be DIC, liver disease, massive blood transfusion, primary blood disorder (e.g. leukaemia).

Abnormal coagulation result

▶ PT ↑ APTT normal

Warfarin, vitamin K deficiency, early liver disease, rarely congenital factor VII deficiency.

▶ PT ↑ APTT ↑

Warfarin overdose, vitamin K deficiency, liver failure, DIC.

▶ PT normal APTT ↑

Unfractionated heparin (UFH), haemophilia A or B, lupus anticoagulant, rarely vWD affects APTT, factor VIII inhibitors are rare but typically prolong APTT.

▶ PT normal APTT normal

Normal PT and APTT do not exclude a significant bleeding tendency, for example effect of low molecular weight heparin, mild factor deficiency, platelet abnormality, or very rare factor deficiency such as factor XIII.

Further investigation

- DIC: check blood film, platelets, thrombin time, fibrinogen, XDPs/D-dimer.
- Vit K deficiency: assay VII and II; give vitamin K and repeat 24h later.
- Liver disease: check LFTs; will not correct to normal with vitamin K.
- Isolated factor deficiency: assay as indicated by PT/APTT results.
- Inhibitor-specific LA tests: check ACL; other factor-specific assays.
- Heparin: ↑ APTT ratio, PT normal if APTT ratio 1.5–2.5, TT ↑, reptilase normal.
- Warfarin: PT prolongation>than APTT, low vitamin K dependent factors.
- vWD: diagnosis of von Willebrand disease requires measurement of vWF level and function. *Note*: bleeding time is neither sensitive nor specific for diagnosis or bleeding tendency.

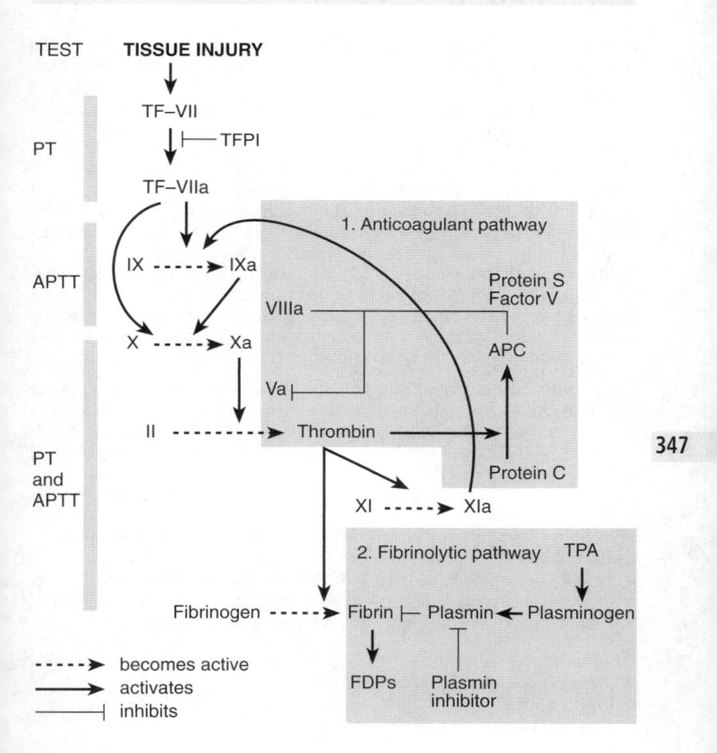

Blood coagulation network
Tissue injury triggers off a cascade of zymogen-to-protease reactions which amplify resulting in thrombin generation and fibrin clot.

Natural anticoagulation network
Natural anticoagulants: Tissue Factor Pathway Inhibitor (TFPI), Antithrombin and Activated Protein C. Thrombin binds to a receptor, thrombomodulin (TM) on the surface of endothelial cells. Bound to TM thrombin loses anticoagulant activity and becomes a potent activator of protein C→Activated PC (APC) with co-factors PS and FV, cleaves and inactivates Factors Va and VIIIa.

Fibrinolytic network
Tissue plasminogen activators (TPA) activate plasminogen to plasmin; this breaks down fibrin releasing degradation products (FDPs, or XDPs when cross-linked) into the circulation.

von Willebrand's disease (vWD) and vWF-related bleeding

Autosomal inherited bleeding disorder due to reduced production of von Willebrand factor (vWF) or production of defective protein, affects both sexes with estimated incidence of 1 per few hundred. First described in 1926 in the Åland Islands in the Baltic, it has a worldwide distribution.

Pathophysiology

vWF, produced in endothelial cells and megakaryocytes, is a protein of 250kDa molecular weight. Initial dimerisation and subsequent removal of propeptide allows polymerisation and secretion of large multimers. The higher molecular weight (HMW) multimers, up to 20×10^3 kDa, are particularly haemostatically active. vWF has two main functions:

1. Its primary haemostatic function is to act as a ligand for platelet adhesion and it is this reduced activity that causes bleeding.
2. It has a secondary function as a carrier protein for factor VIII protecting it from degradation. In most patients with vWD the associated mild reduction in factor VIII level is not the cause of the haemostatic defect.

Many cases of heritable/congenital vWD are currently thought to be caused by genetic mutations at the vWF locus but some may be due to defects in other genes, which affect vWF levels. Increasingly vWF is considered a continuous variable with low levels associated with an increased bleeding tendency.

Many subtypes but for simplicity the disease is classified into 3 main types:

- Type 1—quantitative deficiency of vWF (autosomal dominant).
- Type 2—qualitative deficiency of vWF (autosomal dominant/recessive).
- Type 3—complete deficiency of vWF (autosomal recessive).

Clinical features

- Type 1 is common (70% of cases).
- Type 2 ~25%.
- Type 3 is rare.

The clinical picture varies markedly. Symptoms may be intermittent, due to dysfunction of platelet adhesion e.g. mucocutaneous bleeding, easy bruising, nose bleeds, prolonged bleeding from cuts, dental extractions, trauma, surgery and menorrhagia.

Type 2B causes thrombocytopenia which may present in pregnancy. Usually the picture is consistent within a family. ***Laboratory diagnosis***

- vWF is an acute phase protein—increasing with stress, oestrogens, pregnancy, neoplasm, thyrotoxicosis, etc. vWF levels are dependent on ABO blood group being lower in group O than non-O.
- In type 1 APTT usually normal as are PT and platelets. VIII may be normal or ↓. vWF level and function typically mildly or moderately ↓. Bleeding time is often normal and is no longer used in many haemophilia centres. It has been largely replaced by automated *in vitro* platelet function analysis at high shear rate (PFA-100). When mild, the

condition may be difficult to diagnose as many of the tests are normal, including the VIII and variably the vWF level. Repeat testing is necessary. Family testing is useful.

Classification of von Willebrand's disease

Type	VIII	vWF Ag	vWF activity	RIPA low dose	HMW multimer
1	N/↓	↓	↓	↓/N	N
2A	N/↓	N/↓	↓	↓/N	↓
2M	N/↓	N/↓	↓	↓/N	N
2B	N/↓	N/↓	↓	↑	↓
2N	↓	N	N	N	N
3	↓↓	↓↓	↓↓	↓↓	Usually undetectable

vWF activity measured as ristocetin cofactor activity (Ricof) or collagen binding activity (CBA), which is measured in plasma and is not the same as RIPA (*see below*) which is ability of ristocetin to agglutinate platelet rich plasma.

The main subtypes of type 2 are 2A and 2M. In 2A there is a qualitative defect with absent HMW multimers and in 2M there is a qualitative defect but with HMW multimers present.

RIPA is ristocetin-induced platelet agglutination performed on a patient's platelet rich plasma. Only value of RIPA test is for detection of type 2B when RIPA is increased due to high affinity variant vWF which produces thrombocytopenia and reduced circulating level of VWF

Factor VIII is seldom low enough to cause the joint bleeds seen in haemophilia except in Type 3 which is a severe bleeding disorder.

Type 2N is rare autosomal recessive variant in which the VIII:C carrier function of vWF is reduced. May be misdiagnosed as haemophilia A but clue is that females are affected as well as males and autosomal recessive inheritance.

Management

- Avoid aspirin and NSAIDs.
- Mild bleeding symptoms—easy bruising, bleeding from cuts may settle with local pressure.
- Tranexamic acid (TXA) is a useful antifibrinolytic drug (15mg/kg PO tds).
- TXA mouthwash 5% is useful for dental work.
- Moderate disease and minor surgery
  - DDAVP (0.3mg/kg SC or by slow IV injection/infusion). Fewer side effects with SC route.

  - Most responders have type 1 vWD but may work in some type 2 patients. Avoid in type 2B (may reduce platelets).
- Major surgery, bleeding symptoms or severe disease.
  - If DDAVP insufficient use vWF rich factor VIII concentrate e.g. intermediate purity VIII concentrate, e.g. Alphanate, BPL 8Y, Haemate P.
  - Monitor treatment with VWF:Ricof or VWF:Ag. Bleeding time or PFA-100 (*see below*) may not correct despite good clinical response. Treat post-op for 7–10 days.
- Pregnancy—VIII and VWF rise in pregnancy so rarely presents a problem for type 1. Post-partum vWF falls so watch out for PPH in mod/severely affected women. Give DDAVP or vWF concentrate to maintain levels >30% if clinical problem. In Type 2B abnormal HMW multimers can cause platelet aggregation and thrombocytopenia in pregnancy. Avoid TXA in pregnancy/type 2B as there may be risk of thrombosis.
- Menorrhagia—may be major problem. TXA for first 3 days of the menstrual period helps some patients. Combined oral contraceptive pill is useful. Mirena (hormone impregnated) coil very effective in some patients.

Complications

Vaccination against HBV and HAV recommended for all patients. Inhibitors infrequent—usually type 3 disease.

Natural history

Majority of patients will have type 1 disease which rarely causes life-threatening bleeds; may have little impact on quality of life/life expectancy. Management with vWF rich factor VIII concentrates as for severe haemophilia should enable patients with severe vWD to have good quality of life.

Sadler, J.E. (2003) Von Willebrand disease type 1: a diagnosis in search of a disease. *Blood*, **101**, 2089–2093.

Haemostasis and thrombosis

Haemophilia A and B

Congenital bleeding disorders caused by defective production of factor VIII (haemophilia A) or IX (haemophilia B); sex-linked recessive inheritance. Females carriers are rarely symptomatic. Queen Victoria passed the disease on to her great-grandson, Alexis, son of the Tsar, contributing to the fall of Tsarist Russia.

Pathophysiology

Factor VIII activated by thrombin, and IX activated by the TF/factor VIIa complex, together activate factor X, leading to thrombin generation and conversion of soluble fibrinogen to insoluble fibrin (px). Haemophilia A and B are disorders characterised by inability to generate cell surface-associated factor Xa. Genetic abnormalities include: inversions within intron 22 of factor VIII gene in 50%, point mutations and deletions. Gross gene alterations common in haemophilia A but infrequent in haemophilia B. This may account for low frequency of inhibitors in haemophilia B. Third of haemophilia B patients have dysfunctional molecule.

Carrier detection and antenatal diagnosis now possible in many cases by direct gene mutation detection. Affected family member usually required. Linkage analysis no longer recommended as first line method.

Epidemiology

Haemophilia A occurs in 1:10,000 ♂ in the UK, in ~⅓ cases no family history as new mutation; 5× more frequent than haemophilia B; no striking racial distribution.

Clinical presentation

Haemophilia A and B—clinically indistinguishable. Symptoms depend on the factor level.

Severe disease (plasma level <1%)	Usually presents in the first years of life with easy bruising and bleeding out of proportion to injury
Moderate disease (1–5% factor level)	Intermediate & variable severity
Mild disease (>5%)	May only present after trauma/surgery in later life
General features	Haemarthrosis; spontaneous bleeding into joints (knees>elbows>ankles>hips>wrists) produce local tingling, pain; later—swelling, limitation of movement, warmth, redness, severe pain

Bleeds into muscles, spontaneous bleeding into arms, legs, iliopsoas, or any site—may lead to nerve compression, compartment syndrome, muscle contractures—look for these. Haematuria is common; retroperitoneal and CNS bleeds are life threatening.

Diagnosis
Assess duration, type of bleeding, exposure to previous trauma/surgery and family history. Look for bruising, petechial haemorrhages, early signs of joint damage. Exclude acquired bleeding disorders.

Laboratory tests
PT normal, APTT ↑ depending on degree of deficiency (note: *a normal APTT does not exclude mild disease*). Assay VIII first, then IX. Exclude vWD.

Radiology
Acute bleed—USS or CT scan if in doubt. In established disease—chronic synovitis, arthropathy and other pathological changes seen.

Complications
Chronic arthropathy
Repeated joint bleeds preventable but older patients often have arthropathy.

Development of factor VIII inhibitors
Suggested by ↓ response to concentrates; occurs in 15–25% haemophilia A patients following treatment (IX inhibitors are uncommon; <2%).

Transmission of HBV, HCV and HIV
Transmission high prior to the introduction of viral inactivation of concentrates (1985 in the UK).

HIV management
Prophylaxis against infections and retroviral inhibition have significantly improved prognosis.

HCV
HCV infection of most haemophiliacs treated with pooled human factor concentrates before 1985. Approximately 20% have chronic liver disease. HCV PCR is used to identify patients at higher risk of progressive liver disease. Liver biopsy is not contraindicated if haemophilia management at time of biopsy is optimal. Combined antiviral therapy superior to interferon alone.

Variant CJD
There is no evidence as yet of transmission of vCJD by pooled human blood products.

Haemophilia management
General regular medical and haemophilia review and lifelong support are essential. At presentation establish blood group, liver function and baseline viral status (HIV, HCV, HBV, HAV). Vaccinate against HBV and HAV if not immune. Regularly check inhibitor status, LFTs, FBC. Avoid aspirin, anti-platelet drugs, and IM injections. Early treatment of bleeding episodes is essential. Prophylaxis is preferable to demand treatment for many patients with severe haemophilia. Prophylaxis started in first year or two of life can prevent most if not all joint damage and almost eliminate signif-

icant bleeding. Portacath may be required to deliver prophylaxis. Factor concentrate needs to be administered every 2 or 3 days. If not on prophylaxis home demand treatment is preferable to hospital demand treatment.

Haemophilia A-specific treatment

Mild disease

- Minor bleeds may stop without factor concentrate therapy.
- Tranexamic acid (15–25mg/kg tds oral)—useful for cuts or dental extraction. Do not use when haematuria.
- DDAVP (desmopressin) for minor surgery and bleeds that fail to settle (0.3μg/kg SC or slow IVI/20 min); may also be given by nasal spray. 30 min later take blood sample to check response (if required); plasma level increased 3–4 fold. Reduced response with repeated exposure sometimes observed.
- Cryoprecipitate no longer recommended.

Severe disease

- Factor VIII concentrates are cornerstone of management for severe disease and life-threatening situations.

Products

- Recombinant products are treatment of choice. Second generation recombinants do not contain any human material in product. Human donor-derived products are now subjected to double viral inactivation (solvent-detergent and heat treatment, e.g. 80°C for 72h); good record of viral safety.

  - High and intermediate purity human donor-derived products available for patients not receiving recombinant therapy. No particular advantage for high purity over intermediate except possibly useful in patients with allergic reactions to intermediate purity. High purity previously recommended for HIV +ve patients.
  - Principle of treatment: raise factor VIII to haemostatic level (15–50u/dL for spontaneous bleeds, 40u/dL minor ops; 100u/dL major surgery or life-threatening bleeds).

Formula

1u/kg body weight raises plasma concentration by about 2u/dL. $t_{1/2}$ 6–12h. Spontaneous bleeds usually settle with single treatment if treated early. In major surgery provide cover for up to 10d.

Haemophilia B

- General approach: as for haemophilia A—DDAVP typically of no value.
- Products—recombinant factor IX treatment of choice. If not recombinant then high purity factor IX preferable to intermediate (also known as prothrombin complex concentrate) as high risk of thrombosis with intermediate purity product.

Formula

1u/kg body wt raises plasma concentration 1u/dL; $t_{1/2}$ 12–24h.

Special considerations

Antenatal diagnosis
Carriers can be identified be genetic mutation analysis. Factor VIII: vWF ratio is unreliable. Antenatal diagnosis in carriers with ♂ fetus ideally performed by chorionic villus sample DNA analysis at ~10 weeks gestation to allow termination of pregnancy; rarer nowadays because of improved treatment and prognosis. Issue is complex and counselling/testing should be at comprehensive care centre.

Home treatment has transformed the life of the haemophiliac. Parents, the local GP, the boy himself from age 6–7 onwards, can be trained to give IV factor concentrates at home. Treatment usually starts in first year or two of life and portacath may be needed until age 4 or more.

Prophylaxis—e.g. 3 × weekly injections of concentrate (average dose 15–25u/kg) given at home.

Specialist support—physiotherapy plays key role in preservation of muscle and joint function in patients with haemarthroses. Combined clinics with orthopaedic surgeons, dental surgeons, hepatologists, paediatricians, HIV physicians, and geneticists are required to give comprehensive care.

►► Do not give IM injections when factor is low.

Other congenital coagulation deficiencies

Pathophysiology

Deficiency of other coagulation factors is described but with a prevalence of 1–2 per million is rare *cf.* vWD and haemophilia A and B. Autosomal recessive inheritance, the deficiency either due to reduced synthesis (type 1) or production of a variant protein (type 2). All coagulation factors are produced in the liver and their interaction in the coagulation cascade is shown.

- The $t_{1/2}$ of the factors vary and will determine the frequency and ease of treatment.
- Factor concentrates should be considered when available, e.g. factor XI, factor XIII.
- Recombinant VIIa for factor VII deficiency. The use of recombinant factor VIIa is increasing and it is increasingly used to treat a variety of factor deficiencies and severe platelet function disorders.
- FFP can be used and virally-inactivated plasma should be used when available. FFP is a source of all coagulation factors but large volumes may be required and even with viral inactivation there is risk of disease transmission.

Diagnosis

Conditions rarely produce haemarthrosis, except factor XIII deficiency, and may only present at time of surgery. Clinical and laboratory features of the different conditions are listed.

Treatment

Many patients with inherited coagulation deficiencies will not bleed unless exposed to surgery or trauma, and may seldom require treatment. When bleeding arises or cover for surgery is needed, the aim is to achieve a plasma factor concentration at least as high as the minimal haemostatic value and make sure it does not drop below this until haemostasis is secure.

Specific conditions

Factor XI

Deficiency more common in certain ethnic groups such as Ashkenazi Jews. Clinically of variable severity, often mild; even low factor levels may not produce symptoms whilst significant bleeding can occur with mild deficiency.

Diagnosis

PT normal, APTT normal unless factor XI <40u/dL. Therefore necessary to measure factor XI level to make diagnosis in many cases.

Treatment

Tranexamic acid and DDAVP for oral and dental surgery. Factor XI concentrates sometimes available. Otherwise, use virally-inactivated FFP.

Fibrinogen

Normal range 2.0–4.0g/L. Produced by liver, it is an acute phase protein, raised in inflammatory reactions, pregnancy, stress, etc. Converted into fibrin by the action of thrombin and is a key component of a clot. Abnormalities of fibrinogen are more often acquired than inherited. Inherited defects are usually quantitative and include heterozygous hypofibrinogenaemia or homozygous afibrinogenaemia. Qualitative defects—the dysfibrinogenaemias—are inherited as incomplete autosomal dominant traits with >200 reported fibrinogen variants; defective fibrin polymerisation or fibrinopeptide release may occur. Most patients are heterozygous.

Clinical presentation

Symptoms of bruising, bleeding usually after trauma or operations will depend on the concentration and are more severe when <0.5g/L. Afibrinogenaemia (fibrinogen <0.2g/L) is a severe disorder with spontaneous bleeding, cerebral and gastrointestinal haemorrhage and haemarthrosis. It may present as haemorrhage in the newborn. Recurrent miscarriages occur. Most patients with dysfibrinogenaemia are heterozygous and bleeding symptoms are usually minor; arterial and venous thrombosis is described with some variants.

Diagnosis

↑ PT, APTT and thrombin time; in afibrinogenaemia, the blood may be unclottable. Fibrinogen level measured by Clauss assay. Acquired hypofibrinogenaemia needs to be excluded (DIC, liver disease) and family studies are necessary.

Dysfibrinogenaemia

↑ PT and APTT. Variable abnormalities of thrombin time and reptilase time; fibrinogen-dependent platelet function may be defective. Confirm diagnosis by demonstrating normal chemical/immunological fibrinogen concentrations with reduced functional properties.

Treatment

Fibrinogen has a long $t_{1/2}$ (3–5d), severe deficiency managed by repeated (twice weekly) prophylactic injections with fibrinogen concentrates, FFP or cryoprecipitate. Fibrinogen levels should be raised to 0.5–1.0g/L to achieve haemostasis.

Factor VII

Vitamin K dependent factor playing a pivotal role in initiating coagulation but low level required. The $t_{1/2}$ is short (4–6h). In severe deficiency, bleeding symptoms (similar to haemophilia) occur and spontaneous intracerebral haemorrhage at a young age has been reported.

Diagnosis

↑ PT and normal APTT. Assay factor VII to assess severity.

Treatment

Use factor VII concentrate 1u/kg body wt to elevate plasma conc ~20u/dL or recombinant factor VIIa. For cerebral bleed give a >50u/dL rise and continue treatment for 10d. Very short $t_{½}$ makes management difficult, requiring IV replacement 3–4 ×/24h. If using FFP, give initial IV injection (15mL/kg) and check response.

Other deficiencies

Factor II, V, X deficiencies very rare. Bleeding less severe with factor V deficiency than with factor X or prothrombin deficiency.

Factor XIII (fibrin stabilising factor)

Clinical

Characteristically produces delayed post-operative bleeding (6–24h later). Neonatal umbilical stump bleeding more common than with other deficiencies. High risk of cerebral haemorrhage.

Diagnosis

APTT and PT both normal so will be missed in a bleeding investigation unless specifically looked for by screening test (clot formed with thrombin and stability in acetic acid is measured).

Treatment

Only very low levels required for haemostasis; $t_{½}$ is very long. Severe deficiency should be treated with once-monthly prophylaxis with factor XIII concentrate.

Multiple defects

Rare familial coagulation factor deficiencies described; may be consanguineous parents. Often involves factor VIII and another factor (V>IX>VII). Other combinations seen.

Haemostasis and thrombosis

Vitamin K deficiency

Pathophysiology

Vitamin K (vit K) is a fat-soluble vitamin obtained either by dietary intake (vit K_1) from vegetables and liver, and absorbed in the small gut or produced by bacterial synthesis in the gut and absorbed in the colon (vit K_2). Its essential role in coagulation is as cofactor for the gamma carboxylation of the precursor proteins for factors II, VII, IX, X, protein C and S, all of which are produced in the liver. Until the routine prophylactic administration of vit K, deficiency was common in the neonate, almost exclusively a disease of breast-fed babies because ↓ vit K in human breast milk *cf.* formula feeds, and ↓ synthesis in the neonatal gut.

Clinical features

- Dietary deficiency may arise within a few weeks in patients who are not eating well since body stores are limited and the $t_{1/2}$ of the vitamin is short (days). Coagulopathy due to deficiency common in ITU patients unless vitamin K administered.
- Systemic illness, parenteral nutrition, hepatic or renal failure, hypoalbuminaemia, antibiotics (e.g. cephalosporins) are compounding factors.
- Haemorrhagic disorder of the newborn. Prematurity and maternal intake of anticonvulsants increase the incidence. Usually presents in first few days of life with bleeding (e.g. umbilical stump). Cerebral haemorrhage is rare. A late form seen 3–6 months after birth is rare may be due to liver disease, intestinal malabsorption.

Malabsorption

- Disease of the small gut (e.g. coeliac disease) may lead to clinically manifest vit K deficiency.
- Obstruction of bile flow, either extrahepatic (gallstones, Ca pancreas, or bile ducts) or intrahepatic (liver disease, liver fibrosis) may be associated with overt bleeding or noted on routine coagulation laboratory testing.

Laboratory diagnosis

- Clotting screen shows ↑ PT and APTT.
- Thrombin time and platelet count are normal.
- PT is more prolonged than APTT, and corrects with normal plasma.
- Further investigation (factor assays, PIVKA levels, vit K concentration) rarely required. A therapeutic trial of vit K will confirm diagnosis, with rapid (± 24h) PT correction.

Treatment

Asymptomatic patients—adult dose vit K 10mg IV; repeat as necessary; can be given by mouth in dietary deficiency.

Neonate prophylaxis—1mg IM 1–3 mg PO.

Bleeding patients—in addition to vit K as above, give FFP (10–20mL/kg body wt) for immediate replacement of the clotting factors. PCC (concentrate containing factors II, VII, IX and X) can be used in life-threatening situations.

Natural history

Response to treatment is good but treatment of the underlying condition is necessary to prevent recurrence.

Haemorrhagic disease of the newborn

Haemorrhagic disease of the newborn is caused by deficiency of the vitamin K dependent factors and is a significant cause of bleeding in the neonatal period unless prevented by vitamin K. Two forms described; an early classical and a late form with different aetiology

Pathophysiology

Classical haemorrhagic disease of the newborn is almost exclusively a disease of breast fed babies; incidence may be as high as 1/2500 deliveries in the UK. This is a true deficiency; human milk has less vitamin K than formula milk and there is less bacterial synthesis of vitamin K due to the sterile gut of the newborn. Immaturity of the liver and impaired production of the vitamin K factors may be a contributing factor. The late form ~40–100/million live births also is seen in breast fed babies but is mainly due to malabsorption of vitamin K, secondary to cholestasis, or GIT pathology.

Clinical features

- Early haemorrhagic disease of the newborn presents in the first week of life with bleeding—umbilical cord, the skin, post circumcision bleeding is common; ICH is rare. Presents <24h in haemorrhagic disease of the newborn 2° to maternal drug ingestion (anti-epileptic, anti-TB).
- Late haemorrhagic disease of the newborn has a peak incidence at 2–6 weeks but can occur up to 6 months of age. Underlying cholestatic disease is often present, biliary atresia, cystic fibrosis, α-1 antitrypsin deficiency and diarrhoea are documented causes. About half of cases present with ICH.

Diagnosis—laboratory findings

- PT/APTT—may be markedly prolonged (normal TT, fibrinogen, D-dimer/FDPs low *cf.* DIC).
- Factor assay (II, VII, IX, X) if in doubt. High PIVKA and low vit K—not routinely available tests.
- Correction of coagulation abnormality in ~24h with parenteral vitamin K confirms diagnosis.

Differential diagnosis

- Exclude other causes of bleeding in the neonatal period.
- Thrombocytopenia—platelets are normal in haemorrhagic disease of the newborn.
- DIC—*see below*.
- Congenital disorders e.g. haemophilia.
- Radiological—scan for ICH/internal bleeding as required.

Management

Treatment—general support as indicated by clinical presentation. FFP for immediate correction of bleeding. Vitamin K_1 1mg IV will correct PT/APTT to normal for age—takes ~24 h.

Prophylaxis—1mg at birth will prevent all early and most delayed vit K deficiency in neonate

Because of concerns of cancer risk in neonates given parenteral vitamin K some SCBU give oral vitamin K (2–3mg) to neonates at routine risk, reserving IM for high risk babies (prems/sick/maternal drugs/birth trauma/LSCS birth). Further oral vitamin K at intervals recommended for breast-fed babies, to prevent late onset HDN but is difficult to enforce.

Outcome

Treatment with FFP/vitamin K will correct the abnormal coagulation and stop bleeding. In ICH damage done to CNS leads to death or morbidity in ~⅓ cases particularly likely in late onset HDN.

von Kries, R. (1998) Neonatal vitamin K prophylaxis: the Gordian knot still awaits untying. *BMJ*, **316**, 161–162.

Liver disease

Most coagulation factors, including the vitamin K dependent factors, are made exclusively in the liver. Any damage to the liver may cause rapid reduction in their concentration and coagulopathy because of their short half-life. Associated thrombocytopenia is common in established liver disease, increasing the risk of bleeding.

Pathophysiology

Haemostasis is a fine balance between procoagulant and anticoagulant mechanisms. Because of its central role in the production of these factors, haemostasis is often disturbed in liver disease. Clotting tests become abnormal in liver damage and are useful monitors of liver function. The liver functions as a reticuloendothelial organ, clearing activated coagulation factors from the circulation. Impairment of this function leads to the scene for DIC which is usually low grade but may be fulminant. Fibrinolysis may be decreased in chronic liver disease but is high in liver transplant patients. Dysfibrinogenaemia due to increased sialic acid content of the fibrinogen molecule is described. In obstructive jaundice, impaired bile flow leads to malabsorption of vit K, a fat soluble vitamin. A degree of intrahepatic obstruction secondary to hepatocyte swelling and fibrosis may also have this effect. Thrombocytopenia may be due to portal hypertension, splenic pooling, alcohol, viral infection, drugs or DIC. Altered platelet function with a prolonged bleeding time may occur.

Clinical features

Most patients with established hepatic dysfunction will have an abnormal coagulation profile but may be asymptomatic. Bleeding becomes a problem when other complications arise such as oesophageal varices, thrombocytopenia, surgery, liver biopsy and infection.

Laboratory diagnosis

Coagulation defect	Laboratory diagnosis	Clinical significance
↓ vit K dependent factors	↑PT>>↑APTT	
Fibrinogen		
quantitative defect	Fibrinogen assay	↑ infection, neoplasm, obstruction ↓ severe liver disease
dysfibrinogenaemia	↑ thrombin/reptilase time	uncertain; occurs in cirrhosis
Factor VIII	↑, also vWF Ag	seen in acute viral hepatitis cirrhosis, hepatic failure
Antithrombin	↓ conc (N=80–120iu/dL)	↓ CLD and liver failure
DIC	↑ PT, APTT , F/XDPs ↓ fibrinogen, platelets	low grade common in CLD rarely fulminant

N = normal

Management

Asymptomatic patients do not require treatment other than that directed at the underlying condition. Give vit K to exclude added vit K deficiency. Complete correction of the PT confirms this diagnosis; partial correction indicates combined hepatocellular dysfunction and vit K deficiency. Further doses of vit K for 1–2d may be given.

Liver biopsy—aim to get the INR <1.4 and platelet count >70 × 10^9/L. Check on day of biopsy. Give FFP 10mL/kg ; check INR and repeat FFP dose until PT is satisfactory—not always achieved. PCC contraindicated as may cause DIC and/or thrombosis. Platelet transfusion to 4 platelets to >70 × 10^9/L if necessary.

Active bleeding—blood transfusion as required. Give vit K, FFP, platelets as set out for liver biopsy and monitor the response. FFP only temporary correction; repeat 6–12 hourly as indicated. Surgical manoeuvres to control oesophageal bleeding (Sengstaken tube, etc.) will be explored. DIC is a feature of fulminant liver failure and after liver surgery and transplantation. Control underlying condition, support with platelet/FFP as required. The use of aprotinin, tranexamic acid, AT concentrates, and heparin has varying success.

Natural history

In fulminant liver failure the coagulopathy may be severe contributing to the mortality. The degree of the hepatocellular failure will be the final denominator determining the outcome.

Acquired anticoagulants

The development of inhibitors against coagulation factors is fortunately uncommon other than antiphospholipid antibodies (📖 *p400*). Factor VIII antibodies, either spontaneous or in treated haemophiliacs, are a major clinical problem. Acquired vWD, inhibitors against other coagulation factors and heparin-like inhibitors are all very rare.

Factor VIII inhibitors

Pathophysiology

Spontaneous development of VIII inhibitors in non-haemophiliacs is reported in 1 per million population. Antibody is usually IgG, occasionally IgM or IgA and will neutralise the functional VIII protein. In 15–25% of haemophilic patients antibodies develop as a result of treatment with factor VIII concentrates usually within the first 10–20 treatment exposures. A familial tendency is noted, inhibitors occurring more often in patients with deletions or mutations within factor VIII gene. The antibody acts against part of the amino-terminal component of the A2 domain or the carboxy-terminal part of the C2 domain of the VIII molecule. It may be quantitated by the Bethesda titre (BU; *see below*). Factor IX very rarely (<2%) stimulates antibody formation.

Clinical features

Acquired inhibitors develop in the elderly, during pregnancy, in association with autoimmune and malignant disease, various skin disorders (psoriasis, pemphigus, erythema multiforme) infections, drug therapy (penicillin, aminoglycosides, phenothiazines, etc). Symptoms include bleeding (post-operatively this can cause major problems), easy bruising—haemarthrosis is rare. The mortality is significant, as many as 25% patients with persisting VIII inhibitors will die from bleeding.

15–25% of haemophilia A patients develop inhibitors. In half, inhibitors are transient and low titre, being noted incidentally on review. In half, however, an VIII inhibitor will present a major clinical problem. Suspicion is aroused by bleeding that fails to respond to the usual doses of factor concentrate. Patients may be low (<5BU) or high (>10BU) responders; in the latter, treatment will be difficult.

Laboratory diagnosis

- ↑ APTT with failure to correct with normal plasma.
- Inhibitor assay—patient's plasma reducing the factor VIII in normal plasma over 2h incubation period. Antibody titres reported in BU (Bethesda units). Check titre against porcine VIII as porcine VIII is often an effective treatment.

Differential diagnosis of spontaneous inhibitors—need to exclude non-specific inhibitors e.g. myeloma paraproteins which bind non-specifically to coagulation plasma proteins. Ensure sample not contaminated with heparin.

Management of patients with spontaneous inhibitor

- Severe bleeding—may be life threatening. Suppress inhibitor with prednisolone (1mg/kg/d); may take weeks to work, cyclophosphamide can be added. Treat active bleeding. If no cross-reactivity porcine VIII concentrates can be used if available (50–150u/kg). FEIBA and recombinant VIIa are also effective as 'bypassing agents'.
- Mild bleeding—may respond local pressure, tranexamic acid or DDAVP (📖 *p354*).
- Monitor lab and clinical response.
- Long term immunosuppression may be required.

Management of haemophilic patients with inhibitor

- Asymptomatic patients—observation may be all that is necessary. The inhibitor level may gradually subside; avoid treatment with concentrates to limit exposure to the antigen.
- Mild bleeding—in low responder/low titre patients large (20–100u/kg) doses of human factor VIII are usually effective. If activity against porcine VIII < human VIII this can be more effective.
- High responders/high titre patients—will require bypassing agents such as recombinant factor VIIa or FEIBA.
- Immune tolerance induction—overcomes the VIII inhibitor in about 80% selected patients.
- High responders—need high intensity immune tolerance regimes which may take up to 18 months to work (expensive and may fail to work).

Acquired vWD

Rare disorder presenting in later life, has a variable bleeding pattern similar to the inherited condition. An associated monoclonal gammopathy/lymphoproliferative disorder is common but the condition may be autoimmune or idiopathic. Bleeding symptoms vary from mild to major e.g. catastrophic GI haemorrhage requiring frequent blood transfusion.

Laboratory diagnosis

As type 1 congenital vWD: PT normal; ↓ VIIIC, ↓ vWF antigen, ↓ vWF activity. *In vitro* evidence of the vWF inhibitor not always demonstrable.

Management

High dose immunoglobulin is often effective (1g/kg/day for 2d). Measures used in the treatment of the hereditary condition can be used (DDAVP, vWF-containing factor VIII concentrate e.g. BPL 8Y, Haemate-P, Alphanate) are effective. maintenance IVIg may have a role. Platelet transfusions may help.

Other coagulation inhibitors

Factor IX inhibitors are much less common (<2%) in patients with haemophilia B than A and this is true also of the spontaneously developing IX inhibitors. Immune tolerance with high doses of factor IX concentrate is complicated by hypersensitivity reactions and nephrotic syndrome. Recombinant VIIa is effective for bleeding episodes.

Inhibitors, spontaneous or post-treatment, are reported against most other coagulation factors (V, XI and XII, Prothrombin, XI, VII and X); all are very rare. Factor V antibodies may arise in congenitally deficient patients following treatment or spontaneously following antibiotics, infection, blood transfusion. Post-operative cases may develop as a result of exposure to haemostatic agents contaminated with bovine factor V, e.g. fibrin glue. Most are low titre and transient. Treat with FFP and platelets (a source of factor V).

Heparin-like inhibitors are reported in patients with malignant disease, following chemotherapy (e.g. suramin, mithromycin) and may cause bleeding. Protamine sulphate neutralisation *in vitro* and *in vivo* is a feature of this inhibitor.

Diagnosis

Screening tests (PT, APTT, thrombin time) will give abnormal results depending on the factor involved, with failure to correct with normal plasma. Defining the specific factor requires detailed laboratory workup. Exclude acquired deficiencies e.g. factor X deficiency in amyloidosis.

Treatment

Reserved for actively bleeding patients since acquired inhibitors may not give rise to symptoms. First line treatment is often FFP but large volumes may be required and efficacy may be limited. Some specific concentrates are available. Recombinant VIIa can be considered in many cases. Treatment of the underlying condition may cause the inhibitor to disappear.

Hay, C.R. *et al.* (1996) Recommendations for the treatment of factor VIII inhibitors: from the UK Haemophilia Centre Directors' Organisation Inhibitor Working Party. *Blood Coagul Fibrinolysis*, **7**, 134–138.

Haemostasis and thrombosis

Platelet function tests

Platelets play an essential role in arresting bleeding. Following vascular injury they adhere to subendothelial collagen via the ligand vWF, then stick to each other to form a cohesive mass. Release of internal factors—serotonin, ADP, TXA2, and platelet factor 4 (PF4) induces vascular constriction, and coagulation cascade activation. Finally, together with fibrin they form a thrombus, plugging the hole in the vessel. Within the platelet prostaglandin synthetic pathway, arachidonic acid forms thromboxane A2, a potent platelet aggregant and vasoconstrictor. From platelet activation cessation of bleeding takes 3–5 minutes.

Tests of function

Blood collection needs to be optimal with non-traumatic venepuncture, rapid transport to the lab with storage at room temperature and testing within a maximum of 6h.

Tests in use

Platelet count, morphology, aggregation, and function at high shear rate.

Platelet count

Normal range 150–450 × 10^9/L. Adequate function is maintained even when the count is <⅓ normal level, but progressively deteriorates as it drops. With platelet counts <20 × 10^9/L there is usually easy bruising, petechial haemorrhages (although more serious bleeding can occur).

Morphology

Large platelets are often biochemically more active; high mean platelet volume is associated with less bleeding in patients with severe thrombocytopenia. Reticulated platelets can be counted by new analysers and may prove to be useful in assessing platelet regeneration. Altered platelet size is seen in inherited platelet disorders.

Platelet adhesion

Rarely performed in routine lab practice.

Platelet aggregation

Performed on fresh sample using aggregometer but poor correlation with bleeding tendency except in specific circumstances, e.g. Glanzmann's thrombasthenia, Bernard–Soulier syndrome.

Aggregants

- Adenosine 5-diphosphate (ADP) at low and high concentrations. Induces 2 aggregation waves: primary wave may disaggregate at low conc. ADP; the second is irreversible.
- Collagen has a short lag phase followed by a single wave and is particularly affected by aspirin.
- Ristocetin induced platelet aggregation (RIPA) is carried out at a high (1.2mg/mL) and lower concentrations (0.5mg/dL)and is mainly used to diagnose type 2B vWD.
- Arachidonic acid.
- Adrenaline, not uncommonly reduced in normal people.

For aggregation patterns in the various platelet disorders 📖 p372.

PFA-100
This is an automated machine that measures the ability of platelets to close an aperture at high shear rate. Reproducible on sample with minimal manipulation. Increasingly replacing bleeding time in laboratory practice.

Platelet release
ELISA or RIA are used to measure the a granule proteins β-thromboglobulin (β-TG) and platelet factor 4 (PF4). These are beyond the scope of the routine laboratory.

Practical application of the tests
Main role is in diagnosis of inherited platelet functional defects (📖 *p372*). In acquired platelet dysfunction secondary to causes such renal and hepatic disease, DIC, macroglobulinaemia, platelet function is rarely tested.

Drug induced thrombopathy
Many drugs e.g. aspirin, NSAIDs, corticosteroids, antiplatelet drugs (e.g. dipyridamole), antibiotics (penicillin, cephalosporins), membrane stabilising agents (β-blockers), antihistamines, tricyclic antidepressants, α antagonists, miscellaneous agents (e.g. heparin, alcohol, dextran) may affect platelet function but tests are rarely performed.

Hereditary platelet disorders

All rare. Acquired platelet dysfunction is much more likely to be a cause of bleeding or easy bruising. Two main hereditary qualitative defects are found

1. Defective platelet membrane glycoproteins (GPs). GPIIb/IIIa is a receptor for fibrinogen and other adhesive GPs; also affected is GPIb (specific platelet receptor for vWF). Disorders include Glanzmann's thrombasthenia (abnormal GPIIb/IIIa) and Bernard–Soulier syndrome (BSS)—abnormal GPIb, a specific receptor for vWF with defective adhesion to blood vessels.
2. Abnormalities of platelet granules ie storage pool deficiency (SPD). Either the alpha (α) granules (grey platelet syndrome), the dense granules (May–Hegglin anomaly, Hermansky–Pudlak syndrome, Chediak–Higashi syndrome and the thrombocytopenia-absent radius (TAR) syndrome), or both.

Clinical features

Presenting symptoms of inherited platelet dysfunction: mucocutaneous bleeding (skin, nose, gums, gut) with a positive family history (though not always found). All autosomal recessive. Clinically the bleeding symptoms are similar but may be other clinical features to distinguish the syndromes. Carriers asymptomatic. Menorrhagia may be troublesome. Symptoms may suggest the diagnosis of non-accidental injury in young children. Bleeding in Glanzmann's may be severe and life threatening.

Laboratory findings

- Normal platelet count and size (except for BSS where platelets large and count ↓).
- Abnormal PFA-100. Abnormal platelet aggregation with common aggregants (*see table*).
- Occasionally aggregation is normal.
- Consider aspirin and vWD in the differential diagnosis.

Condition	Platelet		Aggregation with		
	Count	Size	ADP	Collagen	Ristocetin
Thrombasthenia	N	N	absent	absent	N
Bernard–Soulier	L	↑	N	N	Absent
Storage pool disease	N	N	N/abnormal	N/abnormal	N/abnormal
Aspirin ingestion	N	N	N/abnormal	abnormal	N/abnormal
von Willebrand's	N	N	N	N	N/abnormal

N = normal; L = low

Defining abnormality in Glanzmann's thrombasthenia is absent aggregation to both low and high dose ADP and confirmation of membrane defect by flow cytometry with monoclonal antibodies to GPIIbIIIa. Similarly in BSS absent aggregation with ristocetin and confirmation by flow cytometry and monoclonal antibodies to GPIb. In the grey platelet syndrome, the platelet count is often low and the platelets pale, grey and larger than normal.

Treatment

1. Avoid antiplatelet drugs. Use pressure to control bleeding from minor cuts.
2. DDAVP.
3. Tranexamic acid (TXA, 25mg/kg body wt) 8hrly for 7–10d for minor surgery and dental work. TXA mouthwash useful to reduce bleeding from dental work.
4. Platelet transfusions are effective in major surgery and severe bleeding.
5. Recombinant VIIa considered for severe defects, e.g. Glanzmann's.

Osler–Weber–Rendu (OWR) syndrome

Definition

Autosomal dominantly inherited disorder characterised by multiple skin telangiectases. Also known as hereditary haemorrhagic telangiectasia. The basic pathology is a developmental structural abnormality of blood vessels. This results in dilatation and convolution of the venules and capillaries which may be present throughout the body. Theses telangiectases are thin-walled and likely to bleed giving rise to recurrent haemorrhage and anaemia.

Incidence

Rare. ♂ = ♀.

Clinical features

- Presentation may not be until later life.
- Facial and buccal mucosa and nail fold telangiectases.
- Iron deficiency common as a result of bleeding from GIT telangiectases.
- Epistaxis—commonest presenting symptom.
- Menorrhagia.
- Prolonged bleeding after dental surgery.

Diagnosis and investigation

- Recognition of typical telangiectases and family history.
- Beware, another cause of bleeding may co-exist in a OWR patient.
- FBC and film may show iron deficient picture, i.e. microcytic, hypochromic anaemia, ↓ MCV, raised platelets. ↓ serum ferritin.
- Angiography of mesenteric circulation in recurrent bleeding.
- ENT examination.
- CT scan to identify pulmonary AV malformations or desaturation on exercise.

Treatment

- Antibiotics for surgical/dental procedures as risk of cerebral abscess due to bacteraemia and shunting in lungs.
- Observation for iron deficiency.
- Iron replacement therapy.
- Consider interventional procedure e.g. embolisation (if angiography +ve).
- Oestrogen reduces frequency of bleeding episodes.

Prognosis

Generally a benign chronic disorder provided follow-up as above.

Haemostasis and thrombosis

Henoch–Schönlein purpura

Definition

An immune complex disease characterised by a leucocytoclastic vasculitis. Purpura is not of haematological origin.

Incidence and epidemiology

Predominantly affects children aged 2–8 years. Clear preponderance in the winter. Commonly presents 1–3 weeks after upper respiratory tract illness. Various infections, toxins, physical trauma and possibly insect bites, and allergies have all been postulated as triggers of the disease but no clear causation established. May also occur with malignancy.

Clinical features

- Rapid onset usual.
- Classically a palpable purpuric rash over buttocks/legs (extensor surfaces).
- Urticarial plaques and haemorrhagic bullae seen, often bizarrely symmetrical.
- Abdominal pain ?due to mesenteric vasculitis.
- Arthritis, particularly knees and ankles.
- Renal involvement—haematuria ± proteinuria, may lead to either acute or chronic renal failure.

Diagnosis and investigations

- Made by the presence of typical findings above and exclusion of other causes.
- FBC and film normal. Platelet numbers and function are normal. The purpura is not of haematological origin. ESR usually raised.
- Other markers of autoimmune disorders may be present.

Treatment and prognosis

- Spontaneous resolution within a month is commonest outcome in children.
- Long-term sequelae more common in adults e.g. chronic renal failure.
- Steroids may be of benefit particularly if joint pains are troublesome.

Haemostasis and thrombosis

Acquired disorders of platelet function

Acquired disorders may affect platelet–vessel wall interaction and are among the most common causes of a haemorrhagic tendency. These conditions may be associated with a prolonged bleeding time, abnormal platelet aggregation studies and clinical bleeding or bruising.

Drugs that induce platelet dysfunction

- Aspirin.
- NSAIDs.
- β-lactam antibiotics: penicillins and cephalosporins.
- 'Antiplatelet agents': prostacyclin, dipyridamole.
- Heparin.
- Plasma expanders: dextran, hydroxyethyl starch.
- Other drugs: antihistamines, local anaesthetics, β-blockers.
- Food additives: fish oil.

Systemic conditions which affect platelet function

- Renal failure.
- Liver failure.
- Glycogen storage disorders types Ia and Ib.

Conditions causing platelet exhaustion

- Cardiopulmonary bypass surgery.
- DIC.
- Others: valvular heart disease, renal allograft rejection, cavernous haemangioma.

Dysproteinaemias and antiplatelet antibodies

- Multiple myeloma.
- Waldenström's macroglobulinaemia.
- Autoimmune disorders.

Haematological conditions with production of abnormal platelets

- Chronic myeloproliferative disorders.
- Myelodysplasia.
- Leukaemia.

Drugs

Wide range of drugs reported to impair platelet function (most commonly implicated drugs are listed).

Aspirin is commonest cause of clinically significant bleeding, due to irreversible acetylation and inhibition of cyclooxygenase which interferes with formation of thromboxane A2 in the platelet prostaglandin pathway. Effect on bleeding time occurs within 2h of ingestion of 75mg. Aspirin effect may last up to 10d after long term use. Greater effect on clinical bleeding seen in patients who already have bleeding tendency. Laboratory effects on a normal individual is usually mild and there is marked individual variation in the risk of bleeding.

Effects of aspirin

- Easy bruising, epistaxis, haematomas, haemorrhage after surgery especially in patients with a pre-existing bleeding tendency.

- Prolonged bleeding time/abnormal PFA-100.
- Inhibition of platelet release reaction and second wave of platelet aggregation to low concentrations of ADP and collagen.

NSAIDs cause reversible inhibition of cyclooxygenase. Effect on bleeding and platelet aggregation is brief (only as long as circulating drug present) and less likely to cause clinical bleeding in patients without a prior bleeding disorder. *β-lactam antibiotics* affect platelet function by lipophilic attachment to cell membrane in dose-dependent manner. Do so only after sustained high dosage though effect may last 7–10d after discontinuation. Antiplatelet agents, prostacyclin and dipyridamole high cAMP concentration in platelets and inhibit platelet aggregation with little/no effect on bleeding time. A diet rich in *fish oils* (omega-3 fatty acids) can cause mild prolongation of bleeding time. *Ethanol* ingestion can impair *in vitro* platelet function.

Aspirin should be avoided in patients with bleeding tendency. A patient on aspirin should discontinue the drug at least a week prior to a surgical procedure. DDAVP or platelet transfusion should be administered to a patient with severe haemorrhage due to aspirin-induced platelet function defect. In cases with less severe bleeding, discontinuation of the suspected drug is usually effective.

Renal failure—clinical bleeding occurs in patients with uraemia due to chronic renal failure—the former correlates with the severity of the uraemia. Bleeding time does not predict risk of haemorrhage and is not indicated. PFA-100 requires evaluation as a predictor of risk of bleeding in this situation. Associated anaemia also contributes to prolongation of bleeding and correction of anaemia improves the abnormality. Abnormalities of platelet aggregation studies are seen frequently. If haemorrhage occurs in a patient with chronic renal failure, other causes should be excluded before it is attributed to uraemia. Dialysis is mainstay of treatment. DDAVP useful. Conjugated oestrogens improve platelet function.

Liver failure—chronic liver disease, most notably cirrhosis, may be associated with platelet function defects which may be due to abnormalities in the platelet membrane glycoproteins. Abnormalities in bleeding time and platelet aggregation studies may be improved by DDAVP. Haemorrhage in a patient with liver disease is usually multifactorial including decreased levels of coagulation factors, dysfibrinogenaemia, thrombocytopenia due to splenic pooling and DIC.

Conditions causing platelet exhaustion—a number of conditions have been associated with platelet exhaustion (acquired storage pool defect) in which there is laboratory evidence of *in vivo* platelet activation and decreased platelet aggregation in the pattern of a storage pool defect.

- Cardiopulmonary bypass surgery.
- DIC.
- Valvular heart disease.

- Renal allograft rejection.
- Cavernous haemangioma.
- Aortic aneurysm.
- Transfusion reaction.
- TTP and HUS.

Cardiopulmonary bypass surgery—abnormal platelet function and thrombocytopenia are frequently seen in patients subjected to cardiopulmonary bypass surgery. Impaired aggregation studies *in vitro* occur in proportion to duration of the bypass procedure. Believed due to platelet activation and fragmentation in the extracorporeal loop. Platelet transfusion is required in patients with a prolonged bleeding time and excessive haemorrhage after cardiopulmonary bypass surgery.

DIC—platelet exhaustion due to an acquired storage pool defect may occur in DIC due to *in vivo* platelet stimulation and this may cause abnormal platelet aggregation in *in vitro* tests. However, haemorrhage in DIC is multifactorial (📖 *p512*).

Dysproteinaemias—binding of M-proteins to platelet cell membranes in myeloma (particularly IgA) or Waldenström's macroglobulinaemia may result in acquired platelet function defects and less commonly clinical bleeding. Severity of platelet function defect correlates with M-protein concentration. *Note*: haemorrhage is more commonly due to thrombocytopenia or hyperviscosity. Plasmapheresis to remove circulating M-protein may be necessary in bleeding patient in whom the M-protein may be contributory factor through hyperviscosity or impairment of platelet function.

Antiplatelet antibodies—impaired platelet function may be a rare consequence of binding of IgM or IgG molecules to platelet membrane in ITP, SLE and platelet alloimmunisation where the most common result is accelerated platelet destruction and thrombocytopenia. May result in haemorrhagic manifestations at unexpectedly high platelet counts, and in longer than expected bleeding time. If bleeding occurs treatment is that of ITP (📖 *p388*).

Haematological disorders

Myeloproliferative disorders—qualitative platelet disorders occur in association with a prolonged bleeding time and clinical bleeding in MPD. Includes abnormal morphology with decreased granules, acquired storage pool defects, abnormalities of platelet glycoproteins, receptors and arachidonic acid metabolism. Haemorrhage (mucocutaneous) and thrombosis can occur in the same patient. Neither platelet function tests nor degree of thrombocytosis correlates well with risks of bleeding or thrombosis. An increased whole blood viscosity in patients with polycythaemia is clearly related to risk of haemorrhage. There is evidence that that lowering an elevated platelet count to $<600 \times 10^9$/L is associated with a reduced risk of thrombosis. Hydroxyurea is effective. The role of anagrelide is not yet clear. In patients with polycythaemia rubra vera the haematocrit should be kept below 0.44 (♀) or 0.47 (♂). (📖 *p243*).

Myelodysplasia and leukaemia—abnormalities of platelet morphology and *in vitro* aggregation occur in these disorders but haemorrhagic problems are commonly due to thrombocytopenia.

Haemostasis and thrombosis

Numerical abnormalities of platelets—*thrombocytosis*

Defined as platelet count >450 × 10^9/L. May be secondary (or reactive) to another pathological process or it may be due to a myeloproliferative disorder. In MPD it may be associated not only with an increased risk of thrombosis but also with an increased risk of haemorrhage.

Causes of reactive thrombocytosis

- Haemorrhage.
- Surgery.
- Trauma.
- Iron deficiency (📖 *p56*).
- Splenectomy (📖 *p582*).
- Infection.
- Malignant disease.
- Inflammatory disorders (rheumatoid arthritis, inflammatory bowel disease).

Myeloproliferative disorders associated with thrombocytosis

- Primary (essential) thrombocythaemia (📖 *p250*).
- Primary proliferative polycythaemia (polycythaemia rubra vera, 📖 *p240*).
- Chronic myeloid leukaemia (📖 *p164*).
- Idiopathic myelofibrosis (📖 *p256*).

Management

See relevant sections.

Haemostasis and thrombosis

Numerical abnormalities of platelets—*thrombocytopenia*

Defines a platelet count <150 × 10^9/L. May be due either to decreased bone marrow production of platelets or to increased destruction or sequestration of platelets from the circulation (or both). Platelet counts >100 × 10^9/L are not usually associated with any haemorrhagic problems. Purpura, easy bruising and prolonged post-traumatic bleeding are increasingly common as the platelet count falls <50 × 10^9/L. Although there is no platelet count at which a patient definitely will or will not experience spontaneous haemorrhage the risk is greater in patients with a platelet count <20 × 10^9/L and increases further in those with a count <10 × 10^9/L.

Causes of decreased bone marrow production of platelets

- Marrow failure: aplastic anaemia (📖 *p122*).
- Marrow infiltration: leukaemias, myelodysplasia, myeloma, myelofibrosis, lymphoma, metastatic carcinoma.
- Marrow suppression: cytotoxic drugs and radiotherapy, other drugs (e.g. chloramphenicol).
- Selective megakaryocytic: ethanol, drugs (phenylbutazone, co-trimoxazole; penicillamine), chemicals, viral infection (e.g. HIV, parvovirus).

- Nutritional deficiency: megaloblastic anaemia (📖 *p60–62*).
- Hereditary causes (rare): Fanconi's syndrome (📖 *p456*), congenital megakaryocytic hypoplasia, absent radii (TAR) syndrome.

Causes of increased destruction of platelets

Immune

- ITP (📖 *p388*).
- Associated with other autoimmune states SLE, CLL, lymphoma (📖 *p392*).
- Drug-induced: heparin, gold, quinidine, quinine, penicillins, cimetidine, digoxin.
- Infection: HIV, other viruses, malaria.
- Post-transfusion purpura (📖 *p506*).
- Neonatal alloimmune thrombocytopenia (NAIT, 📖 *p448*).

Non-immune

- DIC (📖 *p512*).
- TTP/HUS (📖 *p530*).
- Kasabach–Merritt syndrome.
- Congenital/acquired heart disease.
- Cardiopulmonary bypass (📖 *p378*).

Causes of platelet sequestration

- Hypersplenism (📖 *p392*).

Causes of dilutional loss of platelets

- Massive transfusion (📖 *p524*).
- Exchange transfusion.

Hereditary thrombocytopenia

- Wiskott–Aldrich syndrome, May–Hegglin anomaly, Bernard–Soulier syndrome.

Investigation of thrombocytopenia

- History—drugs, symptoms of viral illness.
- Examination—signs of infection, lymphadenopathy, hepatosplenomegaly.
- FBC—isolated thrombocytopenia or associated disorders.
- Blood film—red cell fragmentation (DIC), WBC differential (atypical lymphocytes/blasts), platelet size (large in ITP and some hereditary conditions), platelet clumps (pseudothrombocytopenia).
- Serology—antinuclear antibody, DAT, monospot, antiplatelet antibodies (unreliable), platelet-associated antibodies (unreliable), HIV serology.
- Routine chemistry—renal disease, hepatic disease.
- BM examination—megakaryocyte numbers, marrow disease or infiltration.

Thrombocytopenia due to decreased platelet production

Diagnosis is confirmed on bone marrow examination, and management is essentially that of the underlying condition. Platelet transfusion may be necessary for the treatment of haemorrhage in patients with bone marrow failure and prophylactic platelet transfusion may be necessary if persistent severe thrombocytopenia ($<10 \times 10^9$/L) occurs.

Haemostasis and thrombosis

Immune thrombocytopenia

These conditions are due to IgG and IgM antibodies which react with antigenic sites (usually GPIIb/IIIa in ITP, platelet alloantigens in post-transfusion purpura and neonatal isoimmune purpura) on the platelet cell membrane, may fix complement and cause accelerated platelet destruction through phagocytosis by reticulo-endothelial cells in liver and spleen. A compensatory increase in bone marrow megakaryocytopoiesis usually occurs which may occasionally prevent or delay the development of severe thrombocytopenia.

ITP

Usually presents with haemorrhagic manifestations, purpura, epistaxis, menorrhagia or bleeding gums but may occasionally be detected in an asymptomatic adult patient on a routine blood test. Intracranial bleeds occur in <1% (associated with platelet count $<10 \times 10^9$/L). Commonest in young adults (♀>♂). The natural history of childhood cases is acute in 90% and usually follows a self-limiting course without treatment. They are often associated with a history of previous viral illness and complete resolution may be expected within 3 months. In adults a chronic course is usual and spontaneous resolution is rare (<5%).

Diagnosis

The platelet count may be $<5–100 \times 10^9$/L. Platelet size often ↑ on the blood film, reflected in ↑ MPV; represents production of young platelets by the reactive bone marrow. Diagnosis of ITP is confirmed by exclusion of a secondary (other autoimmune or drug-induced cause) or hereditary cause of thrombocytopenia in a patient with a normal physical examination, no splenomegaly and normal bone marrow examination. The demonstration of platelet antibodies or increased platelet associated Ig may be confirmatory but neither positive nor negative results are definitive. A small proportion of patients have associated DAT +ve AIHA (Evans' syndrome), most of whom have an underlying disorder (CLL, lymphoma, SLE).

Treatment of ITP

No need to treat mild compensated ITP ($>30 \times 10^9$/L) unless haemorrhagic manifestations. Keep under regular review and advise urgent FBC if haemorrhagic manifestations. Most children do not require treatment—but those in whom chronic ITP develops are treated in the same way as adults. 90% of children eventually recover completely. Aim of therapy of adult ITP is to achieve an improved (preferably normal) platelet count without need for long term maintenance therapy.

Prednisolone

- First-line therapy for most patients.
- Probably ↓ platelet antibody production and interferes with phagocytosis.
- Dose is 1mg/kg/d PO, maintained for at 2 weeks.
- Up to 75% patients will respond but only 15% CR. *Note*: magnitude and speed of response correlates with long term prognosis.
- Once patient has responded, taper prednisolone dose over several months.

- Some patients will maintain an adequate platelet count (>30 × 10^9/L) on discontinuation of steroids or on a low maintenance dose.
- Most adults relapse on tapering the prednisolone dose and require other therapy.

IVIg
- Action: blockade of phagocytes and possible anti-idiotype effect.
- Most ITP patients will have significant platelet rise following administration of 2g/kg over 5d.
- Effect often rapid (within 4d) but usually transient and lasts ~3 weeks (may be prolonged in a minority).
- Increment may be maintained with boosters of 0.4g–1g/kg.
- Relatively non-toxic but expensive.
- Useful in patients
  - refractory to other treatments.
  - who require an urgent increment for surgery and in pregnancy.

Splenectomy
- The only proven curative therapy for ITP (spleen is major site of platelet destruction). Usual pre- and post-splenectomy care (📖 *p582*).
- Indium labelled platelet scan appears to be the only test able to predict those patients who will benefit.
- Consider for patients
  - who fail to respond to prednisolone.
  - requiring prednisolone >10mg/d to maintain acceptable platelet count.
  - who have unacceptable side effects with lower maintenance dose.
- 60–80% of patients achieve at least a partial response to splenectomy.
- A brisk rise in platelet count in the immediate post-operative period is a good prognostic sign.

Immunosuppressive agents
- Act through inhibition of antibody production.
- Effect takes at least 2 weeks (may be up to 3 months).
- May be useful in patients
  - who have failed to achieve an adequate response to splenectomy.
  - in whom splenectomy is contraindicated.
  - in whom an unacceptably high dose of prednisolone is necessary to maintain a 'safe' platelet count.
- Effective in up to 25% refractory patients.
- Azathioprine is the most widely used agent in the UK (max 150mg/d). (maintain neutrophil count >1.0 × 10^9/L and platelet count >30 × 10^9/L.
- May be used with prednisolone to obtain an acceptable platelet count and minimise the toxicity of each agent.
- Cyclophosphamide and vincristine are alternatives.
- Long term therapy carries risk of serious toxicity including MDS and 2° leukaemias with azathioprine and cyclophosphamide.

Danazol

- Effective in ITP.
- Better for elderly (don't use in young ♀).
- May be used as alternative to prednisolone or in combination.
- Normal dose 400–800mg/d for 1–3 months tapering to 50–200mg/d.
- Side effects: virilisation, weight gain and hepatotoxicity.

Other treatments

Intravenous anti-D

- Will produce platelet increment in Rh(D) +ve non-splenectomized patients.
- Role in the management of children with chronic ITP and HIV-infected patients.
- Mode of action is reticuloendothelial blockade.

High dose dexamethasone

- E.g. dexamethasone 20–40mg/d PO for 4 days; repeated 4-weekly.
- May produce a response (less good in patients who have failed splenectomy).

BCSH Guidelines: Investigation and management of ITP in adults, children and in pregnancy can be found at www.bcshguidelines.com/pdf/BJH574.pdf

Haemostasis and thrombosis

Other causes of thrombocytopenia

Gestational thrombocytopenia

Benign thrombocytopenia (platelets >80 × 10^9/L) occurs in 5% of pregnancies. No treatment is indicated

ITP in pregnancy

Fetal thrombocytopenia may occur due to placental transfer of IgG antiplatelet antibodies in a pregnant woman with ITP. Risk of intracranial haemorrhage in fetus during delivery is low although thrombocytopenia <50 × 10^9/L may occur in the fetus in up to 30% of pregnancies in women with previously diagnosed ITP. No good predictor for fetal thrombocytopenia. *Differential diagnosis*: gestational thrombocytopenia (common); count rarely <70 × 10^9/L. Neonatal count normal. Other causes include pre-eclampsia. Treatment with prednisolone, or IVIg should be administered to the mother with thrombocytopenia severe enough to constitute a haemorrhagic risk to her. Avoid splenectomy—high rate of fetal loss. Severe maternal haemorrhage at delivery is rare but may require platelet transfusion, IVIg and possibly splenectomy. Special antenatal treatment of the fetus is unnecessary but avoid prolonged and complicated labour. Ensure paediatric support at delivery and check neonatal platelet count – monitor for several days (delayed thrombocytopenia). IVIg, prednisolone or exchange transfusion may be required.

Other autoimmune thrombocytopenias

E.g. 2° to SLE and lymphoproliferative disorders (esp. low grade NHL and CLL). May present with isolated thrombocytopenia and underlying disorder may only be discovered on further investigation. Often refractory to therapy. Those with lymphoproliferative disorders will require chemotherapy for that condition.

Neonatal alloimmune thrombocytopenia (📖 *p448*)

Post-transfusion purpura (📖 *p506*)

Rare but life threatening. Causes severe haemorrhage due to thrombocytopenia ~1 week after transfusion of blood or blood products. Thrombocytopenia may persist for several days. Occurs most commonly in ♀ and is usually due to antibody to the platelet antigen HPA-1a in an individual lacking this (2% of population) who has been previously sensitised (usually by pregnancy).

Hypersplenism

Thrombocytopenia primarily due to platelet pooling in enlarged spleen. If haemorrhagic complications, consider splenectomy if the underlying cause is unknown or if treatment of underlying disorder has been ineffective.

Non-immune thrombocytopenia due to increased destruction

If haemorrhage occurs platelet transfusion is necessary. Patients with platelet counts >50 × 10^9/L may respond to DDAVP.

Drug-induced thrombocytopenia

Many drugs implicated in idiosyncratic thrombocytopenia, largely through increased destruction—usually immune mechanism. In most cases the patient has been using the drug for several weeks/months and thrombocytopenia is severe (<20 × 10^9/L). Most commonly implicated are heparin, quinine, quinidine, gold, sulphonamides, trimethoprim, penicillins, cephalosporins, cimetidine, ranitidine, diazepam, sodium valproate, phenacetin, rifampicin, PAS, thiazides, (furosemide), chlorpropamide, tolbutamide, digoxin, methyldopa. If drug-induced thrombocytopenia suspected, discontinue the offending agent(s). If the patient is bleeding platelet transfusion should be administered. IVIg may be helpful. Thrombocytopenia usually resolves quickly but may persist for a prolonged period notably that due to gold which may be permanent. Implicated drugs should be avoided by that patient in future.

Thrombophilia

Thrombophilia is a heritable or acquired disorder of the haemostatic mechanism predisposing to thrombosis, typically venous.

Arterial thrombosis is usually the result of atherosclerosis not blood hypercoagulability. Important exceptions are antiphospholipid activity (APL), paroxysmal nocturnal haemoglobinuria and rarely severe hyperhomocysteinaemia. Virchov's triad of vessel, flow and blood is still a useful aide memoire for causes of thrombosis. Testing for heritable thrombophilic is not indicated in patients with arterial thrombosis.

Pathogenesis

Arterial thrombosis (myocardial infarction or stroke) is a major cause of death in people over the age of 40 and is usually secondary to underlying arterial disease, atherosclerosis. Coagulation defects are rarely implicated as significant determinant. Venous thrombosis also is a major cause of morbidity and mortality with an overall annual incidence of 1/1000. Stasis following trauma and surgery is a common aetiological factor as is increasing age. Up to 40% of people >40 may develop deep vein thrombosis (DVT) following orthopaedic or major abdominal surgery; as many as a third of medical patients in ITU may do so. Many medical conditions increase the risk of thrombosis.

Arterial thrombosis	Venous thrombosis
Smoking	Surgery or trauma
Hypertension	Malignant disease
Atherosclerosis	Pregnancy/oral contraceptive pill/HRT
Hyperlipidaemia	Chronic inflammatory bowel disease
Diabetes mellitus	PNH

Clinical features

In many patients with thrombosis an underlying clinical risk factor will be identified.

Who should be referred for investigation?

- Arterial thrombosis—patients <50 years, without obvious arterial disease: test for APL.
- Venous thrombosis
  - Familial thrombosis.
  - Unexplained recurrent thrombosis.
  - Unusual site e.g. mesenteric, portal vein thrombosis.
  - Unexplained neonatal thrombosis.
  - Recurrent miscarriage (=3).
  - VTE in pregnancy and the OCP.

Laboratory investigation

1. Test for underlying medical causes of thrombosis.
2. FBC, ESR, LFTs, autoimmune profile, fasting lipids (arterial disease).
3. Lupus anticoagulant and anticardiolipin antibody titres.

When should tests for heritable thrombophilia be performed?

- When there is evidence of familial venous thrombosis and diagnosis of thrombophilic defect may help determine management of symptomatic patients.
- When case-finding by family studies is likely to reduce risk of VTE at high risk periods in family members.

Heritable defects typically tested for

- Antithrombin.
- Protein C.
- Protein S.
- APC resistance.
- Factor V Leiden.
- Prothrombin gene mutation (*F2* G20210A).
- High factor VIII level.

Conclusion

In most patients with thrombosis, trigger factors will be identified in the history. APL is a relatively common acquired thrombophilic defect detected by lupus anticoagulant activity or elevated anticardiolipin titres. Should be considered in patients with VTE and young patient with arterial thrombosis or those without evidence of atherosclerosis. Testing for inherited thrombophilia is complex, more expensive and only worthwhile in familial thrombosis. A strong family history of VTE will increase the chance of identifying such defects.

British Committee for Standards in Haematology (2001) Investigation and management of heritable thrombophilia. *Br J Haematol* **114**, 512–528.
www.bcshguidelines.com/pdf/BJH512.pdf

Inherited thrombophilia

At present 30–50% patients with thrombosis and a positive family history will have a demonstrable thrombophilic abnormality on testing but this rarely influences clinical management. The frequency of the commonly identified heritable major factors is set out in table.

Defect	Relative risk of VTE	Patients with first VTE	Familial patients with VTE
FVL	2–6	15–20%	10–50%
F2 G20210A	2–4	5%	5-10%
AT deficiency	10	1-2%	4%
PC deficiency	10	1-2%	4%
PS deficiency	4–10	3-6%	6-8%

Activated protein C resistance and factor V Leiden

APC resistance described in 1993 by Dahlback and colleagues. This is the most frequent thrombophilic abnormality in Caucasians (*see above*), ~ 1 per 5000 of population homozygous. APC resistance is due to factor V Leiden mutation in more than 95% of cases.

Pathogenesis

APC inactivates membrane bound factor Va through proteolytic cleavage at 3 specific sites in the heavy chain. >95% cases APCR due to mutation in factor V gene, resulting in glutamine to arginine at position 506 (denoted FV:Q506, or factor V Leiden, FVL). APCR without FVL may be due to other genetic defects, or acquired for example as a result of increased factor VIII concentration.

Clinical features

VTE is increased 2- to 6-fold in heterozygotes and 50- to 100-fold in homozygotes. Most individuals with FVL will not develop thrombosis; other risk factors (e.g. trauma, surgery, OCP, pregnancy) are present in >50% of patients who develop a thrombotic event, and increasing age is a major risk factor. Recent studies indicate little if any value of case-finding in relatives of affected symptomatic patients.

Pregnancy—risk of VTE estimated from personal and family history will determine whether antenatal or postnatal prophylaxis is required..

OCP users have 4 × VTE risk compared to non-users generally. The FVL mutation increase the risk a further 7-fold. Thus the absolute annual VTE risk in women not taking COCs is 0.5/10,000. In women taking COCs the risk is 2/10,000. In women COC users with the FVL mutation the risk is 15/10,000.

The FVL mutation is a minimal risk factor for arterial thrombosis and of no consequence compared to typical risk factors such as smoking, hypertension and hyperlipidaemia.

Laboratory diagnosis
Detected by PCR technique. APC sensitivity test measures prolongation of APTT in response to added activated protein C. A reduced response indicates APC resistance. Positive result is not specific for FVL defect.

Prothrombin gene mutation
A G⟶A nucleotide transition at position 20210 in the 3' untranslated region of the prothrombin gene was reported in 1996. Incidence: 5% patients with first episode of VTE.

Proteins C and S deficiency
Vitamin K dependent factors. Protein S is a cofactor for anticoagulant activity of activated protein C (APC). APC cleaves factors V and VIII on phospholipid surfaces thus limiting thrombin generation. Deficiency results in prothrombotic state and increased risk of VTE.

Less common than FVL, they account for 4–8% of familial thrombosis. Concentrations are low in early life (up to 4 years for PC), following recent thrombosis, vitamin K deficiency, warfarin therapy, in pregnancy (PS) so care must be taken before diagnosing an inherited deficiency. DNA techniques available but not practical for routine diagnosis.

Many patients are asymptomatic and will never have a VTE. Clinically PC and PS deficiency are similar—spontaneous and sometimes recurrent thrombophlebitis and VTE. In neonates with severe deficiency (homozygous) purpura fulminans is life threatening. This is due to microvascular thrombosis (DIC). Skin necrosis may complicate warfarin therapy.

Antithrombin III (AT) deficiency
AT, the main co-factor of heparin and inhibitor of thrombin, was the first major familial defect described (1965). VTE thrombosis risk appears greater than PC/PS deficiency particularly during pregnancy. Homozygous severe AT deficiency is probably incompatible with life.

Homocysteinaemia
Hyperhomocysteinaemia may be due to genetic defects, vit B_{12} or folate deficiency. A severe form (congenital homocystinuria) is associated with arteriosclerosis, thromboembolic disease and mental retardation. Arterial and venous thrombosis is reported in ~10% patients with moderate hyperhomocysteinaemia; may be familial and linked to other thrombophilic defects e.g. PC deficiency. Treatment with folate, vit B_{12} may reduce the hyperhomocysteinaemia but clinical benefit is unproven.

Treatment of thrombophilic states
Treatment often the same in patients with and without laboratory evidence of thrombophilia.

Acute thrombotic event
- Treat appropriately—usually with heparin/warfarin.

- In PC/PS patients make sure heparinisation is adequate—monitor warfarin induction closely to avoid skin necrosis. Patients with AT deficiency do not usually require high heparin doses.
- Duration of anticoagulation following a first event will depend on the severity of the VTE and clinical risk factors for recurrence; each patient needs to be individually assessed. Heritable thrombophilia is not an indication of itself for life-long anticoagulation.

Recurrent thrombosis

- Long-term anticoagulation should be considered

Concentrates

AT and PC concentrates have been used rarely in patients with heritable deficiency during surgical and pregnancy high risk periods but they are not used routinely in the majority of patients.

PC concentrate should be used in fulminant neonatal thrombosis, including purpura fulminans, in severe homozygous deficiency.

Prophylaxis

- Anticoagulation is not recommended for asymptomatic patients.
- Prophylaxis in pregnancy depends on family history and nature of thrombophilic defect. For management of pregnant patient with history of VTE, prophylactic heparin has been successful in subsequent pregnancies.
- High risk situations e.g. surgery, trauma, should be identified and covered with prophylactic SC heparin. Dose will depend on the thrombotic risk. 📖 *p588*
- Patients must be informed of factors that increase thrombotic risk and given an information sheet.
- Patients with an identified thrombophilic defect should be advised of increased risk of VTE with the OCP or HRT.

Counselling

Before embarking on a search for heritable thrombophilia, it is essential that careful thought be given to any possible value for the patient and family.

Natural history

Complicated. At one end of the spectrum, FVL occurs in 3.5% of a healthy population and may give rise to no problems throughout life; at the other PC deficiency causes fatal neonatal purpura fulminans and homozygous AT deficiency is incompatible with life. Thrombophilia has a whole range of clinical problems and new information is accumulating. The patient is best managed in a specialist clinic.

Haemostasis and thrombosis

Acquired thrombophilia

Lupus anticoagulant

The paradoxically named lupus anticoagulant (LA) is arguably the commonest coagulation abnormality predisposing to thrombosis. It is something of a misnomer as it increases the risk of thrombosis not bleeding. It is an IgG /IgM autoantibody and prolongs phospholipid dependent coagulation tests (hence the use of the term anticoagulant); bleeding is very rare despite the prolonged APTT. The LA and other antiphospholipid antibodies (APL) are found in association with arterial or venous thrombosis and/or recurrent fetal loss, the 'antiphospholipid syndrome', first described by Hughes in 1988.

Pathogenesis

APL may be idiopathic or secondary when associated with other disorders. The two main aPL are the LA and the anticardiolipin antibody (ACL) occurring together in most cases but also independently. The antibody specificity is actually to β2-glycoprotein 1 (β2GP1), a phospholipid membrane-associated protein. Rarely antibodies to prothrombin co-exist and can cause hypoprothrombinaemia and bleeding. The mechanism of thrombosis is not clear; APL may act against other vitamin K dependent proteins PC and PS, or possibly the autoimmune state may lead to endothelial damage and/or platelet activation.

Acquired thrombophilia due to APL is a much commoner cause of thrombosis than the congenital defects; the incidence depends on the patient group–e.g. 18% in young stroke patients, 21% young patients with MI. The LA occurs in 1–2% of the population; most patients will not develop thrombosis.

Diagnosis

Clinical features

The LA was first described in patients with SLE—hence its name. Other underlying disorders include the lymphoproliferative disorders, HIV, other autoimmune disorders and drugs (e.g. phenothiazines). The antiphospholipid syndrome (APS) is seen in patients with SLE but is often primary. Thrombosis, the major defining feature, may be arterial (stroke, ocular occlusions, MI, limb thrombosis) or venous (DVT, PE, renal, hepatic and portal veins). Fetal loss may be as high as ~80% in women with APL.

Other clinical manifestations

- Migraine, visual disturbances.
- Thrombocytopenia.
- Livedo reticularis.
- Heart valve disease.
- Myelopathy.
- Catastrophic widespread intravascular thrombosis is reported.

Laboratory diagnosis

1. Must double spin or filter plasma to remove all platelets and prevent false negative result.
2. Coagulation screen: APTT maybe prolonged and does not correct with normal plasma. Normal result does not rule out the condition as

different reagents have different sensitivity. PT usually normal unless hypoprothrombinaemia is present.
4. Dilute Russell's viper venom time (DRVVT).
5. Exner test— kaolin clotting time: platelet extract or excess phospholipid corrects the abnormal test and confirms antiphospholipid defect.
6. aCL is detected using an immunoassay technique and is quantified.
7. Autoimmune profile: ± ANA ± DNA binding.

Treatment

Asymptomatic patients APL positive without thrombosis—no specific action; the risk of thrombosis is estimated at <1% per patient year.

Prophylaxis—probably wise to consider peri-operative thromboprophylaxis.

Antiphospholipid syndrome

Acute thrombotic events—treat as appropriate with heparin/warfarin. Long term anticoagulation is required; target INR 2.5–3.5 depending on clinical risk of recurrence.

Recurrent abortion—subsequent pregnancies have been successfully achieved in women with the antiphospholipid syndrome with combined aspirin and heparin (UFH or LMWH) begun as soon as pregnancy is confirmed. Steroids are not indicated.

Prophylactic anticoagulation—pregnancy in a woman with APL and a past history of thrombosis will require prophylactic anticoagulation with heparin (📖 *p588*).

Natural history

The LA may be transient and spontaneous remissions of the APS are reported. Long term follow-up of these patients is indicated since the clinical manifestations can be severe despite long term anticoagulation.

BCSH Guidelines for the investigation and management of antiphospholipid syndrome. *Br J Haematol* **109**, 704–715 (2000).
www.bcshguidelines.com/pdf/bjh2069.pdf

Anticoagulant therapy

Heparin

LMWH is treatment of choice in most cases as low risk of HITT (heparin-induced thrombocytopenia with thrombosis), given by SC injection and usually does not require monitoring or dose adjustment. Indicated for prevention and treatment of VTE and acute coronary syndromes.

If UFH is given then IV infusion should be monitored by regular APTT measurement, at least once daily. APTT ratio usually maintained at 1.5–2.5 × normal.

HITT is an uncommon complication but high risk of death and limb amputation. Should be considered if 50% reduction in platelet count whilst on heparin therapy. Difficult to confirm diagnosis with lab tests so diagnosis should be made on clinical suspicion. Treatment is to stop all heparin, including flushes, and give direct thrombin inhibitor such as recombinant hirudin or danaparoid (non-heparin activator of antithrombin). HITT can complicate low dose as well as therapeutic doses of heparin.

Warfarin:

Many indications. 1/100 population now taking warfarin. Monitored by INR (International Normalized Ratio) which is a standardised PT ratio. Target INR typically 2.5. Over anticoagulation common. More likely with target INR >2.5 and when other drugs, particularly antibiotics, are prescribed. Avoided by lowest possible target INR, testing within 5–7d of any change in other drug therapy and patient awareness of change in bleeding tendency.

Over anticoagulation due to warfarin increasingly treated with small doses of vitamin K. For example INR >8.0 give 1–2.5mg vitamin K PO.

Note: severe overanticoagulation complicated by major bleeding should be reversed by emergency administration of factor concentrate containing vitamin K-dependent factors, e.g. beriplex. Recombinant factor VIIa may be considered if beriplex or similar concentrate is unavailable. Alternatively FFP can be given but reversal is often incomplete and massive volumes of FFP have to be given.

BCSH Guidelines on oral anticoagulation. *Br J Haematol* **101**, 374–387 (1998).
www.bcshguidelines.com/pdf/bjh715.pdf

Haemostasis and thrombosis

Anticoagulation in pregnancy and post-partum

Pregnancy is a hypercoagulable state with an increased risk of thrombosis throughout and up to 6 weeks post-partum. In addition to increased venous stasis secondary to abdominal pressure and reduced mobility, physiological prothrombotic changes in coagulation take place—*see figure*.

Incidence

The risk of venous thromboembolic events (VTE) increased 10-fold in normal pregnancy ~1/1000 deliveries; fatal PE 10/year in UK is the major cause of maternal death in pregnancy and the puerperium. The risk rises when the pregnancy is complicated (sepsis, prolonged bed rest, advanced maternal age, delivery by LSCS). Previous VTE particularly in pregnancy, inherited/acquired thrombophilia further increase the risk.

Indications for anticoagulation in pregnancy

- Acute VTE presenting in pregnancy.
- Long term anticoagulation for prosthetic heart valves/recurrent VTE.
- Previous VTE, particularly in pregnancy/post-partum.
- Antiphospholipid syndrome (APS).
- Inherited thrombophilia with/without a history of VTE.

General considerations

There are no universally accepted protocols for the management of anticoagulation in pregnancy. There are few controlled studies and much of the information relates to non-pregnant subjects. Both oral anticoagulants and heparin have advantages and disadvantages in pregnancy. LMWH are a significant advance in management.

Warfarin crosses the placenta and is teratogenic in the first trimester. Exposure during weeks 6–12 can cause warfarin embryopathy with nasal hypoplasia, stippled epiphyses and other manifestations. Incidence ranges from <5% to 67% in reported series. Warfarin at any stage of pregnancy is associated with CNS abnormalities and increased risk of fetal haemorrhage *in utero* and at delivery.

Heparin (UFH and LMWH) does not cross the placenta and poses no teratogenic or haemorrhagic threat to the fetus. Maternal complications include haemorrhage (severe in <2%), thrombocytopenia (severe in <1%) and osteoporosis, usually asymptomatic and reversible but rare cause of vertebral fractures. LMWH may have fewer complications *cf.* unfractionated (UF) heparin.

Treatment of VTE presenting in pregnancy

- Heparin 5–7d
  either monitored IV UF heparin; aim for APTT ratio 1.5–2.0
  or therapeutic SC LMWH based on body wt (📖 BNF)
  then monitored therapeutic SC 12-hrly UF heparin or LMWH od or bd
- Heparin requirements vary as pregnancy advances so adjust dose as necessary.
- Continue heparin until delivery; omit heparin during labour.
- Recommence heparin after delivery and start warfarin if desired.

- Continue treatment for at least 6 weeks post-partum; stop heparin once INR in therapeutic range.

Prophylaxis of thromboembolism in pregnancy

National guidelines should be consulted and patients treated in centres with special expertise.

Conclusion

There is an urgent need for controlled trials to establish the appropriate level of anticoagulation in pregnancy. Currently many centres use LMWH for all women except possibly those with prosthetic heart valves because of ease of administration and ↓ risk of complications.

Coagulation changes in normal pregnancy

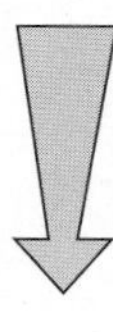

Toglia, M.R. & Weg, J.G. (1996) Venous thromboembolism during pregnancy. *N Engl J Med*, **335**, 108–114.

Immunodeficiency

11

Congenital immunodeficiency syndromes

Incidence: rare, though as knowledge increases there is recognition of an increasing number of inherited defects in the complex human host defence system. The classical life-threatening disorders of specific immunity with major dysfunction or absence of T cells and/or B cells are all diseases that present in childhood, but milder variants may not be recognized until later life. 'Immunodeficiency' is a vague term that is generally taken to encompass also defects in opsonisation and phagocytosis, so can be taken to include neutrophil and macrophage disorders of number, function or both.

Classification of inherited immune deficiency syndromes

- Affecting T cells, B cells and neutrophils.
- Affecting B and T cells.
- Affecting T cells.
- Affecting B cells.
- Affecting neutrophils.

1. Affecting T cells, B cells and neutrophils.

Reticular dysgenesis

An rare autosomal recessive or sometimes X-linked disorder where T cells, B cells and granulocytes are absent. Such children present with serious infection at birth or shortly afterwards. They have no lymph nodes or tonsils, and the usual thymic shadow is absent. Bone marrow is hypoplastic, and there may also be thrombocytopenia and anaemia. It appears to be a pluripotential stem cell failure and carries a dire prognosis. The only curative therapy is BMT.

2. Affecting T cells and B cells (combined immunodeficiency disorders).

Severe combined immunodeficiency—SCID

A mixed group of disorders that all have grossly impaired T- and B-cell function leading to death normally within the first years of life. They can be broadly classified into 5 groups depending on their clinical and pathological characteristics. Reticular dysgenesis (see above) is generally considered to be a SCID variant, accounting for 3% of the total. Other types are:

1. Adenosine deaminase deficiency (16%).
2. T– B– SCID (27%).
3. T– B+ SCID (44%).
4. T+ B+ SCID (9%).

Adenosine deaminase deficiency

A recessively inherited enzyme deficiency. ADA is rate limiting in purine salvage metabolism and is essential for the synthesis of nucleotides in cells incapable of *de novo* purine synthesis—including lymphocytes. The gene for ADA is on chromosome 20q13.4, and many mutations have been defined. Gene deletion leads to very low ADA activity and a profound T and B lymphopenia with early onset of clinical symptoms. Other tissues are involved, and there may be bony defects and neurologic disturbances. A similar rare syndrome is seen with deficiency of the enzyme purine nucleoside phosphorylase. It is less severe and presents later.

Other forms of SCID

SCID with both T-cell and B-cell lymphopenia is a recessive disorder that also occurs without the enzyme deficiencies described above, but the commonest form of the disease is X-linked and shows a lack only of T cells. It appears to be due to a defect in the gene coding for the γ chain of the interleukin (IL)-2 receptor. There are other rare SCID variants where T cells are present but dysfunctional, including MHC class II deficiency, where lymphocytes fail to express MHC class II molecules; and Omenn's syndrome which presents in early infancy with the clinical features of acute widespread graft versus host disease (skin rash, hepatosplenomegaly, diarrhoea, failure to thrive) coupled with persistent infections. It is thought to be due to a failure in T-cell development with inability to recognise self antigens.

Treatment of SCID

- Matched BMT is the treatment of choice for all varieties; a good outcome can be expected in >90%.
- No pre-conditioning needed for matched donors.
- Mis-matched BMT results improving but donor marrow needs careful mature T-cell depletion and patients may need conditioning.
- ADA deficiency can be treated with regular enzyme replacement using a polyethylene glycol-linked ADA preparation.
- ADA deficiency has also been treated with gene replacement therapy, with so far only a transient effect, but the technique shows promise.

Wiskott–Aldrich Syndrome

An X-linked disorder with a triad of (1) eczema, (2) thrombocytopenia with characteristically small platelets, and (3) T- and B-cell dysfunction with susceptibility to infections, particularly otitis media and pneumonia. Due to a mutation in the gene encoding the Wiskott–Aldrich syndrome protein (WASP), important *inter alia* in regulating the cytoskeleton of haemopoietic cells.

- Presents in childhood.
- Tendency to immune cytopenias—compounding pre-existing thrombocytopenia and causing haemolytic anaemia.
- Herpes simplex, EBV, varicella and CMV may be severe and life threatening.
- Greatly increased risk of lymphoid malignancy in adulthood for survivors.
- Splenectomy greatly increases risk of fatal infection.
- Need prophylactic antibiotics and immunoglobulin replacement therapy.
- BMT now treatment of choice; early in childhood if possible.

Ataxia telangiectasia

A recessive disorder with increased chromosome fragility and a single gene defect on chromosome 11q22–23. This affects several systems. The first is neuromotor development with cerebellar ataxia appearing around 18 months of age and progressing to include dysarthria associated with degeneration of the Purkinje cells. Telangiectases appear between 2 and 8 years of age affecting the eyes, face and ears. An immune deficiency is evident affecting both humoral and cellular immunity, though less severe than SCID. Affected children get:

- Sinopulmonary infections.
- Progressive failure of antibody production.
- Hypogammaglobulinaemia.
- CD4+ lymphopenia.
- Small thymus.
- Increased incidence of lymphoid malignancies.

3. Affecting T cells

DiGeorge syndrome

Absence or hypoplasia of the thymus and parathyroid glands with aortic arch anomalies or other congenital heart defects. This congenital anomaly of the 3rd and 4th branchial arches usually presents with hypocalcaemic fits or problems with a heart defect. Total thymic aplasia occurs only in a minority, with severe immunodeficiency and a high risk of transfusion-transmitted GvHD. Most have some T-cell function, and relatively minor problems with impaired immunity for which treatment is supportive.

4. Affecting B cells

X-linked agammaglobulinaemia (Bruton tyrosine kinase deficiency)

Boys with this condition have mutations in the gene for Bruton tyrosine kinase (locus Xq22), resulting in a failure of B-cell development and lack of antibody production. Early infancy is not a problem because of maternally transmitted IgG, but by 2 years of age serious infections become apparent. These include bacterial invasion of the respiratory system, the GI tract, meninges, joints and skin. Viruses, particularly coxsackie and echoviruses, are also a major threat.

- Absent or very low numbers of B cells.
- Absent or low levels of all immunoglobulins.
- Treatment is by regular antibody replacement with polyvalent IVIg.

Hyper IgM syndrome

An X-linked disorder with B-cell dysfunction due to defective T-cell CD40 ligand production and thus lack of signaling to B-cell CD40 receptors. B cells are normal, but receive no instructions to generate isotypes of Ig other than IgM. Low levels of IgG, IgA and IgE result. There is also deficient function of some tissue macrophages and a tendency to develop *Pneumocystis carinii* pneumonia. Treatment is with IVIg replacement therapy and cotrimoxazole prophylaxis.

IgA deficiency

A relatively benign and common disorder affecting 1:500 individuals. They may develop anti-IgA antibodies in serum which can cause urticarial and anaphylactic reactions to blood product infusions. No replacement therapy is needed.

5. Affecting neutrophils, monocytes and macrophages.
Inherited disorders of neutrophil function mostly present in childhood and are described in the paediatric section on congenital neutropenia. Primary functional disorders of monocytes and macrophages are also described in the paediatric section under histiocytic syndromes.

6. Poorly characterised primary immune deficiency syndromes.
There are a number of syndromes where susceptibility to certain types of infection is not associated with a clear pattern of inheritance and where the clinical picture is variable. Few are as severe as the specific syndromes referred to above. They include *chronic mucocutaneous candidiasis*, where there is persistent superficial skin and mucous membrane fungal infection, and where there may be defective T-cell regulation or dendritic cell function. CMC is also associated with a wide variety of autoimmune phenomena, particularly thyroid and adrenal disease, and different patterns of inheritance are seen in different kindreds.

There is also a heterogeneous group of disorders collectively referred to as *common variable immunodeficiency*. Defined by the clinical susceptibility to infection and in the absence of any other apparent cause, this collectively named syndrome is usually a diagnosis of exclusion and presents in adult life. Low rather than absent levels of several isotypes of Ig are usual, and the condition is rarely life threatening.

Acquired immune deficiencies

Clinically important defects in lymphocyte numbers and/or function can be seen as a complication of a variety of acquired diseases. They can also be due to drugs, both those given deliberately to suppress an autoimmune process and those given primarily for other reasons. Similarly neutrophils can be reduced by a large number of acquired disorders and a long list of drugs and toxins. An acquired susceptibility to infection also arises in patients with absent or poorly functioning spleens.

Acquired hypogammaglobulinaemia

Causes

- Malignant lymphoproliferative disorders including CLL and myeloma.
- Immunosuppressive therapy with e.g. azathioprine.
- Maintenance therapy for ALL.
- Nephrotic syndrome.

Clinical features

Bacterial infections—recurrent chest infections (may lead to bronchiectasis), sinus, skin and urinary tract infections common. Fulminant viral infections, especially measles, varicella.

Treatment

- May improve with treatment of the underlying disease.
- IVIg should not be used routinely as prophylaxis.
- High titre specific antibody can be given for serious zoster/varicella infections if available; polyvalent for measles.
- Patients with severe hypogammaglobulinaemia and recurrent infections may be considered for IVIg replacement therapy—give 200mg/kg every 4 weeks.

Acquired T-lymphocyte abnormalities

Reduced numbers

- HIV infection (see following pages).
- High dose steroids.
- ALG.
- Purine analogues especially fludarabine and cladribine.
- Deoxycoformycin (adenosine deaminase inhibitor).
- After allogeneic stem cell transplantation.

Reduced function: Lymphoproliferative disorders, Hodgkin's disease, immunosuppressive agents e.g. cyclosporin and steroids, burns, uraemia.

Clinical features: Increased risk of viral, fungal and atypical infections including HSV, HZV, CMV, EBV, *Candida*, *Aspergillus*, *Mycoplasma*, PCP, toxoplasmosis, TB and atypical mycobacteria.

Treatment: Treat specific infection where possible. Consider prophylaxis against HZV, CMV, PCP and *Candida* in high risk groups e.g. post-allogeneic stem cell transplant.

Combined B- and T-lymphocyte abnormalities

Causes

- Chronic lymphocytic leukaemia.
- Intensive chemotherapy.
- Extensive radiotherapy.
- Severe malnutrition.

Clinical features and treatment

As above.

Neutrophil/macrophage abnormalities

Reduced numbers: *See Neutropenia p136.*

Abnormal function: *See Myelodysplasia p218, Myeloproliferative disorders p237, Histiocytic syndromes p490.*

Clinical features: Bacterial and fungal sepsis.

Treatment: Treat specific infections and consider prophylaxis.

Hyposplenism

Hyposplenism is an acquired immunodeficiency without lymphocyte or neutrophil abnormalities. It arises either following splenectomy, or due to functional deficiency as part of another disorder, especially sickle cell disease, inflammatory bowel disease, and following BMT. It gives rise to susceptibility to overwhelming infection with certain organisms due to lack of the spleen's function as a filter. These include:

- *Streptococcus pneumoniae.*
- *Neisseria menigitidis.*
- *Haemophilus influenzae* type B.
- Falciparum malaria.

The risk of hyposplenic infection is greatest in children in the first 6 years of life. It dwindles thereafter but the risk continues into adult life. All facing splenectomy should be vaccinated against HIB and pneumococcus, and all splenectomised children and young adults (and those with sickle cell disease) should probably take prophylactic penicillin 250–500mg daily.

HIV infection and AIDS

Infection with HIV-1 or HIV-2 produces a large number of haematological effects and can simulate a number of haematological conditions during both the latent pre-clinical phase and once clinical syndrome of AIDS has developed. HIV infection divided into four stages.

Stage 1: primary infection

Entry of HIV-1 or HIV-2 through a mucosal surface after sexual contact, direct inoculation into the bloodstream by contaminated blood products, or IV drug abuse can be followed by a transient febrile illness up to 6 weeks later associated with oral ulceration, pharyngitis, and lymphadenopathy. Photophobia, meningism, myalgia, prostration, encephalopathy and meningitis may also occur. FBC may show lymphopenia or lymphocytosis often with atypical lymphocytes, neutropenia, thrombocytopenia or pancytopenia. Major differential diagnoses are acute viral meningitis and infectious mononucleosis. False +ve IM serology may occur. Specific IgM then IgG antibody to HIV appears 4–12 weeks after infection and routine tests for HIV may be –ve for up to 3 months. However, the virus is detectable in plasma and CSF from infected individuals during this period and the patient is highly infectious.

Stage 2: pre-clinical HIV infection

Although viral titres fall in the circulation at this time there is significant and persistent virus replication within lymph nodes and spleen. The clinically latent period may last 8–10 years and circulating CD4 T-cell count remains normal for most of this period. However, there is a delayed, gradual but progressive fall in CD4 T lymphocytes in most patients, who may remain asymptomatic for a prolonged period despite modest lymphopenia. A number of minor skin problems such as seborrhoeic dermatitis are characteristic of the end of the latent phase.

A patient with latent HIV infection may have isolated thrombocytopenia on routine blood testing. This is due to an immune mechanism and may be confused with ITP as there is frequently ↑ platelet associated immunoglobulin.

Stage 3: clinical symptoms

Marked by onset of symptoms, rising titre of circulating virus and decline in circulating CD4 T-cell count to $<0.5 \times 10^9$/L. Wide variation in individual patient's rate of progression at this stage. A number of minor opportunistic infections are common: oral/genital candida, herpes zoster, oral leucoplakia. Lethargy, PUO and weight loss occur frequently. Deepening lymphopenia (CD4 $<0.2 \times 10^9$/L) invariably present when opportunistic infection occurs. Persistent generalised lymphadenopathy is a condition where lymphadenopathy >1cm at 2 or more extra-inguinal sites persists for >3 months. It is a prodrome to severe immunodeficiency, opportunistic infection and neoplasia.

Stage 4: AIDS

AIDS is now defined as the presence of a +ve HIV antibody test associated with a CD4 lymphocyte count $<0.2 \times 10^9$/L rather than by the development of a specific opportunistic infection or neoplastic complication. This final stage of HIV infection is associated with a marked reduction in CD4 T cells, severe life-threatening opportunistic infection, neoplasia and neurological degeneration. Severity of these complications usually reflects the degree of immunodeficiency as measured by the CD4 T-cell count. However, there is evidence that prophylactic therapy reduces the incidence of complications and newer antiviral therapies slow the progression of this stage.

Haematological features of HIV infection

- Lymphopenia—CD4 lymphopenia may be masked by CD8 lymphocytosis in stage 2; improved by antiviral therapy.
- Neutropenia—marrow suppression by virus or therapy; splenic sequestration.
- Normochromic/normocytic anaemia due to suppression of marrow by virus or therapy. Microangiopathic haemolysis associated with TTP.
- Thrombocytopenia—suppression of marrow by virus or therapy or shortened survival due to immune destruction (may respond to antiviral therapy), infection, TTP or splenic sequestration.
- Bone marrow suppression—direct HIV effect or complication of antiretroviral therapy, ganciclovir, trimethoprim or amphotericin B therapy.
- Bone marrow infiltration—by NHL, Hodgkin's disease, granulomas due to *M. tuberculosis* and atypical mycobacteria or disseminated fungal disease.

Complications of HIV infection

Opportunistic infections

Complications of HIV infection		
Fungal	*Pneumocystis carinii*	pneumonia
	Candida albicans	oro-oesophageal
	Aspergillus fumigatus	pneumonia
	Histoplasma capsulatum	meningo-encephalitis, pneumonia
Mycobacterial	*M. avium intracellulare*	disseminated, intestinal
	M. tuberculosis	pulmonary, intestinal
Parasitic	*Cryptosporidium*	hepatobiliary, intestinal
	Isospora	colon, hepatobiliary
	Toxoplasma gondii	multiple abscesses: CNS ocular, lymphatic
Viral	Cytomegalovirus	retinal, hepatic, intestinal, CNS
	Herpes zoster	mucocutaneous
	Herpes simplex	mucocutaneous
	JC virus	CNS
Bacterial	*Haemophilus influenzae*	meningitis
	Streptococcus pneumoniae	pneumonia, meningitis, septicaemia

Neoplasia

- AIDS-related Kaposi's sarcoma 20–30% of patients; multiple skin lesions; later lymph nodes, mucous membranes and visceral organs ?role of HHV8 (>95% +ve).
- NHL up to 10%; 65% diffuse large B-cell, 30% Burkitt-like; extranodal esp. small bowel and CNS; primary effusion lymphomas; aggressive. ?role of EBV(100% +ve in 1° CNS NHL).
- Cervical carcinoma.
- Anal carcinoma.
- Hodgkin's disease; advanced stage, extranodal sites.

Direct effects of HIV infection

- Bone marrow suppression: dysplastic appearance; pancytopenia.
- Small bowel enteropathy; malabsorption syndrome.
- CNS; dementia, myelopathy, neuropathy.

Immunodeficiency

Therapy of HIV infection

Infection prophylaxis	
Drugs	**Activity against**
Fluconazole/itraconazole	Oro-oesophageal candidiasis ± cryptococcal meningitis
Trimethoprim	*Pneumocystis carinii*, ± ocular/CNS toxoplasmosis
Dapsone/nebulised pentamidine	*Pneumocystis carinii*
Rifabutin/azithromycin/clarithromycin	*M. avium-intracellulare*
Acyclovir	HSV and HZV
?Ganciclovir	CMV

Antiviral therapy

- Nucleoside class of viral reverse transcriptase (RT) inhibitors have been widely used both as single agents and in combination: zidovudine (AZT), didanosine (ddl), zalcitabine (ddC), stavudine (d4T), lamuvidine (3TC) and abacavir.
- Specific therapy is followed within hours by rapid clearance of virions from the circulation and subsequently by reappearance of circulating T cells and a rising count over several days. Viral resistance develops with time, especially to single agent treatment.
- Non-nucleoside class of reverse transcriptase inhibitors used in combination therapy: nevirapine and efavirenz.
- Protease inhibitors interfere with virus assembly and have dramatic effects on viral load: saquinavir, ritonavir, indinavir, amprenavir, nelfinavir.
- The most effective antiretroviral therapy uses a combination of two nucleoside RT inhibitors plus either a non-nucleoside RT inhibitor or one or two protease inhibitors .and is currently recommended for all patients with stage 3 and 4 disease.

Treatment of complications	
Oro-oesophageal candidiasis	Systemic fluconazole or amphotericin then lifelong prophylaxis
Pneumocystis pneumonia	High dose co-trimoxazole or pentamidine then lifelong prophylaxis
Tuberculosis	Multi-agent therapy (drug resistance common) ± lifelong isoniazid prophylaxis
Fungal pneumonia	Amphotericin B then lifelong prophylaxis
CMV pneumonitis/retinitis	Ganciclovir/foscarnet then lifelong prophylaxis
CNS toxoplasmosis	Pyrimethamine then lifelong prophylaxis.
Cryptococcal meningitis	Amphotericin/fluconazole
AIDS-related Kaposi's sarcoma	Limited disease: local DXT, cryotherapy, intra-lesional vincristine, interferon-α; advanced disease: combination chemotherapy such as adriamycin, bleomycin and vincristine (ABV), liposomal daunorubicin, paclitaxel
Non-Hodgkin's lymphoma	Poor prognosis; combination chemotherapy (often standard regimens at reduced dosage due to toxicity) 50% response, median survival <9 mo; CNS lymphoma particularly poor prognosis; palliative dexamethasone DXT

Paediatric haematology

12

Blood counts in children

Blood counts in children are often different from adults, to varying degrees at different ages. The differences are greatest during the neonatal period.

Red cells

The relatively hypoxic intrauterine environment means that the newborn is polycythaemic by adult standards, a phenomenon that self-corrects during the first 3 months of life by which time the normal infant is anaemic relative to adults. Neonatal red cells are also macrocytic by adult standards, a feature that also disappears during the first 6 months as HbA replaces HbF.

- Neonatal red cells show much greater variation in shape than those from adults, particularly in premature babies—alarming microscopists more used to adult blood films.
- Occasional nucleated red cells are normal in the first 24–48h of life.
- Iron lack is common around 12 months of age due to increased demand from ↑ red cell mass and (often) poor oral intake—cows' milk has virtually no iron content. The MCV falls to what would be abnormally low levels for adults as a reflection of this.
- In healthy premature neonates all these red cell differences may be exaggerated, with a nadir Hb at 2–3 months of 8–9g/dL in those with birth weight 1–1.5kg.
- Children have slightly lower Hb than adults until puberty.

White cells

The most striking difference between children and adults is the high lymphocyte count in infants and young children. This means that the normal differential WBC in those <4 years shows more lymphocytes than neutrophils. Otherwise most of the changes in white cell counts seen in children are similar to those seen in adults and due to the same causes, with a few exceptions:

- Healthy term babies show a transiently raised neutrophil count in the first 24h after birth ($7–14 \times 10^9$/L) which returns to the normal (adult) range by 48h.
- Immature neutrophils (band cells and myelocytes) may comprise 5–10% of the total WBC in healthy neonates.
- Sick neonates with bacterial infections commonly show a paradoxical neutropenia, with or without an increased band cell count.
- Black children have lower neutrophil counts that other ethnic groups.
- Lymphocytoses with very high counts occur in children with specific infections—notably pertussis.

Platelets

Platelet counts in children are essentially the same as adults as far as the lower limit is concerned, but there is greater volatility at the upper end and infants tend to produce high counts ($>500 \times 10^9$/L) as part of an acute phase reaction more frequently. There is a statistically significant fall in the upper limit (95th centile) from 4 years onwards from around 500 to reach 350–400 by the end of childhood.

Cord blood platelets are less reactive to aggregating agents *in vitro* and have other features of hypofunction compared with mature platelets.

Normal blood count values from birth to adulthood

(source *Pediatric Hematology* 2E; eds. Lilleyman, Hann and Blanchette; Churchill Livingstone, London 1999).

Age	Hb (g/dL)	MCV (fL)	Neuts	Lymph	Platelets
Birth	14.9–23.7	100–125	2.7–14.4	2–7.3	150–450
2 weeks	13.4–19.8	88–110	1.5–5.4	2.8–9.1	170–500
2 months	9.4–13.0	84–98	0.7–4.8	3.3–10.3	210–650
6 months	10.0–13.0	73–84	1–6	3.3–11.5	210–560
1 year	10.1–13.0	70–82	1–8	3.4–10.5	200–550
2–6 years	11.5–13.8	72–87	1.5–8.5	1.8–8.4	210–490
6–12 years	11.1–14.7	76–90	1.5–8	1.5–5	170–450
Adult ♂	12.1–16.6	77–92	1.5–6	1.5–4.5	180–430
Adult ♀	12.1–15.1	77–94	1.5–6	1.5–4.5	180–430

Neuts, neutrophils; lymph, lymphocytes and platelets, all × 10^9/L

Other haematological variables in childhood

There are important differences in the concentration of various clotting factors during early infancy as described on p690. Other laboratory investigations where children differ include:

- Reticulocyte counts low in the first 8 weeks of life as neonatal polycythaemia corrects itself.
- HbF comprises 75% of the total Hb at birth, 10% at 5 months, 2% at 1 year and <1% thereafter.
- Some red cell enzymes (G6PD, PK, hexokinase) have greater activity (150–200% of adult values) in neonatal RBC.
- The lower limit of normal for serum ferritin at 1 year (12.5mg/L) is 50% of the LLN at 12 years (25mg/L).
- B_{12} and folate levels are around 2× higher in infants and younger children than adults.

Red cell transfusion and blood component therapy—special considerations in neonates and children

Babies in Special Care Baby Units are now amongst the most intensively transfused of our hospital patients.

- To replace blood losses of investigative sampling.
- To alleviate anaemia of prematurity.

Note:
- Hb estimation alone is an inadequate assessment.
- Hb reduction with symptoms, e.g. failure to thrive, is needed to justify transfusion.
- Generally, neonatal Hb <10.5g/dL + symptoms—transfuse; if neonate requiring O_2 support, aim for Hb 13.0g/dL.

Source of blood

Directed donations from 'walking donors' (including donations from relatives) cannot be regarded as safe as microbiologically-screened volunteer donor blood—therefore not recommended.

Small volume transfusions

QUAD 'pedipacks' (SAGM blood) ensure that 4 transfusions possible from a single donor and so ↓ donor exposure in infant needing multiple transfusions.

Pre-transfusion testing

Maternal and neonatal samples should be taken and tested as follows:

Maternal samples
1. ABO and Rh group.
2. Antibody screen.

Infant samples
3. ABO and Rh group.
4. DAT.
5. Antibody screen (if maternal sample unavailable).

Note: Provided no atypical antibodies are present in maternal or infant serum and the DAT on the infant's cells is –ve, a conventional cross-match is unnecessary. Small volume replacement transfusions can be given repeatedly during the first 4 months of life without further serological testing. Transfusion centres may specifically designate a supply of low anti-A, B titre group O Rh (D) –ve blood for use in neonatal transfusions. After the first 4 months, compatibility testing should conform to requirements for adults.

Exchange transfusions

- To prevent kernicterus caused by rapidly rising bilirubin.
- Most commonly needed in haemolytic disease of the newborn.
- Plasma-reduced red cells (Hct 0.50–0.60).

- For small volume transfusions, age of red cells does not matter. For exchange transfusions within 5d of collection. ([K^+] levels rise in older blood).
- Transfusion should not take >5h/unit due to risk of bacterial proliferation.
- Volumes of 5mL/kg/h usually safe.

Special hazards

- GvHD: in congenitally immunodeficient neonates immunocompetent donor T lymphocytes can cause GvHD—rare.
- Need to irradiate all blood products in these children. Also irradiate if first degree relatives used as donors.
- CMV infection: particular risk in low birth weight babies, or immunocompromised children undergoing transplantation. CMV seronegative donations should be used. Alternatively use (modern) leucodepletion filter to reduce risk.
- Hypocalcaemia—rare now, due to change of additive.
- Citrate toxicity, also rare nowadays due to improvements in additive.
- Rebound hypoglycaemia, induced by high glucose levels of blood transfusion anticoagulants.
- Thrombocytopenia—dilution, DIC.
- Volume overload.
- Haemolytic transfusion reactions in necrotising enterocolitis. Thought to be due to the 'T' antigen on baby's RBCs becoming exposed due to action of bacterial toxin entering the blood from diseased gut. Anti 'T' is present in almost all donor plasma.

Use of 4.5% albumin

Use controversial, but may be helpful after large volume paracentesis, as fluid replacement in therapeutic plasma exchange, or in nephrotic syndrome resistant to diuretics. There are better products for resuscitation and volume expansion. Should NOT be used in nutritional protein deficiency or chronic hypoalbuminaemia (e.g. cirrhosis or protein-losing enteropathy). Risk of infection transmission minimal but not zero.

Use of immunoglobulin

Intravenous polyvalent immunoglobulin widely used as replacement therapy in immunodeficiencies, for Kawasaki disease to prevent the formation of coronary microaneurysms, and also as non-specific agent for reticuloendothelial blockade in immune cytopenias, chiefly (and usually unnecessarily) in childhood ITP. Can get immunoglobulin with particularly high titre against RSV, HZV and hepatitis B. Usually this is for intramuscular use only and should not be given IV due to risk of complement activation. IVIg has transmitted hepatitis C in the past due to poor virus inactivation procedures, so should not be used in trivial conditions.

Use of FFP

Available in aliquots of 50mL. Must be ABO and Rh compatible. Infused via filter. Main indication—DIC. No need for CMV screening, or irradiation. Dose: 10–15mL/kg. Check PT and APTT. Repeat as necessary. May need cryoprecipitate also (📖 p524, 654), if evidence of ↓ fibrinogen (<1.0g/L). Both contain untreated plasma, so potential infection risk, though FFP should be virus-inactivated in future.

Use of platelets

- Thrombocytopenia more hazardous in neonates, so prophylactic transfusion if count $<30 \times 10^9$/L.
- Reserve for children with marrow failure and counts $<10 \times 10^9$/L otherwise:
  - Only use in *immune* thrombocytopenia for life-threatening bleeding.
  - Then use massive 'swamping' dose to overwhelm antibody.
  - One dose (one paediatric platelet concentrate) contained in ~50mL 'fresh' plasma, available either from apheresis or buffy coat derived.
  - Check increment 1h later if no clinical response.
  - Care with volume overload.
  - Must be administered within 2h of receipt on ward.
  - Irradiate for immunosuppressed children.
  - Refractoriness can arise due to alloimmune antibodies.

Use of granulocytes

- Severely infected neonates may develop profound neutropenia.
- Usually respond to antibiotic therapy.
- Granulocyte transfusions very rarely given because of lack of effect, risk of CMV and toxoplasmosis and respiratory distress syndrome.
- Blood products now routinely leucodepleted to reduce risk of CMV transmission.

Paediatric haematology

Polycythaemia in newborn and childhood

As in adults, polycythaemia in children may be relative or absolute (📖 p240, 248). The condition is usually secondary and most commonly seen as a clinical problem in neonates or older children with congenital cyanotic heart disease or high-affinity abnormal haemoglobins. Primary polycythaemia is very unusual in childhood; benign familial erythrocytosis is a very rare autosomal dominant self-limiting condition of unknown aetiology.

Pathophysiology

Polycythaemia is physiological in the neonatal period with ↑ Hct (range 42–60% in cord blood) persisting in the first few days of life. Pathological polycythaemia is defined in the neonate as Hct >65% (Hb >22.0g/dL), is uncommon (<5% of all births) and usually due to hypertransfusion or hypoxia.

Causes of polycythaemia in the newborn

- Relative—dehydration, reduced plasma volume.
- Hypertransfusion—delayed cord clamping, maternofetal, twin to twin.
- Hypoxia—placental insufficiency, intrauterine growth retardation.
- Endocrine—congenital adrenal hyperplasia, thyrotoxicosis.
- Maternal disease—toxaemia of pregnancy, DM, heart disease, drugs e.g. propranolol.
- Other miscellaneous conditions such as Down syndrome.

Clinical features

Hyperviscosity may give rise to vomiting, poor feeding, hypotonia, hypoglycaemia, lethargy, irritability and tremulousness. On examination—plethora, cyanosis, jaundice, hepatomegaly. Complications include intracranial haemorrhage, respiratory distress, cardiac failure, necrotising enterocolitis and neonatal thrombosis.

Diagnosis

- Clinical presentation may suggest the diagnosis e.g. anaemic twin.
- FBC (free-flowing venous sample) ↑ neonatal Hct >65%.
- Hypoglycaemia, hypocalcaemia, unconjugated hyperbilirubinaemia.
- Hb studies for excess HbA—? maternal haemorrhage.
- Radiology: CXR shows ↑ vascularity, infiltrates, cardiomegaly.

Management

- Supportive—IV fluids, close observation for complications.
- Exchange transfusion—partial with FFP/albumin to ↓ Hct<60%.

$$\textbf{Vol of exchange (mL)} = \frac{\textbf{Blood vol} \times \textbf{(observed} - \textbf{desired Hct)}}{\textbf{observed Hct}}$$

Treatment

As required for associated abnormalities.

Outcome

Provided the condition is identified early and appropriate measures taken to reduce the hyperviscosity, the outcome should be good.

Neonatal anaemia

Intrauterine conditions require a state of polycythaemia. Congenital anaemia is present with cord blood Hb <14.0g/dL in term babies. In the healthy infant, Hb drops rapidly after birth (📖 *Blood Counts in Children p690*) and by end of the neonatal period (4 weeks in a term baby), the mean Hb may be as low as 10.0g/dL. With ↑ RBC destruction, there is a concomitant ↑ in serum bilirubin. Thus complex changes occur in this period making distinction between physiology and pathology difficult.

Pathophysiology

In normal full term babies, red cell production ↓ in the first 2–3 months of life. RBC survival shortens; reticulocytes and erythropoietin production ↓; iron, folate and vitamin B_{12} stores are normal. Anaemia in the neonate may be due either to *impaired production* of RBCs or to *increased destruction* or *loss*.

Impaired production	Increased destruction	
Anaemia of prematurity	Overt or concealed haemorrhage; repeated venepuncture	
Infection		
α thalassaemia	**Haemolytic anaemia**	
DBA	***Non-immune***	***Immune***
Fanconi anaemia	TORCH infection	Rh/ABO HDN
CDA	Congenital RBC abn.	Maternal autoimmune haemolytic anaemia
	Drugs, MAHA	

TORCH, toxoplasmosis, rubella, CMV, herpes simplex; DBA, Diamond–Blackfan anaemia; CDA, congenital dyserythropoietic anaemia; Rh/ABO HDN, rhesus/ABO haemolytic disease of the newborn; MAHA, microangiopathic haemolytic anaemia.

Blood loss during delivery is common, in ~1% severe enough to produce anaemia. Infection is also a significant cause of anaemia; primary haematological disorders are rare. Anaemia in premature infant is almost invariably present, induced and multifactorial. Jaundice arises in 90% healthy infants making interpretation of a raised bilirubin (📖 *hyperbilirubinaemia, p444*) a critical piece of the jigsaw when investigating an anaemic neonate.

Clinical features

History may make the diagnosis. Check events at time of delivery, past obstetrical history, maternal and family history. Non-specific symptoms—lethargy, reluctance to feed, failure to thrive—all may indicate anaemia.

Laboratory tests

- FBC and reticulocytes.
- MCV and RBC morphology, bilirubin and Kleihauer (on mother)

Interpret as follows:

- – Reticulocyte count normally very low in first 6 weeks of life.
- – ↑ haemolysis, blood loss.
- – +ve Kleihauer suggests fetomaternal bleed (quantitate amount).
- – Bilirubin ↑ (unconjugated).
- – Check DAT: +ve in immune haemolytic anaemia (except ABO HDN).

  - Negative in other haemolytic anaemias, including ABO HDN).
  - Bilirubin ↑ (conjugated/mixed look for hepatobiliary obstruction/dysfunction).
- Blood film
  - *Note*: ↑ polychromasia, occasional NRBC, poikilocytes and spherocytes day 1–4 in healthy babies.
  - RBC morphology may suggest congenital spherocytosis, other RBC membrane disorders or HDN.
- ↓ MCV—α thalassaemia syndromes.
- ↑ WBC—?reactive, ?congenital leukaemia.
- Neutropenia—?sepsis, ?marrow failure.

Anaemia of prematurity

Anaemia is an almost invariable finding in the premature infant. By week 3–4 of life the Hb may be as low as 7.0g/dL in untreated infants. In a study of very low birth weight infants (750–1499g) 75% required blood transfusion. A number of factors are causal.

Pathogenesis

- RBC production and survival are ↓.
- Erythropoietin production very low in the first few weeks.
- Iatrogenic from repeated blood sampling (depletes the RBC mass and Fe stores—by 4 weeks the premature baby may have had its total blood volume removed).

Clinical features

The increased oxygen needs and metabolic demand of the premature baby makes them less able to tolerate ↓ Hb. Over 50% infants <30 weeks gestation develop tachycardia, tachypnoea, feeding difficulties and ↓ activity when anaemic. High HbF level and ↑ O_2 affinity exaggerates the hypoxia.

Treatment

- Delayed cord clamping increases Fe stores.
- Close control of blood sampling is important.
- Transfusion indications will vary in neonatal units—decide on clinical grounds, particularly if ventilated. The following are guidelines only:
  - Prems <2 wk with Hb <14.0g/dL, Hct <40%.
  - Prems >2 wk, Hb <11.0g/dL, Hct <32%.
- A rising reticulocyte count in some centres is used as a sign to withhold transfusion.
- Some studies have shown better weight gain in transfused infants (not confirmed by others).
- Fe supplementation (2mg/kg/d PO) after first 2 weeks and until iron sufficient.
- Erythropoietin—controversial. It can be effective but its indiscriminate use is not encouraged. Large randomised trials have shown it to have an effect, but its expense makes cost effectiveness a concern and modern neonatal practice has already reduced the need for transfusion making it less necessary. Its best use is probably reserved for transfusion avoidance in infants weighing <1000g. A suitable regimen would be 200–250u/kg SC × 3/week between day 3 and week 6.

Natural history

Despite the growing safety of blood and its ready availability and convenient packaging to reduce donor exposure, blood transfusion carries definite risks and is to be avoided. It is likely that in affluent societies the use of erythropoietin will increase, despite its limited effect.

Paediatric haematology

Haemolytic anaemia in the neonate

Normal red cell life span in term infants is <80 days, in pre-term infants <50 days. Red cell 'cull' in first month with jaundice is physiologic. Pathological haemolysis, when present, is most commonly due to isoimmune HDN secondary to fetomaternal blood group incompatibility in Caucasian populations. In other ethnic groups G6PD deficiency and congenital infection are major causes.

Pathophysiology

Physiological haemolysis occurs soon after birth and there is a marked drop in the Hb and RBC count in the first weeks of life. Neonatal RBCs are more susceptible to oxidative stress and there is altered RBC enzyme activity compared to adult RBC and reticulocytes. So pathological haemolysis occurs in the neonatal period more than at any other time.

Causes of haemolytic anaemia

Haemolysis may be due to intrinsic defects of the RBC, usually congenital, or to acquired extracorpuscular factors which may be immune or non-immune as described below.

Clinical features

- Pathological jaundice may be clinically obvious at birth or within 24h (distinguishing it from the common physiological anaemia which occurs >48h after birth, 📖 *Hyperbilirubinaemia, p444*).
- Anaemia may be severe depending on cause.
- Infections are common cause of hyperbilirubinaemia (📖 p444) with specific clinical findings. *In utero* infections (TORCH) do not usually cause severe jaundice *cf.* post-natal bacterial sepsis where jaundice may be striking and associated with MAHA.
- Splenomegaly at birth indicates a prenatal event; when noted later it may be secondary to splenic clearance of damaged RBC and is non-specific.
- Kernicterus is the major complication of neonatal hyperbilirubinaemia.
- Family history and drug history may be informative.

Laboratory diagnosis of haemolysis

- ↑ unconjugated bilirubin with anaemia is hallmark of haemolytic anaemia.
- ↑ reticulocytes (haptoglobins are unreliable in the newborn).
- Blood film—may show RBC abnormalities e.g. spherocytes, elliptocytes, fragmented cells.
- DAT, if +ve indicates immune haemolysis; –ve does not rule this out—especially consider ABO HDN.
- Heinz body test—positive in drug-induced haemolysis, G6PD deficiency and occasionally other enzyme disorders.
- Intravascular haemolysis—look for haemoglobinuria/haemoglobinaemia.

Paediatric haematology

Congenital red cell defects

Pathophysiology

The neonate is uniquely disadvantaged when it comes to handling pathological haemolysis because of hepatic immaturity and altered enzyme activity. Thus congenital defects of the RBC commonly present in the newborn except for defects involving the β globin chain (e.g. SCD, β thalassaemia) which become clinically manifest several weeks after birth but can be diagnosed *in utero*, or in the neonatal period if suspected. HS is the commonest congenital haemolytic anaemia in Caucasian populations; half present in the neonatal period. Worldwide, G6PD deficiency occurs in 3% population; neonatal presentation is common in Mediterranean and Canton peoples. α thalassaemia is incompatible with life causing hydrops fetalis (all 4 α globin genes deleted), or may present as HbH disease (3 of the 4 α globin genes deleted) with mild to moderate haemolysis in neonate.

Hereditary RBC defects in neonatal haemolytic anaemia

- Membrane defects
  - Hereditary spherocytosis, hereditary elliptocytosis and variants e.g. stomatocytosis and pyropoikilocytosis (Afro-Americans).
- Haemoglobin defects
  - αδβ thalassaemia.
  - Unstable haemoglobins (e.g. HbKöln, HbZurich).
- Enzyme defects
  - Glycolytic pathway; pyruvate kinase and other enzyme deficiencies.
  - Hexose monophosphate shunt; G6PD deficiency, other enzymes.

Clinical features

Congenital haemolytic anaemia with mild or moderate unconjugated hyperbilirubinaemia. No gross excess of bile pigments in urine (old collective name for these diseases was 'acholuric jaundice'), ± hepatosplenomegaly. A +ve family history is common but not invariable.

Laboratory investigation

May be difficult to diagnose in neonate, especially if post-transfusion. Often have to wait until clinically stable some weeks/months later.

- Exclude acquired disorders, and immune lysis (DAT).
- RBC morphology is one key to diagnosis and further investigation, but spherocytes not specific for HS.
- Further tests for suspected
  - Membrane defect (osmotic fragility, autohaemolysis, membrane chemistry).
  - Hb defect; Hb electrophoresis, HbF, A_2 measurement.
  - Enzyme defect; Heinz body prep, screening tests for specific enzymes, G6PD, PK.
- Heinz body test +ve
  - Drug or chemical induced in neonate without hereditary defect.
  - Enzyme deficiency: G6PD commonest but consider others.
  - Unstable Hb.
  - α thalassaemia.

Outcome

Given supportive management including transfusion if necessary, most problems due to congenital red cell defects other than haemoglobinopathies will improve during the first weeks and months of life as the infant matures.

Acquired red cell defects

These may be either immune or non-immune. Main cause of the latter will be underlying infection either acquired *in utero* or in the days following delivery. Drug-induced haemolysis in the newborn is rare.

Pathophysiology

Neonatal RBCs have ↑ sensitivity to oxidative stress due to altered enzyme activity, and are more liable to be destroyed by altered physical conditions, mechanical factors, toxins and drugs than adult RBC. Infection acquired *in utero* post-natally is a common cause of mild to moderate haemolytic anaemia. The mechanism is multifactorial, and includes ↑ reticuloendothelial activity and microangiopathic damage. Drug-induced haemolysis and Heinz body formation is occasionally noted as a transient phenomenon in normal neonatal RBCs as a result of chemical or drug toxicity but is much more often seen when there is an underlying RBC defect such as G6PD deficiency.

Acquired RBC defects causing congenital haemolytic anaemia

- Infection
  - Congenital TORCH infections (TOxoplasmosis, Rubella, Cytomegalovirus, Herpes simplex), also rare but serious are malaria (can cause stillbirth) and syphilis.
  - Post-natal, either viral or (more commonly) bacterial.
- Microangiopathy—2° to severe infections ± DIC, also Kasabach–Merritt syndrome (giant haemangioma with haemolysis and thrombocytopenia).
- Drug or chemically induced.
- Infantile pyknocytosis (📖 *Vitamin E deficiency, below*).
- (Rare) metabolic disease such as Wilson's disease, galactosaemia.

Clinical features

Congenital infections: all rare with adequate antenatal care. Most infants with herpes simplex will be symptomatic with DIC and hepatic dysfunction—haemolysis is not a major finding. Haemolytic anaemia is also mild in CMV and rubella infections but 50% infants with toxoplasmosis will be anaemic (may be severe).

Post-natal infections: viral, bacterial and protozoal (congenital malaria can be delayed for some days or weeks or it can be acquired early in life). Anaemia can be severe and associated with DIC.

MAHA 2° to toxic damage to the endothelium is rare in the neonate outside the context of DIC and sepsis, and is seen in burns and (classically) in the Kasabach–Merritt syndrome—a visible or covert giant haemangioma with haemolysis, RBC damage and profound thrombocytopenia.

Drugs/chemical exposure are more likely to cause Heinz body haemolysis in premature babies or those with G6PD deficiency. Incriminating agents include sulphonamides, chloramphenicol, mothballs, aniline dyes, maternal intake of diuretics and, in the past, water-soluble vitamin K analogues. Vitamin E (a potent antioxidant) has a number of RBC stabilising activities. Now rare due to dietary supplements, deficiency used to be seen occasionally in premature infants, following oxygen therapy and diets rich in polyunsaturated fatty acids. Clinical findings included haemolysis, pre-tibial oedema and CNS signs. Acanthocytosis/pyknocytosis of the RBC is characteristic, and this may have been the main cause of infantile pyknocytosis.

Infantile pyknocytosis: indicates the diagnostic feature of this uncommon acquired disorder. Haemolysis with increased numbers (>6–50%) of pyknocytes (irregularly contracted RBCs with multiple projections) in the peripheral blood. Cause unknown, though may be associated with vitamin E deficiency. Anaemia may be severe and present at birth, and is most striking at ~3 weeks (Hb <5g/dL reported). Exchange transfusion occasionally required but the condition spontaneously remits by ~3 months. Its self-limiting nature and ill-understood pathology means that it may not be a distinct clinical entity.

Metabolic disorders—rare.

Laboratory investigation

Criteria set out above will establish the diagnosis of haemolytic anaemia. A +ve DAT points to an immune process—probably Rh/ABO disease. If non-immune, further tests to look for a congenital abnormality.

The diagnosis may be made by

- Peripheral blood findings.
- Heinz body positive—?chemical/drug-induced haemolysis.
- RBC enzyme screen to exclude G6PD or PK deficiency.
- Hb electrophoresis to exclude Hb defects.

Often no definitive cause is found and the HA will be presumed 2° to underlying systemic illness.

Management

1. General supportive measures for hyperbilirubinaemia (📖 *p444*).
2. Treatment of specific conditions
   - Haemolytic disease of the newborn—📖 *p440*.
   - Neonatal infection as appropriate.
   - Exchange transfusion almost never needed.

Outlook

Prognosis is that of the underlying condition. Anaemia will usually respond as the condition is brought under control.

Haemolytic disease of the newborn (HDN)

Arises when there is blood group incompatibility between mother and fetus. Maternal Abs produced against fetal RBC antigens cross the placenta and destroy fetal RBCs. Most commonly caused by the rhesus D antigen, but maternal passive immunisation with rhesus (Rh) D immunoglobulin (anti-D) introduced in the late 1960s transformed the outlook. Despite this, HDN due to anti-D and other red cell antibodies (e.g. anti-c, anti-Kell) still remains an important cause of fetal morbidity.

Pathogenesis

Placental transfer of fetal cells→maternal circulation is maximal at delivery; the condition does not usually present in the firstborn (*Note*: ABO incompatibility is an exception). Previous maternal transfusion, abortion, amniocentesis, chorionic villus sampling (CVS) or obstetric manipulations can cause antibody formation. Maternal IgG crosses placenta, reacts with Ag +ve fetal RBCs.

Rh HDN classically presents as jaundice in first 24h of life.

Mild HDN may go unnoticed and presents as persistent hyperbilirubinaemia or late anaemia weeks after birth.

Severe HDN may result in a macerated fetus, fresh stillbirth or severely anaemic, grossly oedematous infant (hydrops fetalis) with hepatosplenomegaly 2° to compensatory extramedullary haemopoiesis *in utero*.

Kernicterus: Neurological damage secondary to bilirubin deposition in the brain, depends on a number of factors including the unconjugated bilirubin level, maturity of the baby, the use of interacting drugs.

Diagnosis

Rh HDN is the commonest cause of neonatal immune haemolysis; routine antenatal screening should identify most cases prior to delivery allowing appropriate action.

In suspected case at delivery *cord blood* is tested for
- ABO and Rh (D) group.
- Presence of antibody on fetal RBCs by DAT.
- Hb and blood film (spherocytes, increased polychromasia, NRBCs).
- Serum bilirubin (↑).

***Maternal blood* is tested for**
- ABO and Rh (D) group.
- Serum antibodies against fetal cells (by indirect antiglobulin test, IAGT).
- Antibody titre.
- Kleihauer test—detects and quantitates fetal RBCs in maternal circulation.

Diagnostic findings include
- DAT +ve haemolytic anaemia ± spherocytosis in the infant.

- Maternal anti-D, or other anti Rh antibody—the next most common to produce severe disease is anti-c.

ABO HDN

Theoretically should occur more frequently since ~1 in 4/5 babies and mothers are ABO incompatible. Usually occurs in group O mothers who may have high titres of naturally occurring IgG anti-A or B, and with a boost to this during pregnancy haemolysis can occur.

Clinical features

First pregnancies are not exempt, but condition is usually mild. Presentation is later than with Rh HDN (2–4d, but may be weeks after birth).

Diagnosis

May be difficult—DAT commonly and puzzlingly –ve, but offending antibody can be eluted from infant RBC.

Antibody studies

Maternal high titre anti-A/B almost always in a group O mother cord-blood/infant's serum-an inappropriate antibody (e.g. anti-A in a group A baby).

Other blood group antibodies

Can occasionally produce severe HDN; anti-Kell in particular. Serological testing will establish diagnosis. Maternal autoimmune haemolytic anaemia may produce a similar picture to alloimmune HDN where the auto-antibody cross-reacts with the infant RBC. Usually the diagnosis will have been made antenatally. Severity in infant varies depending on maternal condition.

Management—prevention

Routine antenatal maternal ABO and Rh D grouping and antibody testing carried out at booking visit (~12–16 weeks).

If antibody positive repeat at intervals to check the antibody titre.

If antibody negative and Rh D negative repeat at ~28 weeks' gestation. Establish if paternal red cells heterozygous, homozygous or negative for the specific Ag.

Anti-D prophylaxis

- 250iu IM during pregnancy to Rh D negative women without antibodies to cover any intrauterine manoeuvre or miscarriage.
- After delivery, a standard dose of 500iu anti-D within 72h unless baby is known to be Rh (D) –ve.
- If Kleihauer test result shows a bleed of >4mL give further anti-D.

Treatment of affected fetus—before delivery

Treatment depends on past obstetric history, the nature and titre of the antibody and paternal expression of the antigen. The fetal genotype can be established by CVS, fetal blood sampling and PCR.

Examination of the amniotic fluid to assess the degree of hyperbilirubinaemia is indicated with a poor past history (exchange transfusion or stillbirth in previous baby) and high titre (1:8–1:64) of an antibody likely to cause severe HDN (e.g. anti-D, anti-c or anti-Kell). The amniotic fluid bilirubin at optical density 450nm dictates treatment according to the Liley chart (opposite), which estimates the blood concentration.

Options include intrauterine transfusion (IUT) if fetus is not deemed mature enough for delivery (check lung maturity on phospholipid levels) or induction of labour if it is. Intensive maternal plasmapheresis may be useful to reduce antibody titre. Advances in management of very premature babies are such that nowadays IUT rarely performed.

After delivery

- Full paediatric support—metabolic, nutritional and respiratory.
- If unconjugated hyperbilirubinaemia not a problem, treat anaemia (*note*: cord blood Hb <14.0g/dL) by simple transfusion.
- Exchange transfusion with Rh (D) neg and (if possible) group specific blood for:
  - A severely affected hydropic anaemic baby.
  - Hyperbilirubinaemia (bilirubin level at or near 340mmol/L (20mg/dL) or rapidly rising level e.g. >20mmol/h) in first few days of life.
  - Signs suggesting kernicterus—exchange transfusion may have to be repeated.
- Phototherapy to reduce the bilirubin level.
- Follow-up required—late anaemia can be severe particularly if exchange transfusion has not been carried out.

Outcome

With modern techniques, the outlook is good even for severely affected infants.

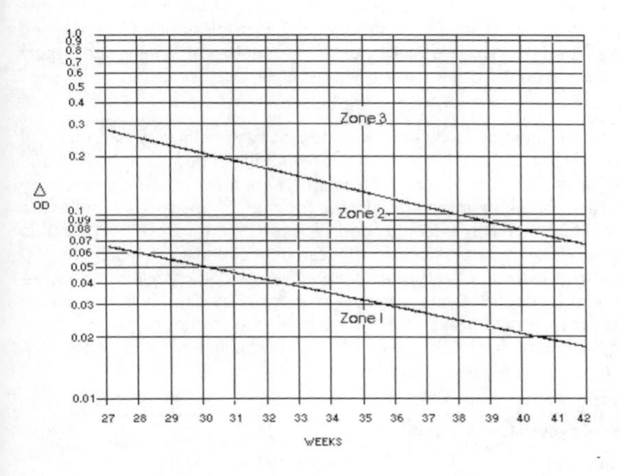

Liley chart

The amount of bilirubin can be quantitated by spectrophotometrically measuring absorbance at 450nm wavelength in a specimen of amniotic fluid that has been shielded from light. The results (delta 450) are plotted on a 'Liley' curve, which is divided into three zones.

A result in **Zone I** indicates mild or no disease. Fetuses in zone I are usually followed with amniocentesis every 3 weeks. A result in zone II indicates intermediate disease. Fetuses in low **Zone II** are usually followed by amniocentesis every 1–2 weeks. A result above the middle of Zone II may require transfusion or urgent delivery.

Hyperbilirubinaemia

Bilirubin results from the breakdown of haem, mostly Hb haem. It may be unconjugated water insoluble pre-hepatic (a mark of excessive RBC breakdown) or conjugated soluble post-hepatic (↑ in cholestasis). Unconjugated bilirubin ↑ in most neonates and is usually physiological; conjugated hyperbilirubinaemia, on the other hand, is almost always pathological.

Pathophysiology

Physiological jaundice is defined as a temporary inefficient excretion of bilirubin which results in jaundice in full-term infants between the 2nd and 8th day of life. Occurs in ~90% of healthy neonates. Hepatic immaturity and ↑ RBC breakdown overloads the neonate's ability to handle the bilirubin which is mainly unconjugated. The bilirubin is rarely >100μmol/L, though between 2–5 days occasionally can be >200 in a term baby or 250 in a healthy pre-term. Levels much above this need investigation. Reaches a maximum by days 3–6 and usually ↓ to normal by day 10. In premature neonates it may take longer to settle. HDN due to blood group incompatibility accounts for ~10% cases of hyperbilirubinaemia and about 75% of those requiring exchange transfusion.

Causes of hyperbilirubinaemia

Unconjugated	Conjugated
Physiological jaundice	Mechanical obstruction
Haemolytic anaemia	Bile duct abnormalities
Haematoma	(e.g. atresia, cysts)
Polycythaemia	Hepatocellular disorders
Biochemical defects	Hepatitis

Clinical features

- *Note: clinical jaundice in the first 24h of life is always pathological.*
- Presenting after this, the jaundice may/not be pathological—usually not. Inadequate food/fluid intake with dehydration can aggravate the physiological bilirubin. A higher concentration is acceptable for the full-term breast-fed baby (serum bilirubin 240μmol/L) than bottle-fed baby (190μmol/L).
- Jaundice in an active healthy infant is likely to be physiological.
- In a sick infant the underlying cause of the jaundice may be clinically evident—e.g. infection, anaemia, shock, asphyxia, haemorrhage (may be occult).
- Physical examination—hepatosplenomegaly is pathological.
- Maternal history (drugs, known condition) and family history may help.

Laboratory investigation

- FBC, reticulocyte count and film-?haemolytic anaemia.
- Serum bilirubin—?conjugated or unconjugated
  - Unconjugated hyperbilirubinaemia.
    DAT, maternal and neonatal blood group serology.
    Infection evaluation including TORCH.
    Thyroid function.

Reducing substances.
- Conjugated hyperbilirubinaemia.
  Abdominal USS, bile pigments in stool, liver pathology.
- Further investigation as determined by results and clinical picture.

Management
- General—adequate hydration, nutrition, other supportive measures.
- Treat underlying cause—antibiotics, metabolic disturbances.
- Haemolytic anaemia—blood transfusion.
- Specific phototherapy (light source with wavelength between 400–500mm) effective in treating most causes of unconjugated hyperbilirubinaemia. *Note*: contraindicated in conjugated hyperbilirubinaemia.
- Exchange transfusion—the indications are complex. Main indication is severe haemolytic anaemia and is used in full-term infants when the bilirubin is >340μmol/L and at a lower concentration in premature infants.
- Hyperbilirubinaemia due to mechanical obstruction may need surgery.

Outcome
In most infants hyperbilirubinaemia resolves by 2 weeks. When pathology has been excluded the commonest cause of prolonged hyperbilirubinaemia persisting beyond this period is breastfeeding. In 20% healthy breast-fed infants the bilirubin is still significantly ↑ at day 21. Kernicterus is not a complication but the condition causes concern before it spontaneously remits.

Neonatal haemostasis

Neonates can develop bruising and/or purpura due to defects in platelets, coagulation factors or both. Coagulation tests should be interpreted with caution because in the term infant the concentration of vitamin K-dependent proteins (II, VII, XI and X together with protein C and protein S) are 50% of normal adult values, contact factors (XI, XII, PK and HMWK) are 30–50% of adult concentrations, and all are lower in pre-terms. Factors VIII, V and vWF are normal. Thrombin inhibitors antithrombin (AT, previously called antithrombin III) and HCII are ↓ but α2-M is ↑. Platelet count is the same as adults in both term and pre-term infants. There are technical problems in obtaining uncontaminated (heparin from catheters or IV lines) and adequate venous samples from neonates, causing *in vitro* inhibition or pre-test activation of clotting factors or dilution due to short sampling and thus excess anticoagulant. All can give spurious results.

Pathophysiology

Haemostatic and fibrinolytic system in neonates is immature. Sepsis, liver disease, necrotising colitis and RDS can precipitate DIC easily. Thrombocytopenia can be caused by DIC and also immune mechanisms or marrow failure.

Disorders causing bleeding in neonates

Inherited (rare)	Acquired (common)
Haemophilia	DIC (sepsis, necrotising colitis, hypoxia, RDS)
von Willebrand's disease (only type 3)	Vitamin K deficiency
Other inherited factor deficiencies	Liver disease
Inherited thrombotic disorders	Acquired thrombotic disorders
Glanzmann's thrombasthenia	Neonatal alloimmune thrombocytopenia Maternally derived ITP Endogenous ITP Aplasia Leukaemia

Clinical features

- Petechiae indicate problems with small vessels or platelets, bruises can be due to platelet deficiencies and/or coagulation disorders.
- Oozing from multiple venepunture sites in sick infants usually indicates generalised haemostatic failure and DIC.
- Haemorrhagic disease of the newborn due to functional vitamin K deficiency presents in 3 forms with bruising, purpura and GI bleeding in otherwise well babies; early (within 24h) usually due to maternal drugs such as warfarin, classical (days 2–5) in babies who have not been given adequate vitamin K prophylaxis and who have been breast fed and late, a variant of the classical form (i.e. insufficient vitamin K, breast-fed) arising at 2–8 weeks and with a higher morbidity and ↑ incidence of ICH.

- Thrombosis usually catheter related, can be rarely associated with AT III deficiency or homozygous protein C and protein S deficiency (neonatal purpura fulminans—a life-threatening condition with widespread peripheral gangrene).
- Haemophilia and other coagulant deficiencies can cause large haematomas but rarely cause trouble in the neonatal period except factor XIII lack—typically presents with bleeding from the umbilical stump.
- In well babies, petechiae and bruises with thrombocytopenia suggests immune basis—antibody usually from mother (alloimmune or autoimmune). Rarely, infants under a month can develop endogenous ITP.
- Clear symptoms of thrombocytopenia with normal platelet count suggests major functional defect—Glanzmann's.
- Marrow failure due to infiltration, aplasia.

Neonatal alloimmune thrombocytopenia (NAIT)

Occurs when mothers form alloimmune antibodies against fetal platelet-specific antigens that their own platelets lack. These antibodies react with fetal platelets *in utero* causing thrombocytopenia which can be severe, and in some cases life threatening in late pregnancy and early life. A more serious condition with greater morbidity than thrombocytopenia due to maternal autoantibodies against platelets—i.e. where the mother has ITP.

Pathophysiology

In >90% cases the mother will be HPA-1a (old term PLA1) –ve with anti-HPA-1a antibodies against the HPA-1a +ve fetus; only 2% population are HPA-1a –ve (i.e. homozygous HPA-1b). Incidence of NAIT is 1/1000 pregnancies and accounts for 10–20% cases of neonatal thrombocytopenia. Other antigens may be involved e.g. HPA-5 (Br) and HPA-3 (Bak) are the commonest.

Clinical features

- Commonly presents in first born infant and recurs in 85–90%.
- Maternal platelet count normal with no past history of ITP.
- Bleeding manifestations in 10–20% evident within the first few days of life e.g. umbilical haemorrhage, petechiae, ecchymosis, internal haemorrhage, intracranial haemorrhage (ICH).
- Baby's platelet count ↑ to normal over the next 2–3 weeks as the antibody is cleared.
- Haemorrhage *in utero* with fatal ICH in ~1% cases.

Laboratory diagnosis

Baby	**Parents**
Severe thrombocytopenia platelets $<20 \times 10^9$/L in 50%	Mother's platelet count normal
BM has megakaryocytes ++ (not usually necessary)	Serology: Mother's platelets usually HPA-1a –ve
	Rarer Ab include anti-HPA-3a, HPA-5b, HPA-4 (Yuk/Pen)
	Mother's serum contains anti-platelet antibody
	(*Note*: antibody titre cannot predict degree of thrombocytopenia in fetus in subsequent pregnancies)
	Father's platelets carry offending antigen

Management

Of bleeding neonate: transfuse platelets –ve for Ag (usually HPA-1a –ve); use random donor platelets in an emergency. Maternal platelets (*irradiated*) are a good source. Repeat platelet transfusion PRN. IVIg as for

ITP can be used in exceptional cases (response within days). Close observation (ICH is potentially lethal—screen using USS).

Of subsequent pregnancies: cordocentesis *in utero* at ~24 weeks; take 1–3mL blood for platelet count and phenotype. If affected, treatment needs to be started immediately.

Options

1. *In utero* CMV –ve compatible platelet transfusions at 2–4 weekly intervals (depending on severity and history). Invasive and technically demanding. Keep platelet count >50 × 10^9/L (platelets ↓ rapidly so frequent follow-up mandatory).
2. Maternal administration of IVIg (1g/kg) weekly from ~24 weeks onwards: check fetal platelet count ~4 weeks later and again near term; response variable—around 75% respond—transfuse platelets if non-responsive. Check cord blood at birth and treat as necessary.

Outcome

With aggressive treatment the outcome is good, death *in utero* and ICH occur rarely. A history of a previous ICH correlates with severe thrombocytopenia in subsequent pregnancies.

Congenital dyserythropoietic anaemias

A rare group of inherited lifelong anaemias with morphologically abnormal marrow erythroblasts and ineffective erythropoiesis. Three clinically distinguishable types are recognised where inheritance may be recessive (types I and II) or dominant (type III). A number of families have been described that share some features but do not fit with the typical patterns.

Pathophysiology

Ineffective erythropoiesis (cell death within the BM); RBC survival in PB is not much reduced (III). Abnormal serological and haemolytic characteristics (type II CDA) and membrane abnormalities are described but as yet no defining shared defect in all cases of CDA.

Type	Bone marrow	Blood findings	Inheritance
I	Megaloblastic + intranuclear chromatin bridges	Macrocytic RBC	Recessive
II (HEMPAS)*	Bi/multinuclearity with	Normocytic RBCs pluripolar mitosis Lysis in acidified serum (not autologous serum)	Recessive
III	Giant erythroblasts with multinuclearity	Macrocytic	Dominant

*Hereditary erythroblast multinuclearity with positive acidified serum test; commonest form, found in ~66% cases

Clinical features

- Age of presentation variable; but usually in older children (>10 years). Can rarely present as neonatal jaundice and anaemia.
- Anaemia—in type I, Hb 8.0–12.0g/dL; type II anaemia may be more severe, patient may be transfusion dependent. Type III (rare) anaemia is mild/moderate.
- Jaundice (2° to intramedullary RBC destruction).
- Gallstones.
- Splenomegaly common.

Laboratory diagnosis

- Peripheral blood—normocytic/macrocytic RBC with anisopoikilocytosis.
- WBC and platelets usually normal; reticulocytes slightly ↑.
- BM appearance—striking, showing ↑ cellularity with excess abnormal erythroblasts.
- Type II shows positive acidified serum test.
- ↑ Serum ferritin due to ↑ Fe absorption; haemosiderosis can occur without transfusion dependence. Type III very occasionally Fe deficient due to intravascular haemolysis and haemosiderinuria.

Differential diagnosis

- CDA variants—not all CDA falls neatly into 3 subtypes on BM findings, serology or clinical features.
- PNH—acidified serum test is +ve with heterologous and autologous serum. In HEMPAS +ve with heterologous serum only.
- Other megaloblastic/dyserythropoietic anaemias—including vitamin B_{12} and folate deficiency.
- Primary/acquired sideroblastic anaemia.
- Erythroleukaemia (M6 AML).

Treatment

- Mostly unnecessary.
- Avoid blood transfusion if possible (iron overload)—iron chelation as necessary.
- Splenectomy not curative but may decrease transfusion requirements.
- Type I may respond to high dose IFN-α; not recommended as routine therapy.

Natural history

Severity of CDA varies considerably and many patients have good quality of life with no therapy. Haemosiderosis is a long term complication which may impact on survival.

Congenital red cell aplasia

Diamond and Blackfan first described congenital red cell aplasia in infants in 1938 giving rise to the name of Diamond–Blackfan anaemia (DBA). Incidence now estimated to be 4–7/million live births.

Pathophysiology

Probably always due to an as yet undefined germline genetic mutation, either inherited or arising in the affected infant. Familial patterns with both autosomal dominant and recessive inheritance have been described. Surviving sporadic cases (i.e. non-familial) have transmitted the disease to their children. Nature of underlying defect not known. Gene(s) involved not yet identified despite multiple associated developmental abnormalities. Anaemia likely to be due to intrinsic RBC progenitor cell defect rather than one of the microenvironment. ↓ sensitivity of these cells to Epo and other cytokines described.

Clinical features

- Usually presents in the first year of life: in 25% at birth and 90% <6 months of age. Rarely presents >1 year.
- Mildly affected individuals may rarely be detected as older children or adults during family studies.
- Associated physical anomalies in 50%; abnormal facies with abnormal eyes, webbed neck, malformed (including triphalangeal) thumbs, other skeletal abnormalities, short stature, congenital heart lesions, renal defects.
- Anaemia usually severe and child commonly transfusion dependent.
- Susceptibility to infection is not ↑.
- Hepatosplenomegaly absent.
- Family history is +ve in only 10–20% cases; most are sporadic.
- ↑ risk of AML in long survivors; ~5% in biggest series reported to date.

Laboratory diagnosis

- Hb ↓, reticulocytes ↓, MCV ↑ (> normal for age), WBC and platelets not ↓.
- Red cells—normal morphology, have ↑ i antigen positivity, ↑ ADA activity.
- HbF ↑, Epo ↑, serum Fe/ferritin ↑.
- BM findings—usually absent erythroid precursors; other cell lines normal.
- No evidence of parvovirus infection.
- Radiological investigation to define other congenital defects.

Differential diagnosis

- Transient erythroblastopenia of childhood (📖 *following section*; later presentation, transient, no other defects).
- Drugs, malnutrition, infection.
- Haemolytic anaemias in hypoplastic phase, with parvovirus B19, delayed recovery in HDN.
- Megaloblastic anaemia in aplastic phase.

Treatment

- Prednisolone 2mg/kg PO in divided doses, slowly ↓ over weeks; 70% respond well. Titrate to lowest dose to maintain Hb >7g/dL. Many achieve this on almost homeopathic doses despite true dependence. Around 10% need high dose maintenance and have trouble with side effects. 30% steroid resistant (try high dose methylprednisolone).
- Transfusion dependency usual in those who cannot be maintained on very low dose steroids. Need chelation to prevent iron overload. Use CMV –ve leucocyte-depleted packed RBC.
- Splenectomy not helpful (unless hypersplenism).
- Bone marrow transplantation worth considering for transfusion dependents with suitable donor; risk stratification as for severe thalassaemia (iron overload). Complicated decision due to chance of spontaneous remission even after years of transfusion dependency.

Natural history

Spontaneous remission in 10–20% (even after several years). Median survival estimated at 30–40 years, though data patchy. Death due to haemosiderosis, complications of steroid therapy, or evolution of AML or aplastic anaemia. BMT may offer better outlook. DBA Registry established in 1993 is prospectively gathering new data.

Acquired red cell aplasia

Isolated failure of erythropoiesis. Most commonly transient—either due to parvovirus B19 infection or transient erythroblastopenia of childhood (TEC). Acquired pure red cell aplasia (PRCA) seen in adults with or without thymoma and probably autoimmune in nature (📖 *p122*) virtually unknown in childhood, though very occasionally seen in adolescents.

Parvovirus B19 infection

Clinical features

- Causes transient reticulocytopenia and (occasionally) neutropenia and thrombocytopenia in otherwise healthy individuals.
- In children with increased red cell turnover for any reason (compensated haemolysis, ineffective erythropoiesis) or those with reduced red cell production (marrow suppression or hypoplasia) can produce dramatic falls in Hb.
- Can affect any age.
- Self-limiting as infection subsides following antibody response, 7–10d.
- In immunosuppressed children (e.g. chemotherapy, HIV) anaemia can occasionally become chronic with persisting viraemia.

Pathogenesis

Parvovirus shows tropism for red cells through the P antigen, and is cytotoxic for erythroid progenitor cells at the colony forming stage (CFU-E) *in vitro*.

Transient erythroblastopenia of childhood

Pathogenesis

Serum and cellular inhibitors of erythropoiesis and defective bone marrow response to stimulating cytokines have been demonstrated. The condition may be idiopathic or associated with viral infection. It is uncommon but not excessively rare and there may be many subclinical cases where a blood count is not done.

Clinical features

- Boys and girls equally affected: age range 6 months to 5 years; most commonly around 2 years.
- Typically a previously well young child presents with symptoms and signs of anaemia, sometimes but not invariably following an infection. Onset is insidious and the child becomes listless and pale—or just pale.
- Associated infections are usually viral (EBV, mumps), preceding the onset of TEC by some weeks.
- Fever is rare.
- Pallor may be striking.
- No lymphadenopathy or hepatosplenomegaly.
- No physical abnormalities.

Laboratory diagnosis

- Normocytic, normochromic anaemia which may be severe (Hb <5g/dL).
- Reticulocytes absent unless in early recovery phase; WBC and platelets usually normal.
- Blood film shows no abnormality other than anaemia.
- Biochemical profile normal.

- Bone marrow shows normocellular picture with absent erythroid precursors. Iron content is normal.
- No karyotypic abnormalities.
- Exclude parvovirus infection (📖 *p454*).
- No other investigation is of diagnostic help.

Differential diagnosis

- Exclude acute blood loss and anaemia of chronic disease.
- Exclude common ALL.
- Diamond–Blackfan anaemia (*see previous section*). Usually presents within the first 6 months of life and other abnormalities (skeletal malformation, short stature, abnormal facies) are commonly present.
- Parvovirus infection (*see above*).

Treatment

Blood transfusion should be avoided but may be necessary if symptomatic.

Natural history

Spontaneously remits (if not then diagnosis probably wrong) commonly within 4–8 weeks but may be up to 6 months. Relapse is rare. There are no long-term sequelae or associations.

Fanconi's anaemia

First described by Fanconi in 1967, Fanconi's anaemia (FA) is a clinically heterogeneous disorder usually presenting in childhood with the common feature being slowly progressive marrow failure affecting all 3 cell lines (RBC, WBC and megakaryocytes) and manifest by peripheral blood pancytopenia and eventual marrow aplasia. It is a recessively inherited disorder with several different germline genetic mutations involving at least 8 genes, 4 of which have been identified and characterised, and all of which are on different chromosomes.

Pathophysiology of Fanconi's anaemia.

FA affects all cells of the body and the cellular phenotype is characterised by increased chromosomal breakage, hypersensitivity to DNA cross-linking agents such as diepoxybutane (DEB) and mitomycin C (MMC), hypersensitivity to oxygen, increased apoptosis and accelerated telomere shortening. The increased chromosomal fragility is characteristic and used as a diagnostic test. Apart from progressive marrow failure, 70% of FA patients show somatic abnormalities, chiefly involving the skeleton. 90% develop marrow failure and survivors show an increased risk of developing leukaemia, chiefly AML. Rarely, FA can present as AML. There is also an increased risk of liver tumours and squamous cell carcinomas.

Clinical features

- Autosomal recessive inheritance: in 10–20% the parents are related.
- Phenotypic expression of the disease varies widely, though similar in any given kindred. Most commonly presents as insidious evolution of pancytopenia, presenting in mid-childhood with a median age of presentation of 9 years. Cell lines affected asynchronously; isolated thrombocytopenia may be first manifestation, lasting 2–3 years before other cytopenias occur.
- 10% present in adolescence or adult life, 4% present in early infancy (<1 year).
- Disorders of skin pigmentation common (60%)—café-au-lait spots, hypo- and hyperpigmentation.
- Short stature in 60%, microcephaly and delayed development in >20%.
- Congenital abnormalities can affect almost any system—skeletal defects common, >50% in the upper limb especially thumb, spine, ribs.
- Characteristic facies described—elfin-like, with tapering jaw line.

Diagnosis

Laboratory findings

- Pancytopenia and hypoplastic marrow—patchy cellularity.
- Bone marrow may also show dyserythropoietic morphology.
- Anaemia varies in its severity and may be macrocytic (MCV 100–120fL).
- Excessive chromosomal breaks/rearrangements in culture of peripheral blood lymphocytes challenged with clastogens (DEB or MMC) is the defining abnormality, and can be used on fetal cell culture for antenatal diagnosis.
- Direct probing for mutations in the FA genes that have been identified and characterised permits molecular diagnosis in around 80% of patients, but is complex and slow.

- Further investigation for systemic congenital abnormalities is indicated.

Differential diagnosis
- Acquired aplastic anaemia (📖 *p122*).
- Other congenital or inherited childhood marrow failure syndromes—*see following page*.
- Bloom's syndrome—clinically like Fanconi's anaemia with similar congenital defects, spontaneous chromosomal breaks and a predisposition to leukaemia but without pancytopenia, or bone marrow hypoplasia. Autosomal recessive. Characteristically have photosensitivity and telangiectatic facial erythema. Genetic mutation mapped to chromosome 15q26.

Treatment

General
- Supportive—blood transfusion with iron chelation as required.
- Treatment of associated congenital anomalies where necessary.

Specific
- Combined therapy with steroids (moderate dosage alternate days) and androgens (oxymethalone 2–5mg/kg/d). Most patients respond to treatment but eventually become refractory.
- Haemopoietic growth factors may offer temporary relief from neutropenia and anaemia.
- BMT is potentially curative, but FA patients hypersensitive to conditioning agents cyclophosphamide and radiation. Using low doses, matched sibling grafts give 70% actuarial survival at 2 years; unrelated donor results less good but improving. Early survivors showed ↑ risk of tumours, especially head and neck.
- Much interest in gene therapy. Early trials have occurred, but no major therapeutic success. Theoretically should be possible to transduce patient stem cells from those with known mutations with the appropriate wild type FA gene, and for these stem cells to have a natural growth advantage over FA cells. So far responses have been disappointing and short-lived.

Outcome

Median survival of conventional treatment responders who do not undergo BMT is ~25 years. Non-responders have a median survival of ~12 years. Death most commonly due to marrow failure, but 10–20% will develop MDS or AML after a median period of observation of 13 years.

Rare congenital marrow failure syndromes

Amegakaryocytic thrombocytopenia (congenital amegakaryocytic thrombocytopenia)

Presents in infancy (usually at birth or within 2 months) with profoundly ↓ platelets and associated physical signs (petechiae and bruising). Around 40% of affected children also have other congenital abnormalities—chiefly neurologic or cardiac. Developmental delay is common. The marrow completely lacks megakaryocytes and the disorder evolves to severe aplastic anaemia in around 50% of sufferers, usually in the first few years of life. Has none of the unstable DNA features of Fanconi's anaemia (*see previous page*). Also quite distinct from the syndrome of thrombocytopenia with absent radius (TAR syndrome, *see below*) since it is a trilineage problem with a much greater mortality. Usually sporadic, but familial cases occur and disorder thought to be inherited. No gene yet identified.

Outlook

Without BMT, mortality from bleeding, infection or (occasionally) progression to leukaemia near 100%.

Amegakaryocytic thrombocytopenia with absent radii (TAR syndrome)

- Usually diagnosed at birth because of lower arm deformity due to bilateral radial aplasia.
- No hyperpigmentation.
- Isolated thrombocytopenia with other cell lines normal.
- Bone marrow lacks megakaryocytes; has adequate WBC/RBC precursors.
- No chromosomal breaks in cell culture.
- Autosomal recessive; no gene yet identified.
- Thrombopoietin ↑; platelets gradually increase as child grows.
- Bleeding problems greatest in infancy.
- Supportive therapy only needed.

Outlook

Usually good, with problems receding as childhood proceeds. Occasional patients continue to have problems with ↓ platelets. No ↑ malignancy.

Dyskeratosis congenita

- Inherited disorder of mucocutaneous and haemopoietic systems.
- Clinical triad of skin pigmentation, leucoplakia of the mucous membranes, dystrophic nails and, in 50% patients, severe aplastic anaemia develops, usually in the second decade.
- Usually sex-linked inheritance through single gene at Xq28, though 15% autosomal so phenotype dependent on more than 1 gene.
- Other congenital and immunological abnormalities described.
- Chromosome fragility on challenge with DEB or mitomycin C normal—important to distinguish DC from Fanconi's anaemia (*see previous page*).
- Despite this some evidence of DNA instability; results of BMT for aplastic anaemia in DC patients poor, perhaps because of this.
- Anecdotal reports of good response to haemopoietic growth factors.

Outlook

10% develop cancers before the age of 40—mostly epithelial, but also MDS/AML. Life expectancy depends on development of aplasia or malignancy. 30% survive to middle age.

Kostmann's syndrome (congenital neutropenia)

- Autosomal recessive.
- Severe neutropenia with neutrophils $<0.2 \times 10^9$/L.
- Marrow shows maturation arrest at promyelocyte/myelocyte stage.
- High risk of severe infection in untreated state.
- Not due to germline mutation in G-CSF receptor gene, though abnormal receptor may be present in myeloid precursors.
- 90% will respond to pharmacological doses of G-CSF and continue to do so for years.
- Up to 10% develop AML/MDS—role of G-CSF not clear, but probably complication of disease revealed by longer survival.

Diagnosis

Distinguish from cyclical neutropenia (by observation); benign congenital neutropenia (by WBC) and reticular dysgenesis a severe inherited immunodeficiency with congenital lack of all white cells, including lymphocytes.

Outlook

Good provided response to G-CSF satisfactory and maintained. Non-responders may need BMT.

Shwachman–Diamond syndrome

- Congenital exocrine pancreatic insufficiency; chronic diarrhoea, malabsorption and growth failure associated with neutropenia.
- Bone marrow failure not usually trilineage, though platelets and red cells can be involved.
- Bone marrow varies—may be dysplastic/hypo/aplastic.
- Probably autosomal recessive, but no gene yet identified.
- Psychomotor delay common.

Diagnosis

- Exclude cystic fibrosis (by normal sweat test).
- Exclude Fanconi's anaemia (by normal chromosome fragility).
- Pearson's syndrome clinically similar with severe pancreatic insufficiency but with anaemia rather than neutropenia and marrow shows ring sideroblasts and vacuolisation of red and white cell precursors.

Treatment

- Supportive with pancreatic enzymes, G-CSF and antibiotics.
- Greatly increased risk (up to 30%) of progression to MDS/leukaemia (AML > ALL).
- Limited experience with BMT for aplasia/leukaemia; may be increased risk of cardiotoxicity—ventricular fibrosis seen at autopsy in 2/5 patients who died post BMT.

Outlook

Depends on development of severe aplasia or leukaemia; long survivors few if so. Pancreatic insufficiency improves as childhood progresses.

Seckel's syndrome—bird-headed dwarfism

- Rare autosomal recessive disorder with (proportionate) very short stature and mental deficiency.
- Facial features fancifully described as bird-like.
- Gene(s) responsible unknown.
- Progression to aplastic anaemia common, clinically similar to Fanconi's anaemia (*see previous page*) but chromosome fragility normal.

Infantile osteopetrosis

- Pancytopenia can arise in this autosomal recessive disorder where the marrow cavity is obliterated with cortical bone due to a functional deficiency of osteoclasts.
- It is a primary marrow failure in the sense that there is no marrow, but is a failure of the microenvironment rather than haemopoietic stem cells.

Outlook

Poor due to cranial compression, and children usually die in early childhood unless successful allogeneic BMT can replace normal osteoclast function.

Paediatric haematology

Neutropenia in childhood

Apart from primary marrow failure due to aplastic anaemia or other marrow failure syndromes (📖 p122) or marrow suppression due to antineoplastic, immunosuppressive or antiviral chemotherapy, neutropenia can also arise as an immune phenomenon, a cytokine mediated problem or due to cyclic or non-cyclic disturbances of the homeostasis of neutrophil production.

Pathophysiology

- Commonest cause of a clinically important low neutrophil count in children ($<0.5 \times 10^9$/L) is myelosuppression due to drugs.
- Primary marrow stem cell failure failure either involving all cell lines or granulopoiesis alone is rare.
- Neutropenia can also be due to less serious inherited deficiencies of neutrophil production where neutropenia can be variable or cyclical and the problem seems to be one of production control rather than primary stem cell failure.
- Probably due to cytokine disturbances, several microbial infections can cause paradoxical neutropenia, particularly in neonates but also in older children.
- Autoimmune causes of neutropenia can arise in infancy or later in childhood.
- Isoimmune neutropenia in the newborn—due to maternal anti-neutrophil antibodies and analogous to HDN.

Homeostatic disorders

Cyclic neutropenia: Rare. Neutropenia arising every 21d lasting 3–6d. Counts may fall $<0.2 \times 10^9$/L. Associated with episodes of fever, malaise, mucous membrane ulcers, lymphadenopathy. Serious infection can arise and deaths May improve after puberty. Usually positive family history when problem encountered in childhood. Treatment supportive with antibiotics. G-CSF may be useful.

Chronic benign neutropenia: More common. Persistent rather than cyclical, though often variable without clear periodicity. Neutrophil count usually $>0.5 \times 10^9$/L, so clinically mild or silent. May have autosomal dominant or autosomal recessive family history. Variable severity, often mild with few problems. To be distinguished from severe congenital neutropenia (📖 *Kostmann's syndrome, p459*) by milder clinical course and (usually) later presentation. Therapy not usually necessary.

Infections causing neutropenia		
Viruses	**Bacteria**	**Others**
RSV	Tuberculosis	Rickettsiae
Malaria	Typhoid/paratyphoid	
Influenza	*E coli* (neonates)	
Measles		
Varicella		
HIV		

Autoimmune neutropenia (AIN)

Infant form of isolated autoimmune neutropenia occurs within 1st year of life; demonstrable autoantibodies. Not familial; girls>boys. Self-limiting and usually relatively benign. Therapy supportive. Steroids not usually needed and can increase infection risk. IVIg has been used.

Older children may get

- Isolated AI neutropenia.
- Neutropenia as part of Evans' syndrome (📖 *p388*).
- Neutropenia as part of multi-system AI disease—lupus erythematosus
- Immune neutropenia following allogeneic BMT.
- Felty's syndrome (rheumatoid arthritis with splenomegaly and hyper-splenic cytopenias—📖 *p17*) may also be associated with neutrophil autoantibodies.
- All are potentially more serious and complicated than the infant form and may require immunosuppression as well as supportive therapy.

Isoimmune neutropenia of the newborn

- Maternal antibodies to fetal neutrophil antigens cross the placenta and give rise to neutropenia in the newborn child.
- Most commonly antibodies directed at neutrophil-specific antigens NA1 and NA2. (Maternal HLA antibodies do not cause trouble because antigens expressed on many tissues so quickly absorbed.)
- Estimated incidence up to 3% of newborns, so may be more common than generally appreciated; perhaps because usually clinically mild and neutropenia thought to be acquired due to drugs/infection.
- Condition resolves by 2 months as antibody disappears.
- Severely affected babies may show recurrent staphylococcal skin infections. Therapy supportive. Need for exchange transfusion very rare.
- Diagnosis based on serology.

Prognosis of neutropenia

Whatever the cause, severe neutropenia ($<0.2 \times 10^9$/L) is serious and incompatible with long survival if prolonged. It requires careful expert management.

Disorders of neutrophil function

Acquired
Mild defects arise in many clinical situations; following some infections, associated with drugs (steroids, chemotherapy) and systemic disease (malnutrition, diabetes mellitus, rheumatoid arthritis, CRF, sickle cell anaemia)—here the underlying condition will dominate the clinical picture.

Congenital
Inherited defects rare but several important and disabling syndromes occur in children.

Pathophysiology
Neutrophils produced in BM are released into circulation where they survive for only a few hours. Fundamental role is to kill bacteria. Do this by moving to site of infection drawn there (chemotaxis) by interaction of bacteria with complement and Ig (opsonisation) and engulf them (phagocytosis). Killing is accomplished by H_2O_2 generation, release of lysosomal enzymes, neutrophil degranulation (respiratory burst). Several enzyme systems are involved (MPO, cytochrome system, HMP shunt). In the neonate neutrophil function is defective (↓ chemotaxis, phagocytosis, motility) particularly if premature, jaundiced. Killing is normal.

Classification
Disorders of all aspects of neutrophil function are described and there is no consensus as to how best to classify them. All are rare. In several of the best described conditions multiple defects are present.

Classification

↓ Chemotaxis	↓ Opsonisation	↓ Killing
Lazy leucocyte syndrome	Complement C_3 deficiency	Chronic granulomatous disease
Hyper IgE syndrome		MPO deficiency
Chediak–Higashi syndrome		
↓ Specific neutrophil granules		

Clinical features
All congenital syndromes are rare and diagnosis of the specific defect difficult. Few haematological/immunological labs are set up to perform the required range of tests. Specialist referral for diagnosis and treatment is indicated and may be able to alter the otherwise grim prognosis in many of these conditions.

Lazy leucocyte syndrome: Leucocyte adhesion deficiency due to ↓ HMW membrane glycoproteins. Rare. Autosomal recessive. ↑ Recurrent infections often in oral cavity, delayed wound healing. Lab features: ↑ neutrophil count, normal BM, abnormal chemotaxis on Rebuck skin window test. The condition is relatively mild. Treatment is of specific infections with the need for prophylaxis in some patients.

Hyperimmunoglobulin E syndrome: Also known as Job's syndrome (📖 *Old Testament*) because of recurrent staphylococcal abscesses. Autosomal recessive inheritance, associated with atopic dermatitis and other autoimmune phenomena. Bacterial/fungal infection, chronic dermatitis. Lab features: ↑ IgE, ↑ eosinophils.

Complement deficiency: Autosomal recessive inheritance of C_3 deficiency, homozygotes have severe recurrent bacterial infection, particularly encapsulated organisms.

Chronic granulomatous disease (CGD): Though rare, commonest life-threatening inherited neutrophil functional defect. More than one disorder. Most are sex linked and boys affected 7× more frequently than girls, but 3 autosomal mutations recognised. Presents in early life but also in adults; carriers asymptomatic. Multiple skin and visceral abscesses, systemic infection (pneumonia, osteitis etc.)—bacterial/fungal, lymphadenopathy, hepatosplenomegaly. Lab features: nitro blue tetrazolium (NBT) test (an index of defective respiratory burst) +ve. Specific mutational analysis now possible for earlier and prenatal diagnosis. Outlook better than it used to be. Improved by aggressive antibiotic policy and IFN-γ. BMT little used due to improving outlook with conservative/prophylactic treatment. Early results poor. Prospect of gene therapy attractive but awaits development.

Chediak–Higashi syndrome: Rare autosomal recessive disorder. Multiple defects. Partial oculocutaneous albinism, recurrent infection, lymphadenopathy, peripheral neuropathy and cerebellar ataxia. A fatal accelerated phase occurs in ~85%, usually in the second decade, with lymphocytic infiltration of liver/spleen/nodes/BM, pancytopenia.

Lab findings
- ↓ Hb, ↓ neutrophil count, ↓ platelet count.
- Characteristic giant greenish grey refractile granules in neutrophils (also lymph inclusions).
- Treatment is supportive. High dose ascorbic acid may help some patients. Anecdotal reports of successful BMT.

Myeloperoxidase deficiency:
Autosomal recessive. Commonest of neutrophil dysfunction conditions (1:2000) but also least serious. Often asymptomatic. Manifest in diabetics with recurrent infections—commonly *Candida albicans*. Good prognosis.

Lab findings
- ↑ neutrophil/monocyte peroxidase on histochemical analysis.
- Automated cell counters using MPO activity to count neutrophils may show spurious neutropenia.

Childhood immune (idiopathic) thrombocytopenic purpura (ITP)

ITP occurring in children differs from the adult form of the disease (📖 *p388*) in two ways—first, most cases are of abrupt onset and rapidly self-limiting, and secondly those that progress to chronicity have a lower morbidity and mortality.

Epidemiology

Incidence of ITP in children overall around 4–5 per 100,000 per year. 10–20% become chronic—i.e. last >6 months.

Pathophysiology

Thrombocytopenia mediated by antibodies opsonizing platelets that are then destroyed by the reticuloendothelial system. Antibodies can be part of immune complexes non-specifically attached to platelet Fc receptors (as in typical acute childhood ITP) or true autoantibodies usually targeted at glycoproteins IIb/IIIa and Ib (as found in up to 75% of chronic childhood ITP and commonly in adults).

Clinical features

- Onset of bruising ± petechiae abrupt (80–90%) or insidious (10–20%).
- May have gingival and oral mucosal bleeding or epistaxis.
- Life threatening bleeding extremely rare.
- Child otherwise perfectly well.
- May have history of recent infection; specific (rubella, varicella) or non-specific (URTI).
- Can follow vaccination.

Laboratory diagnosis

- Isolated thrombocytopenia; blood count otherwise normal.
- Marrow shows abundant megakaryocytes and is otherwise normal (not necessary to investigate unless clinical course or presenting features unusual).
- Platelet antibody studies difficult to perform and not necessary in most cases since they do not alter management.
- Exclude EBV infection (infectious mononucleosis).
- Exclude multisystem autoimmune disease (ACL, ANA, positive DAT test)—not necessary unless disease becomes chronic.
- Exclude underlying immunodeficiency syndrome (HIV, Wiskott–Aldrich).

Differential diagnosis

- Congenital or familial thrombocytopenias.
- Leukaemia or aplastic anaemia.
- Other rare thrombocytopenias (e.g. type IIB vWD).
- Multisystem autoimmune disease—Evans' syndrome (AIHA + immune thrombocytopenia), systemic lupus erythematosus.
- Immune thrombocytopenia associated with immunodeficiency due to other disease—HIV infection, Hodgkin's disease, Wiskott–Aldrich syndrome.

Management

Newly presenting

Seldom require urgent therapy though this is frequently given, either polyvalent IVIg 0.8g/kg (single dose) or prednisolone 4mg/kg. Never justified in the absence of obvious bleeding since neither therapy without risk. Simple observation for spontaneous recovery should be preferred.

Chronic

No therapy is needed based on platelet count alone. Absence of symptoms and signs is sufficient. Excessive restriction of activities is seldom justified. Open access to expert help and advice provides reassurance to families and teachers. If therapy required to control symptoms (recurrent nosebleeds, menorrhagia) try local measures or hormonal control. Regular IVIg or steroids seldom effective and may produce more problems than untreated disease. For the most difficult cases (very rare) splenectomy still worth considering, though post-splenectomy mortality may be > than that of untreated ITP. Newer therapies include danazol and rituximab, though experience still anecdotal and long-term risks not yet evaluated.

Life-threatening haemorrhage or other emergency

Risk of life-threatening haemorrhage very small (<1/1000 in first week after diagnosis) though is a function of a platelet count $<10–20 \times 10^9$/L and the time exposed to this. Risk consequently rises in rare children with chronic unremitting severe disease for >1–2 years for whom more adventurous therapy (splenectomy, rituximab) can be contemplated, though risk still small and those of treatment may be higher. If a large intracranial (ICH) or other catastrophic bleed occurs, this can be dealt with by simultaneous massive platelet transfusion, IVIg, IV methylprednisolone and (if the diagnosis is beyond doubt) emergency splenectomy. Mortality of major ICH less than 50% given active therapy.

Outlook

Most children with ITP recover irrespective of therapy, usually within weeks or occasionally within months. Even 75% of those whose problem persists for >6 months eventually spontaneously remit, sometimes several years later. It is very rare for children to carry ITP into adult life and beyond, and the occasional individuals who do are unlikely to much troubled by it or to develop autoimmune disease of other systems.

Guidelines for the investigation and management of idiopathic thrombocytopenic purpura in adults, children and in pregnancy (2003) *Br J Haematol*, **120**, 574–596.

Haemolytic uraemic syndrome

Characterised by a triad of *microangiopathic haemolytic anaemia* (MAHA), *renal failure* and *thrombocytopenia*. More common in children than adults and of two types; the more common epidemic form and the less common sporadic form closely related to thrombotic thrombocytopenic purpura (TTP)—a disease primarily of adults that also rarely occurs in children. TTP has the same triad of signs with two others—fever and neurologic disturbances (📖 *p530*)

Pathogenesis

HUS usually occurs in outbreaks and in 90% is due to *Escherichia coli* 0157 and other verocytotoxin-producing *E coli*. Food sources of the infection include uncooked/under-cooked meats, hamburgers and poor food hygiene. The verocytotoxin causes endothelial damage, particularly of the renal endothelium, leading to the formation of fibrin-rich microthrombi and MAHA.

Clinical features

- Young children (<4 years) are especially prone to the disease.
- Acute onset with a history of abdominal pain and bloody diarrhoea.
- Onset of ↓ urine output heralding renal failure occurs days later.
- In ~10% onset is non-epidemic and insidious—can be associated with chemotherapy/TBI.
- Other symptoms: anaemia (may be severe), jaundice, bruising, bleeding.
- Absence of fever and neurologic signs distinguish it from TTP.

Laboratory findings

- MAHA may be severe.
- Film shows fragmented RBCs/schistocytes/spherocytes.
- Thrombocytopenia.
- Coagulation tests: PT/APTT—usually normal; fibrinogen and F/XDPs also normal. Reduced large vWF multimers.
- Proteinuria and haematuria.
- Biochemical evidence of renal failure.
- Stool culture may be +ve for *E coli*.

Differential diagnosis

- TTP (📖 *p530*).
- Other causes of MAHA and renal failure.

Complications

- ARF⟶CRF rare but more likely in older children and those with sporadic insidious onset HUS.
- Microvascular thrombosis and infarction of other organs.

Treatment

- Renal failure—fluid restriction, correct electrolyte imbalance.
- If anuria persists >24h—dialysis as necessary.
- Blood transfusion for anaemia.
- Platelet transfusion rarely needed—may ↑ thrombotic risk.
- Severe persistent disease may require plasmapheresis as for TTP (📖 *p530*).
- Specific treatment: none of proven value.

Outcome

Epidemic HUS has a good prognosis, patients usually recover and it rarely recurs. CRF does occur occasionally. Insidious onset HUS has a poorer prognosis. Overall mortality ~5%.

Childhood cancer and malignant blood disorders

Epidemiology

In Europe 1 child in 600 develops cancer before the age of 15. Annual incidence 1:10,000; ~1200 new cases/year in UK. Pattern of childhood cancers is very different from that seen in adults: carcinomas are rarely seen. Overall, childhood cancer is slightly more common in boys than girls.

- *Leukaemias* account for about 35% of the total: 80% are some type of ALL, 15% some type of AML. 5% chronic myeloid leukaemias, (adult and juvenile types) or myelodysplastic syndromes. CLL does not occur in children.
- *Brain tumours* are commonest solid malignancies, 25% of the total. Different tumour types from adults; commonest medulloblastoma in posterior fossa.
- *Embryonal tumours* 15%, seen almost exclusively in children. Include neuroblastoma, nephroblastoma (Wilms' tumour), rhabdomyosarcoma, hepatoblastoma.
- *Bone tumours* 5% osteosarcoma, Ewing's sarcoma.
- *Lymphomas* 9%—NHL and Hodgkin's disease. NHL in children closely related biologically to ALL; low grade disease very rare.
- Remainder of cases are mainly germ cell and primitive neuroectodermal tumours (PNETs), including retinoblastomas.

Aetiology

- Childhood cancer generally represents aberrant growth and development rather than defective repair and renewal from which most adult tumours arise.
- Growths arising in infancy are mostly congenital and the genetic mutations concerned arise *in utero*. Causes of such mutations and those arising later in childhood largely unknown.
- Although isolated cases are attributable to high dose radiation (e.g. thyroid cancer in Chernobyl survivors), there is no convincing link to levels of background radiation or electromagnetic fields.
- Population mixing studies have suggested that patterns of exposure to infection may contribute to some cases of ALL in the peak years of incidence (2–6 years).
- Childhood cancer rarely familial, but study of retinoblastoma (rare tumour that is commonly familial) has led to better understanding of tumour suppressor genes; germline mutation in one allele of *RB* gene in affected families only gives rise to tumours in cells where there is an acquired mutation in the other, healthy, wild type allele (the 'two hit' hypothesis).
- Cancer arising in older children may still be due to intrauterine event as concordance studies in identical twins with ALL have shown identical genetic mutations in malignant cells some years after birth. This suggests twin⟶twin transfer of potentially malignant clone through shared circulation.

Haematological effects of non-haemic tumours (*for leukaemias, lymphomas and MDS see following sections*)

- Marrow infiltration may be evident at the time of presentation (most commonly neuroblastoma, less commonly Ewing's sarcoma, rhabdomyosarcoma).
- Associated with anaemia, occasionally other cytopenias. Blood count hardly ever normal if marrow involved.
- Peripheral blood may show leucoerythroblastic picture, but not as commonly in adult cancers metastasising to bone marrow.
- Non-haemic tumours appear on cytomorphology as poorly differentiated fragile blast cells, often in sheets or clumps (unlike leukaemic blasts).
- Marrow infiltration may arise as a late event in terminally progressive disease in other tumours, including CNS malignancies, PNETS and germ cell tumours.

Investigations in suspected childhood cancer

Haematology

- FBC and film. Leukaemia usually reflected in the blood count: ↑ or ↓ WBC, ± thrombocytopenia and anaemia. Blasts often present. In a small percentage, blood count entirely normal. With other malignancies there may be signs of marrow infiltration (*see above*), anaemia or no abnormalities at all.
- BM aspirate and trephine if blood count abnormal. In children generally done under GA. Bilateral samples needed in the staging of neuroblastoma.

Biochemistry

- Full biochemical profile.
- Urinary catecholamines for neuroblastoma (easy test to do in unexplained bone pain).
- Tumour markers: α-FP, βHCG in hepatoblastoma or germ cell tumours.

Radiology

- CXR for mediastinal mass (mandatory pre-anaesthetic).
- Abdominal USS.
- CT/MRI scan of primary lesion. CT chest/abdomen may be required for staging. In young children sedation/general anaesthetic usually needed for CT/MRI scans.

Histology

- Solid tumours need adequate biopsy material for diagnosis taken under general anaesthetic.

Genetics

- Fresh tumour material from all childhood cancers should be sent for cytogenetic and molecular genetic studies. Information from these is increasingly being used in risk-stratifying therapy and in predicting outcome.

Specialist centres for treatment and investigation

Children with suspected malignancy should be referred to a specialist centre for investigation and initial treatment. Thereafter, shared care may be carried out nearer to home at a local hospital. Most children across the country receive treatment as part of a national trial or protocol. This is co-ordinated by the United Kingdom Children's Cancer Study Group and similar groups in other countries, and the success of such trials and studies is one of the reasons for the improved outlook for childhood cancer. Overall long-term survival is ~60%.

Late effects

It is estimated that soon 1:1000 adults will be survivors of childhood cancer. Long term follow-up clinics are needed to monitor growth, fertility, side effects from drugs (e.g. cardiotoxicity) and psychological well-being. There is an increased risk of further malignancy developing which varies according to both the primary diagnosis and treatment used.

Paediatric haematology

Childhood lymphoblastic leukaemia

Lymphoblastic leukaemia ('acute' is superfluous, but disease widely known as ALL) is a group of clonal malignancies all arising in developing lymphocytes. There is more overlap with lymphomas than in adults. Commonest malignant disease in childhood (35% of all cancers). Incidence 4–5/100,000 children per year with a peak incidence between 2–6 years of age.

Aetiology

Many cases thought to be due to antenatal mutations in developing B-cell clones; Majority of cases B-cell derived, occur between 2 and 6 years, and may be abnormal response to infection where exposure to pathogens delayed or precipitated by population mixing. Evidence implicating background ionising or electromagnetic radiation now discredited. Cause of T-ALL unknown.

Pathophysiology

- ~80% childhood ALLs arise in developing B lymphocytes; ~20% in developing T cells. Acquired genetic mutations found in the various sub-types are growing in number as the molecular biology of leukaemia unravels.
- In early B cells commonest mutation is a fusion between the *TEL* gene at 12p13 and the *AML1* gene at 21q22—arises in 20% overall; other common mutations are t(1;19)(q23;p13.3)—8% overall, t(9;22)(q34;q11.2) *BCR-ABL* (Philadelphia chromosome); 5% overall.
- ~30% have 'high hyperdiploidy' (>50 chromosomes per cell) with or without translocations; 7% show hypodiploidy.
- Infants (<18 months) frequently have a mutation of the *MLL* gene on chromosome 11 involving a range of fusion partners; most commonly *AF4* on chromosome 4.
- The above changes mark biologically different types of precursor B-derived ALL in terms of clinical features and response to treatment.
- 1–2% of ALLs have features of mature B cells and a mutation where the *MYC* gene is translocated adjacent to the Ig heavy chain locus—t(8;14). Also called Burkitt-type as the cell biology is similar to that of Burkitt's lymphoma.
- T-ALL shows greater genetic diversity than B-derived disease but 12 recurring cytogenetic abnormalities now defined and under study. Clinical importance yet to be defined.
- ALL also classified by immunophenotyping using antibody cell markers for various differentiation antigens designated clusters of differentiation (CD), numbered according to their order of discovery. Immunophenotypes so defined include early pre-B (60%), pre-B (20%), transitional pre-B (1%), B-ALL (1%) and T-ALL (18%).

Clinical features

- Commonly presents insidiously in three ways, separately or combined.
- Signs of marrow failure—often anaemia predominates, with extreme pallor and listlessness (60%); also bruising/petechiae (40%).
- Hepatosplenomegaly and lymphadenopathy ('lymphomatous' features) 10–20%.
- Bone pain mimicking irritable hip(s) or juvenile rheumatoid 10–20%.

Laboratory features
- Usually pancytopenia with circulating blast cells indicates diagnosis.
- Confirmed by bone marrow examination and classified by immunophenotyping and cytogenetic/molecular genetic analysis.
- In sick children with very high blast cell counts classification studies can be carried out on peripheral blood, but marrow always preferred.
- Peripheral blood count may show cytopenias without obvious blasts (aleukaemic picture) when differential diagnosis is aplastic anaemia.
- Kidney/liver function usually normal, but ALLs with high blast counts and rapid cell turnover may have tumour-lysis organ dysfunction before therapy (urate nephropathy with ↑ urea, creatinine and ↓ urine output).

Treatment of newly diagnosed disease
- All modern protocols have common elements of remission induction (RI), consolidation/intensification (C/I), CNS directed treatment and continuing (maintenance) therapy with or without delayed intensification (DI).
- RI drugs include dexamethasone, vincristine and asparaginase.
- C/I and DI drugs include anthracyclines, cytarabine, cyclophosphamide asparaginase and thioguanine.
- CNS therapy is intrathecal cytarabine and methotrexate (radiotherapy now reserved for those with active CNS infiltration only).
- Maintenance therapy is a 2–3 year schedule of daily thiopurine (6-mercaptopurine) and weekly oral methotrexate.
- ALL is the only human malignancy that requires such a drawn-out chemotherapy module, immunosuppressive rather than antineoplastic.
- B-ALL is an exception; it does not respond to conventional ALL therapy, does not need maintenance and is treated on a 6 month intensive lymphoma schedule (📖 *p478*).
- Treatment is usually risk-directed based on biological features of the disease with more intensive schedules reserved for those with adverse prognostic factors (*see below*).
- BMT rarely used as first-line therapy.

Outlook
98% overall will remit on modern therapy, 75–80% overall will become long term disease-free survivors—figures vary according to prognostic factors (*see below*). >90% long term survivors in low risk disease.

Treatment of relapse
- Some 20–25% of children will relapse; either on treatment or after its completion.
- Outlook depends on length of first remission; very bleak if relapse on treatment.
- Salvage therapy more successful if relapse >2 years off therapy.
- Relapsed T-ALL more difficult to treat successfully than other types.
- Treatment includes intensive chemotherapy with the addition of podophyllins, anthracycline analogues and fludarabine.

- BMT reserved for those who show slow-to-clear residual disease by PCR amplification of unique disease-specific Ig or TCR gene rearrangements, those who relapse on treatment and those with relapsed T-ALL.

Prognostic factors

- Several features of ALL predict response to current standard therapies and are used to stratify treatment. Infants <1 year have a poor outlook, and older children >10 years do less well than those 1–10 years.
- High presenting WBC ($>100 \times 10^9$/L) in boys marks high risk, as do some genetic features (*MLL* gene rearrangements, *BCR-ABL* fusion genes, hypodiploidy).
- All children with T-ALL , and all with slow disease clearance during the first few days of therapy, are excluded from being classified as low risk.
- Low risk B-precursor ALL is that which shows none of these features.

Late effects of therapy

With ↑ long survivors, late effects of therapy are becoming more important. Most morbidity seen after TBI given for BMT.

Problems include

- Growth failure due to CNS damage from radiation.
- Intellectual deficit due to CNS damage from radiation.
- Precocious puberty (girls > boys) after cranial radiation.
- Infertility (boys > girls) not dependent on radiation.
- Obesity (girls > boys) not dependent on radiation.
- 7–10 fold ↑ risk of brain tumours not dependent on radiation.

Paediatric haematology

Childhood lymphomas

Lymphomas account for around 8–10% of all childhood cancers (this equates to around 1 per 100,000 children per year). Around 30–35% are Hodgkin's disease, the rest non-Hodgkin lymphomas.

Hodgkin's disease

Clinical features

Uncommon <5 years; incidence increases during the early teenage years. The disease is biologically the same as that of adults and the histological classification is identical (*for more details* 📖 *p208*), though mixed cellularity disease may be more common in the young. Staging is also similar to adults (📖 *p210*), but overall children and adolescents have a greater proportion of low-stage disease (I and II). Stage IV accounts for <10% of childhood cases.

Treatment and outcome

Treatment is so successful that most efforts are currently directed at reducing toxicity and late effects. Radiotherapy for stage I disease is being attenuated, and some therapists have abandoned it as first line treatment and rely on chemotherapy alone. Chemotherapy regimens in turn are evolving (to avoid or minimise alkylating agents and their effect on fertility and anthracyclines with their potential for cardiotoxicity), but at present the traditional drugs are still being used with or without involved field radiotherapy, particularly in stage III or IV disease.

The outlook for even stage IV disease is good, given the best current regimen of chemotherapy and involved field radiotherapy, and over 80% should achieve long term EFS.

Non-Hodgkin's lymphoma

Childhood non-Hodgkin's lymphomas are a heterogeneous group of tumours quite different from those seen in adults. Virtually all are disseminated, high-grade diffuse malignancies of immature B or T lymphocytes, and many are closely related to subtypes of ALL that occur in this age group.

Classification of NHL has always been confusing, but the Revised European American Lymphoma system is currently preferred. This maps disease in children into 6 categories:

1. ***Burkitt's lymphoma, Burkitt-like lymphoma, high grade B-cell disease.*** Different manifestations of biologically very closely related diseases and pathologically indistinguishable from B-ALL. ~45% of the total. Characteristic 'starry sky' histological pattern and deeply basophilic blasts on Romanowsky stains with prominent vacuoles (FAB L3 features). Associated with chromosomal translocation involving *MYC* locus on chromosome 8 and Ig heavy chain gene on 14 (or less commonly with a κ or λ light chain gene on 2 or 22) with resultant dysregulation of *MYC* gene transcription; the *MYC* product functions as a transcription factor.
2. ***Precursor B lymphoblastic lymphoma.*** Indistinguishable pathologically from common ALL. ~5% of the total. Commonly presents as a solitary subcutaneous swelling, typically on the scalp.

3. ***Precursor T lymphoblastic lymphoma***. Indistinguishable pathologically from T-ALL. ~20% of the total. 66% have mediastinal involvement. Marrow involvement common in advanced disease; so may be classified as T-ALL rather than stage IV NHL.
4. ***Diffuse large B-cell lymphoma***, including primary sclerosing mediastinal form; no leukaemic counterpart, accounts for ~3–4% of the total. Chiefly abdominal. Occasionally mediastinal. Has some features of Burkitt's but no *MYC* gene mutation.
5. ***Peripheral T-cell lymphoma unspecified***; no leukaemic counterpart. Skin involvement. Retrospective review shows most so classified to be type 6 (*large cell anaplastic, see below*). Poorly defined entity hardly ever seen in children.
6. ***Large cell anaplastic, T or null cell type***. No leukaemic counterpart. More frequently recognised, and complex biological features gradually becoming better understood. ~15% of the total. Used to be diagnosed as peripheral T-cell lymphomas or 'malignant histiocytosis'. Biological hallmarks are Ki-1 (CD30)+, also t(2;5).

Around 9 % childhood NHLs defy classification and <1% adult type follicular lymphomas will occasionally arise in older children.

St Jude staging system for childhood NHL

A staging system for childhood NHL has been developed, though therapy is increasingly being directed more by the biology of the disease rather than its anatomical distribution or extent. Staging affects prognosis only within given tumour type.

St Jude staging system for childhood NHL	
Stage I	Single tumour (extranodal or single nodal anatomic area), excluding mediastinum or abdomen
Stage II	Single extranodal tumour with regional node involvement = 2 nodal areas on the same side of the diaphragm 2 single extranodal tumours ± regional node involvement on same side of the diaphragm Primary GIT tumour, usually ileocaecal, ± involvement of associated mesenteric nodes
Stage III	2 extranodal tumours on opposite sides of the diaphragm = 2 nodal areas above and below the diaphragm Presence of 1° intrathoracic tumour (mediastinal, pleural or thymic) Presence of extensive primary intra-abdominal disease Presence of paraspinal or epidural tumours, regardless of other sites
Stage IV	Any of the above with initial CNS and/or bone marrow involvement

Treatment

Burkitt's lymphoma/B-ALL: Short 6 month course of pulsed intensive high dose therapy (vincristine, steroids, methotrexate, cyclophosphamide, anthracyclines and etoposide) including CNS treatment. No maintenance treatment needed.

B precursor lymphoblastic: If isolated to one site, 6 month program of ALL-type therapy may suffice, else treat as common ALL with extended maintenance (📖 *lymphoblastic leukaemia p475*).

T precursor lymphoblastic: Treated as T-ALL (📖 *p161*).

Diffuse large B-cell lymphoma: Treated as Burkitt's lymphoma.

Large cell anaplastic Ki-1+: Skin, CNS and mediastinal involvement and splenomegaly are adverse features. Best therapy undefined but usually treated with short intensive Burkitt-like regimens. EFS is around ~75% (high risk cases ~60%).

General points on therapy/outlook

- Surgery usually indicated for the complete resection of a localised abdominal primary tumour when possible.
- Low-dose involved field radiotherapy indicated for airway or spinal cord compression. Mediastinal irradiation for persistent local disease.
- Given best current therapy, the outlook for most patients is good with around 80% EFS for childhood lymphomas overall.

Paediatric haematology

Childhood acute myeloid leukaemia

Acute myeloid leukaemia in children accounts for ~15% of all malignant blood disorders, with around 80–90 new cases arising in the UK each year. Unlike ALL, the disease is classified on morphological grounds using the FAB classification, as is AML in adults (📖 *p150*). The frequency of the different subtypes differs in children, however. M6 AML is very rare whereas M7 (megakaryocyte derived AML) is more common—especially in children with Down syndrome.

Proportion of children with *de novo* AML by FAB type

	M0	M1	M2	M3	M4	M5	M6	M7
% of total	2	18	29	8	16	17	2	8

Pathophysiology

AML is a clonal neoplasm arising from developing blood cells affecting all haemopoietic cell lines, most commonly granulocyte or monocyte precursors but also occasionally involving immature erythroblasts or megakaryocytes. Apart from primary, *de novo* disease for which no cause can be identified, some cases of AML are due to chemotherapy given for other diseases (secondary AML), and some arise in children with predisposing syndromes where the risk is greatly increased and where specific subtypes of AML may develop.

- Secondary AML caused by topoisomerase II inhibitors (e.g. etoposide) has a latency of 1–3 years and is of FAB type M4/M5 with a characteristic *MLL* gene mutation.
- Secondary AML caused by alkylating agents (e.g. cyclophosphamide) has a latency of 4–6 years, a myelodysplastic phase and loss or deletions of chromosomes 5, 7 or both.
- Down syndrome children are 20 times more likely to develop leukaemia than normal children; infants are more likely to develop M7 AML, older Down children develop ALL.
- Other conditions predisposing to AML in children are Fanconi's anaemia and Bloom's syndrome (📖 *p457*), dyskeratosis congenita, Kostmann's syndrome and Shwachman–Diamond syndrome (📖 *p459*), Diamond–Blackfan anaemia (📖 *p452*), and neurofibromatosis.

Apart from the specific changes in secondary AMLs (*see above*), clonal chromosome abnormalities are found in blasts from ~90% of those with *de novo* disease. Two-thirds of these are non-random, and many are associated with characteristic clinical and biological features.

Commonest genetic mutations in childhood AML

Abnormality	Involved genes	FAB type	Frequency	Clinical features
t(8;21)	*ETO; AML1*	M2	10–15%	Extramedullary chloromas good outlook
t(15;17)	*PML; RARA*	M3	5–10%	Coagulopathy responds to retinoids
Inv16(p13q32)	*MYH11; CBFB*	M4eo	7–10%	Extramedullary deposits good outlook
t(9;11)	*AF9; MLL*	M4/M5	7–10%	Infants, CNS disease poor outlook
t(1;22)	N/K	M7	2–3%	Secondary myelofibrosis Down syndrome

Laboratory features

- Peripheral blood shows a variety of abnormalities—usually pancytopenia with circulating blasts.
- WBC seldom >50 × 10^9/L though can occasionally be very high with symptoms of leucostasis—deafness, confusion and impaired consciousness.
- Bone marrow usually shows heavy overgrowth of blasts with different morphology depending on FAB type. Auer rods (abnormal elongated primary granules seen on Romanowsky stains in cytoplasm of malignant myeloblasts) are diagnostic of AML and are not found in health. Seen in all types of AML except M6 and M7, most common in M1/2/3, particularly M3.
- Cytochemistry may help; non-specific esterase positive in M4/M5 AML, not other types and myeloperoxidase positivity can help distinguish between poorly differentiated AML and ALL. M7 AML may develop extensive marrow fibrosis making aspiration difficult; trephine histology needed.
- Genetic abnormalities common in blast cells (*see above*).
- Immunophenotyping less important that in ALL, though essential for immediate diagnosis of M7 AML which has no distinguishing morphological or cytochemical features. CD antigens expressed vary according to FAB type; CD33 strongly +ve in all, CD13 in M2/3; CD4 in M4/M5 and CD41/61 in M7. M6 disease expresses glycophorin A.

Clinical features

Children with advanced AML are commonly more sick than those with ALL. They can present with bleeding, haemostatic failure and/or septicaemia as manifestations of marrow failure and profound neutropenia. Extramedullary chloromas (solid deposits of malignant cells) arise in around 10% of cases. They may precede marrow failure (or even detectable marrow infiltration). They can arise internally around the spine or spinal cord, causing pressure symptoms and mimicking non-haemic solid tumours. They are more common in AML with t(8;21). Peri-orbital chloromas are also not unusual in infants with M4/M5 AML.

Treatment and outlook

Outcome of therapy for childhood AML has shown a dramatic improvement over the last 15 years. From a dismal outlook in the 1970s through around 30% EFS in the 1980s we have now achieved >50% EFS at the turn of the 21st century. This has been due to increasingly intensive chemotherapy and parallel improvements in supportive treatment for the secondary marrow failure it produces.

The principle of treatment is to ablate marrow with chemotherapy to the point that endogenous recovery occurs within 4–6 weeks and to repeat the process with different drug combinations 4 or 5 times, giving a total treatment time of around 6 months. Results using this approach have improved for children in the best risk groups to the point where allogeneic BMT is no longer considered the consolidation treatment of choice even if a matched donor is available.

- Drugs used in remission induction include daunorubicin, etoposide, cytarabine and mitoxantrone (mitozantrone).
- Drugs used in post induction and consolidation treatment include amsacrine, high-dose cytarabine, L-asparaginase, etoposide and mitoxantrone (mitozantrone).
- Good risk patients are those with t(8;21), t(15;17) and inv (16)—together accounting for around 20–25% overall; standard risk patients are those without good risk genetic changes but that respond well and remit after one course of chemotherapy (65% overall), and poor risk are those without good genetics who have residual disease at the start of course 2 of treatment (around 10% of the total).
- Long term EFS for good risk children is around 75–80%, for standard risk around 60–65%, and for poor risk around 15%.
- Allogeneic BMT as consolidation therapy of first remission is reserved for children in standard and poor risk groups. It is also used as a salvage strategy for good risk patients who relapse.
- The role of autologous stem cell rescue following myeloablative conditioning in children with AML has not been established.
- The need for skilled supportive therapy confines AML therapy to specialist units.

Paediatric haematology

Childhood myelodysplastic syndromes and chronic leukaemias

Myelodysplastic syndromes of childhood present a different spectrum of disease from that seen in adults. All are rare. The FAB classification of adult MDS (📖 *p220*) has been translated to paediatric disease, but sits uncomfortably and is of limited use clinically or in understanding the complex biology of this diverse group of clonal disorders of marrow function. The proportion that map to the various adult categories is shown below.

Adult *vs.* childhood MDS based on the FAB classification

Category	% Adults	% Children
Refractory anaemia (RA)	28	24
Refractory anaemia with ring sideroblasts (RARS)	24	<1
Refractory anaemia with excess blasts (RAEB)	23	16
Refractory anaemia with excess blasts in transformation (RAEB-t)	9	5
Chronic myelomonocytic leukaemia (CMML)	16	50
Unclassifiable	0	4

- Many children with MDS have a monocytosis which results in their being classified as CMML, also the clinical features and outlook for childhood CMML are quite different.
- RARS is virtually never seen in children.

Individual disorders

Refractory anaemia: Children with a clonal genetic marker in the marrow who present with refractory anaemia usually progress to RAEB and AML. Those without such a marker probably do not have MDS but some other cause of erythropoietic failure.

RAEB and RAEB-t: Many of the RAEB syndromes in children arise in those with pre-existing disease like Down syndrome, trisomy 8, neurofibromatosis type 1, Fanconi's anaemia, Kostmann's syndrome, Diamond–Blackfan anaemia and Shwachman–Diamond syndrome (*see previous section*). All these diseases predispose to leukaemia, and RAEB is merely part of the evolution of AML. A substantial proportion of childhood MDS in the RA or RAEB category is also induced by previous chemotherapy as a prodrome to secondary AML. In other words all paediatric cases of RAEB/RAEB-t are best regarded as AML and treated as such if the diagnosis is not in any doubt.

- Down syndrome children have a particular predisposition to develop M7 (megakaryoblastic) AML in the first few years of life. This is commonly preceded by a RAEB prodrome where the marrow is hard to aspirate through secondary sclerosis. The decision when to start therapy is difficult, but the overall outlook is potentially good with EFS >50%.

Transient abnormal myelopoiesis (TAM): Down children also have a predisposition to develop a transient blast cell overgrowth in infancy that looks like frank leukaemia with blasts in the peripheral blood. It is completely self-limiting within days or weeks and is not associated with marrow failure, arising alongside normal haemopoiesis. There is no genetic abnormality in the marrow apart from trisomy 21. It is important that chemotherapy is withheld in what is regarded as a temporary stem cell instability. Rarely the problem can arise in non-Down children, where trisomy 21 is found in the bone marrow only.

JCMML (juvenile chronic myelomonocytic leukaemia): Originally called juvenile chronic myeloid leukaemia to distinguish it from adult type chronic myeloid leukaemia (*see below*), this pernicious disease still has a high mortality. It is now recognised to be a clonal disorder, with all marrow cell lines involved. It has several distinctive clinical and haematological features.

- Stigmata of fetal erythropoiesis; high HbF, ↑ red cell i antigen expression and carbonic anhydrase activity, ↑ MCV.
- Modest ↑ WBC; average 30–40 × 10^9/L, with evident monocytosis, blasts 5–10%, and occasionally a basophilia.
- Marrow appearances unremarkable; modest ↑ blasts.
- Thrombocytopenia; sometimes profound.
- Skin rashes; butterfly distribution on face.
- Increasing hepatosplenomegaly.
- Associated with neurofibromatosis type 1. May be present in >10% of cases.
- Poor outlook with progression associated with wasting, fever, infections, bleeding and pulmonary infiltrations.

Monosomy 7 syndrome: Conventional cytogenetic analysis of the marrow in JCMML shows no abnormality in the classic syndrome, though there is a subvariety (or similar condition that may nevertheless be biologically distinct) where monosomy 7 is found. Whether this is a different disorder is not clear. Apart from the different genetics, monosomy 7 syndrome and JCMML have several features in common. However, monosomy 7 children may have:

- A longer prodrome with RA or RAEB and no monocytosis.
- They may respond to AML chemotherapy (JCMML responds poorly and seldom remits).
- They may remain stable for years without therapy.
- They respond better to BMT (JCMML achieve <40% EFS even with BMT).

Adult-type chronic myeloid (granulocytic) leukaemia (ATCML, see Adult CML p164): More common than JCMML, though still rare, ATCML arises in around 1 in 500,000 children per year (20 in whole of UK). Tends to affect older children (60% >6 years) though it has been reported in a 3 month old infant.

- Associated with Ph chromosome and t(9;22) *BCR-ABL* fusion gene in all haemopoietic cells exactly as seen in adults.
- Natural history exactly the same as the disease in adults with benign phase and eventual progression to accelerated acute phase.
- Only curative therapy is allogeneic BMT, but impressive remissions of so far unknown length are now being achieved with novel tyrosine kinase inhibitor, STI571 (imatinib). This is set to replace the conventional management of the chronic phase with α-interferon or hydroxyurea, but at present is reserved for those who fail to respond to IFN or those entering the accelerated phase.

Paediatric haematology

Histiocytic syndromes

Monocytes are formed in the marrow and move through the peripheral blood into the tissues where they become histiocytes, either in the mononuclear phagocytic system (MPS) or the dendritic cell system (DCS). MPS cells are *antigen processing*, are predominantly phagocytic and include many organ-specific cells such as Kupffer cells and pulmonary alveolar macrophages. DCS cells include tissue-based Langerhans cells (LC) which are *antigen presenting*. There is a variety of syndromes where histiocytes proliferate and malfunction and some of these carry a high mortality. A few are clonal neoplasms but most are produced by cytokine disturbances. In 1991 a new classification of histiocytic syndromes was set out as shown:

Histiocytic syndromes	
Class I	*Disorders of dendritic cells*
	Langerhans cell histiocytosis
	(previously known as histiocytosis X)
Class II	*Disorders of macrophages*
	Haemophagocytic syndromes
	Haemophagocytic lymphohistiocytosis (HLH)
	Primary (genetic)
	Secondary (to infection or malignant disease)
	Sinus histiocytosis with massive lymphadenopathy
	Histiocytic necrotising lymphadenitis
Class III	Malignant histiocytic disorders
	Malignant histiocytosis
	Monocytic leukaemias

Class I: Langerhans cell histiocytosis (LCH)

Cellular destructive tissue infiltration with LC. These are well differentiated large cells (15–25μm) with an indented nucleus and inconspicuous nucleolus; they are not phagocytic. Other reactive cells (granulocytes, eosinophils, macrophages) are often present. Diagnostic criteria of LC include the presence of Burbeck granules on electron microscopy and immunochemical positivity for CD1A. The aetiology of LCH remains unclear. Despite some evidence of clonality (not itself evidence of malignancy), no genetic mutations have been identified and the disorder is not regarded as a form of cancer.

Clinical features: LCH is primarily a disease of the very young with a peak incidence of 1–3 years. It can present in a variety of ways, from a small bone lesion heavily admixed with eosinophils (eosinophilic granuloma), through multiple lytic bone lesions, exophthalmos and diabetes insipidus (Hand–Schuller–Christian disease) to multiple tissue infiltration involving skin, liver, lung bone and bone marrow (Letterer–Siwe disease). The eponymous terms are no longer used for what is now regarded as a common pathology and the overarching term LCH is preferred. This is staged on the basis of the number of organ systems showing infiltration, and virtually any can be involved. The skin rash of LCH is characteristically in skin folds and scaly with red/brown papules. It may be mistaken for nappy rash. Systemic symptoms including fever and weight loss are common in advanced disease. It can be staged as follows:

Stage A Involvement of bones ± local nodes and adjacent soft tissue.
Stage B Skin ± mucous membranes involvement, ± related nodes.
Stage C Soft tissue involvement—not stage A, B or D.
Stage D Multisystem disease with combinations of A, B, C.

Diagnosis
Based on tissue biopsy. Skeletal survey to define extent of disease; also bone scan, MRI. Urine osmolality studies for diabetes insipidus. BM aspirate and biopsy if anaemic or other cytopenias present.

Treatment
Local curettage of any isolated lesion, with or without intra-lesional steroids. Stable and symptomless disease can be simply observed for spontaneous resolution. Options for widespread disease include steroids and chemotherapy—rarely radiotherapy. Indications for chemotherapy include organ dysfunction and/or disease progression/recurrence. Drugs commonly used include steroids, vinblastine or etoposide, singly or combined.

Outcome
Generally good, but widespread organ involvement with dysfunction and progression indicates a poor prognosis. Overall mortality 15–20%. Long term sequelae include pulmonary/liver fibrosis, diabetes insipidus, growth failure. Risk of malignant disease increased, chiefly leukaemias and lymphomas.

Class II: macrophage functional disorders—haemophagocytic syndromes

Primary (genetic)
Primary haemophagocytic lymphohistiocytosis (HLH) is an autosomal recessively inherited disease of infants and young children (>50% <1 year) also known as familial erythrophagocytic lymphohistiocytosis (FEL) due to the striking degree of marrow red cell phagocytosis. The gene defect is not known, and the pathology of the condition is unclear apart from cytokine dysregulation and high concentrations of IL-1 and 2, GM-CSF and TNF. CNS involvement common. Laboratory investigation shows peripheral blood cytopenias, hypertrigliceridaemia and hypofibrinogenaemia. Histopathology shows histiocyte/lymphocyte infiltration and haemophagocytosis in BM, nodes and spleen.

Treatment and outcome: Seldom effective, steroids, chemotherapy, ALG, cyclosporin A, BMT. Disease usually rapidly fatal.

Secondary

- Clinical and laboratory picture is similar to primary (genetic) HLH. Distinction between the two may be difficult.
- Affects more older patients, often immunocompromised.
- Commonly associated with underlying viral/bacterial infection when called infection-associated haemophagocytic syndrome (IAHS).
- Triggered by a wide variety of infections including (especially) EBV and malaria. Also associated with some malignancies (usually involving T cells) and lipid infusions.

Treatment and outcome: Good survival rates if underlying infection easily treatable. Otherwise has high mortality.

Class III: Malignant histiocytosis

Monocyte-derived acute leukaemias account for 10% of AMLs arising in children. What used to be called 'malignant histiocytosis' with hepatosplenomegaly, fever, wasting and pancytopenia and tissue infiltration with large monocytoid cells is now recognised as a lymphocyte-derived lymphoma (large cell anaplastic, CD30+, 📖 *p198*). It is doubtful whether true histiocyte-derived malignancies other than AML occur in children.

Paediatric haematology

Haematological effects of systemic disease in children

Non-haematological disease in children can produce a variety of haematological effects specific to the disease, to childhood, or both. Some of the more striking examples are listed below.

Wilson's disease: Genetic defect in copper metabolism that occasionally presents as a brisk non-immune haemolytic anaemia without specific features. More commonly presents with liver dysfunction, neurological symptoms or renal disease.

Cyanotic congenital heart disease: Commonly associated with mild thrombocytopenia for ill-understood reasons.

Mast cell disease: Abnormal accumulations of mast cells in the skin or internal organs. Mast cell leukaemia does not occur in children. Commonest manifestation is urticaria pigmentosa in infants. Bullous or urticarial lesions eventually become infiltrated with mast cells. Marrow involvement rare. The cells produce histamine and cause itching. Condition resolves by adulthood.

Juvenile rheumatoid arthritis: Classically the anaemia of chronic inflammatory disease—a defective marrow response to anaemia in a variety of chronic inflammatory disorders primarily due to cytokine mediated inhibition of erythropoiesis rather than deficiency of erythropoietin. True iron deficiency also occurs due to NSAID therapy. Neutropenia may arise, either immune mediated or due to hypersplenism.

Systemic lupus erythematosus: Commonly associated with immune cytopenias (all cell lines) and anticardiolipin antibodies. May also produce marrow hypoplasia.

Epstein–Barr virus infection: Infects CD21 positive B lymphocytes and other tissues including nasopharyngeal epithelium. Primary infection in the immunocompetent may be asymptomatic in the early years of childhood but in adolescence produces the syndrome of infectious mononucleosis ('glandular fever') associated with a striking atypical lymphocytosis. Occasionally there are associated self-limiting immune cytopenias—especially thrombocytopenia. The majority of adults harbour the latent virus in B cells. EBV in some cellular immune deficiency states (such as X-linked lymphoproliferative disease also known as Purtilo's or Duncan's syndrome) can produce a fatal infection with uncontrolled lymphoproliferation and infection associated haemophagocytosis (📖 *HLH, p491*).

Parvovirus B19 infection: Causes 'fifth disease' in infants and young children with the characteristic 'slapped cheek' rash on the face. More importantly shows trophism for marrow erythroblasts and causes temporary red cell hypoplasia. This causes very low Hb concentrations in children with chronic haemolysis. Persistent viraemia can arise in the immunosuppressed and can cause transfusion dependency.

TORCH infections: A miscellaneous group of congenital infections—TOxoplasmosis, Rubella, Cytomegalovirus, Herpes simplex and syphilis. All can cause neonatal anaemia and thrombocytopenia.

Leishmaniasis: The Mediterranean type of visceral leismaniasis primarily affects young children under 5. Infected sand flies transmit parasites that develop in macrophages and the child presents often several weeks or months later with fever and progressive pancytopenia and hepatosplenomegaly. Fatal if untreated but responds well to pentavalent antimony or amphotericin B.

Hookworms (ankylostoma): Are a common cause of iron deficiency in tropical underdeveloped countries. Infestations may be heavy with each worm consuming up to 0.2mL blood per day.

Tapeworms: A rare cause of vitamin B_{12} deficiency in societies that eat raw fish—Baltic states, Japan and Scandinavia, due to infestation by *Diphyllobothrium latum.*

Kawasaki disease: An acute multisystem disease of young children, presumed to be infective but no organism has so far been identified. Presents with conjunctivitis, rashes, reddening of the mucous membranes, hands and feet with desquamation and lymphadenopathy. Coronary artery aneurysms develop in ~20%; fatal in 3%. Haematological manifestations include anaemia (normochromic normocytic), neutrophilia, and a striking secondary thrombocytosis that may linger after the acute phase has passed. Treatment is with aspirin and high dose IVIg.

Nutritional disorders

Iron deficiency: Occurs in apparently healthy children (*cf.* adults where main cause is blood loss). Linked to rapid growth and poor intake the first 2 years of life and again at adolescence. Cows' milk is a poor source of iron. Cereals inhibit its absorption Premature infants run out of iron by 2 months of age.

Protein-calorie malnutrition: Covers adequate calories with protein lack (kwashiorkor) and simple calorie lack (marasmus)—or both. Chiefly in undeveloped countries, but also occasionally in vegan families, with gastrointestinal disease or other chronic illness. Concomitant iron or folate deficiency may be present. Normochromic normocytic anaemia is usual.

Scurvy: Occasionally seen in infants due to poor intake with fruit juices being boiled. Pseudoparalysis due to painful legs. Petechial, periorbital or subdural haemorrhages can arise. Bleeding tendency due to loss of vascular integrity with collagen deficiency.

Poisons

Lead poisoning:
Inhibits haem synthesis and the activity of pyrimidine-5'-nucleotidase, causing hypochromic anaemia with basophilic stippling of red cells and ring sideroblasts in the bone marrow. Also causes abdominal pain. Commonest in toddlers eating flakes of old lead-based paint.

Sodium chlorate: A common weedkiller, also a powerful oxidising substance causing acute intravascular haemolysis and renal failure if ingested.

Nitrates, aniline dyes, nitrobenzene and azo compounds: Can all cause methaemoglobinaemia. If >20% metHb formed, exchange transfusion may be needed.

Storage disorders

Gaucher's disease: Inherited (autosomal recessive) disorder resulting in deficiency of the enzyme glucocerebrosidase (β-glucosidase) Most common form has accumulated glycolipid in macrophages of spleen, liver and bone marrow. May be diagnosed at any time during life depending on severity. Some cases are not identified until adulthood. Clinical presentation is highly variable. Symptoms and signs of presentation may include anaemia, fatigue, thrombocytopenia, petecchiae, bruising, bleeding, leucopenia, splenomegaly, hepatomegaly, bone pain, bone crisis, osteonecrosis, bone marrow infiltration, generalized osteopenia, Erlenmeyer flark deformity of long bones, growth retardation, abdominal pain episodes, gammopathies, haematological malignancy (esp. multiple myeloma). Diagnosis by assay of deficient enzyme, but characteristic (not diagnostic, *see below*) Gaucher cells evident in bone marrow (laden macrophages with appearance of crumpled tissue paper). Enzyme replacement therapy is the standard of care and is shown to effectively redress or control haematological, visceral and skeletal manifestations.

Niemann–Pick (N-P) disease: Though rare, commonest cause of foamy macrophages in marrow of affected patients. Caused by the inherited deficiency of sphingomyelinase resulting in accumulation of sphingomyelin. Four types of Niemann–Pick disease have been defined, type A (classic N-P disease) presents in the first year of life with developmental delay, neurodegeneration and death within 3 years; type B with visceral rather than CNS involvement also presents in infancy and is also progressive and fatal but spares the CNS; type C presents later in childhood but then shows neurodegeneration with death in the 2nd or 3rd decade; and type 4 patients simply store sphingomyelin in viscera without ill health and live to adulthood.

Marrow and blood cells in storage disorders: The foamy macrophages seen in the marrow of N-P patients vary between types and are not in any way diagnostic or specific. Foamy macrophages are also seen in several other storage disorders and a variety of other clinical circumstances. Pseudo-Gaucher cells are seen in chronic granulocytic leukaemia, thalassaemia and some atypical mycobacterial infections. Several storage disorders produce vacuolation of peripheral blood leucocytes, particularly lymphocytes, and this is also a non-specific finding. Diagnosis always rests on the appropriate enzyme assay.

Paediatric haematology

Haematological emergencies 13

Septic shock/neutropenic fever

▶▶ One of the commonest haemato-oncological emergencies.

- May be defined as the presence of symptoms or signs of infection in a patient with an absolute neutrophil count of $<1.0 \times 10^9$/L. In practice, the neutrophil count is often $<0.1 \times 10^9$/L.
- Similar clinical picture also seen in neutrophil function disorders such as MDS despite normal neutrophil numbers.
- ***Beware***—can occur without pyrexia, especially patients on steroids.

Immediate action

▶▶ Urgent clinical assessment.

- Follow ALS guidelines if cardiorespiratory arrest (rare).
- More commonly, clinical picture is more like cardiovascular shock ± respiratory embarrassment viz: tachycardia, hypotension, peripheral vasodilatation and tachypnoea. Occurs with both Gram +ve (now more common with indwelling central catheters) and Gram –ve organisms (less common but more fulminant).
- Immediate rapid infusion of albumin 4.5% or Gelofusin to restore BP.
- Insert central catheter if not *in situ* and monitor CVP.
- Start O_2 by face mask if pulse oximetry shows saturations <95% (common) and consider arterial blood gas measurement—care with platelet counts $<20\times 10^9$/L—manual pressure over puncture site for 30 mins.
- Perform full septic screen (*see guidelines on IV antibiotics, p552*).
- Give the first dose of first line antibiotics immediately e.g ureidopenicillin and loading dose aminoglycoside (ceftazidime or ciprofloxacin if pre-existing renal impairment). Follow established protocols.
- If the event occurs while patient on first line antibiotics, vancomycin/ciprofloxacin or vancomycin/meropenem are suitable alternatives.
- Commence full ITU-type monitoring chart.
- Monitor urine output with urinary catheter if necessary—if renal shutdown has already occurred, give single bolus of IV frusemide (furosemide). If no response, start renal dose dopamine.
- If BP not restored with colloid despite ↑ CVP, consider inotropes.
- If O_2 saturations remain ↓ despite 60% O_2 delivered by rebreathing mask, consider ventilation.
- ***Alert ITU giving details of current status.***

Subsequent actions

- Discuss with senior colleague.
- Amend antibiotics according to culture results or to suit likely source if cultures negative (*see p554, 556*).
- Check aminoglycoside trough levels after loading dose and before second dose as renal impairment may determine reducing or withholding next dose. Consider switch to non-nephrotoxic cover e.g ceftazidime/ciprofloxacin.
- Continue antibiotics for 7–10d minimum and usually until neutrophil recovery.
- If cultures show central line to be source of sepsis, remove immediately if patient not responding.

Haematological emergencies

Transfusion reactions

Rapid temperature spike (>40°C) at start of transfusion indicates transfusion should be ***stopped*** (suggests acute intravascular haemolysis).

If slow rising temperature (<40°C), providing patient not acutely unwell, slow IVI. Fever often due to antibodies against WBCs (or to cytokines in platelet packs).

▶ Immediate transfusion reaction

Intravascular haemolysis (→haemoglobinaemia and haemoglobinuria). Usually due to anti-A or anti-B antibodies (in ABO mismatched transfusion). Symptoms occur in minutes/hours.

Immediate transfusion reaction or bacterial contamination of blood

Symptoms	Signs
Patient restless/agitated	Fever
Flushing	Hypotension
Anxiety	Oozing from wounds or venepuncture sites
Chills	Haemoglobinaemia
Nausea and vomiting	Haemoglobinuria
Pain at venepuncture site	
Abdominal, flank or chest pain	
Diarrhoea	

If predominantly extravascular may only suffer chills/fever 1h after starting transfusion—commonly due to anti-D. Acute renal failure is *not* a feature.

Mechanism

Complement (C3a, C4a, C5a) release into recipient plasma→smooth muscle contraction. May develop DIC (*see p512*); oliguria (10% cases) due to profound hypotension.

Initial steps in management of acute transfusion reaction

- Stop blood transfusion immediately.
- Replace giving set, keep IV open with 0.9% saline.
- Check patient identity against donor unit.
- Insert urinary catheter and monitor urine output.
- Give fluids (IV colloids) to maintain urine output >1.5mL/kg/h.
- If urine output <1.5mL/kg/h insert CVP line and give fluid challenge.
- If urine output <1.5mL/kg/h and CVP adequate give furosemide (frusemide) 80–120 mg.
- If urine output still <1.5mL/kg/h consult senior medical staff for advice.
- Contact Blood Transfusion Lab before sending back blood pack and for advice on blood samples required for further investigation.

Complications

Overall mortality ~10%.

Haematological emergencies

Immediate-type hypersensitivity reactions

May occur soon (30–90min) after transfusion of blood/component. Antibody often unknown but in some cases is due to antibody directed against IgA (in recipients who have become sensitised).

- Mild reaction: urticaria, erythema, maculopapular rash, periorbital oedema.
- Severe reaction: bronchospasm.
- Hypotension.

Management
- Stop transfusion immediately.
- Change giving set.
- IV colloids to maintain BP/circulatory volume.
- Give
  - **epinephrine (adrenaline)** **1:1000 1mL IM stat**
  - **hydrocortisone** **100mg IV stat**
  - **chlorphenamine (chlorpheniramine)** **10mg IV stat**

Febrile transfusion reactions

Seen in 0.5–1.0% blood transfusions. Mainly due to anti-HLA antibodies in recipient serum or granulocyte-specific antibodies (e.g. sensitisation during pregnancy or previous blood transfusion). Less common now that all blood is leucodepleted after donation.

Treatment
- Slow down rate of transfusion.
- Antipyretic.

Delayed transfusion reaction

Occurs in patients immunised through previous pregnancies or transfusions. Antibody weak (so not detected at pretransfusion stage). 2° immune response occurs—antibody titre ↑.

Symptoms/signs
- Occur 7–10d after blood transfusion.
- Fever, anaemia and jaundice.
- ± haemoglobinuria.

Management
- Check DAT and repeat compatibility tests.
- Transfuse patient with freshly cross-matched blood.

Haematological emergencies

Bacterial contamination of blood products

Uncommon but potentially fatal adverse effect of blood transfusion (affects red cells and blood products e.g. platelet concentrates). Implicated organisms include Gram –ve bacteria, including *Pseudomonas*, *Yersinia* and *Flavobacterium*.

Features

- Fever.
- Skin flushing.
- Rigors.
- Abdominal pain.
- DIC.
- ARF.
- Shock.
- Cardiac arrest.

Management—as per *Immediate transfusion reaction*

- Stop transfusion.
- Urgent resuscitation.
- IV broad-spectrum antibiotics if bacterial contamination suspected.

Post-transfusion purpura

Profound thrombocytopenia occurring 5–10d after blood or platelet transfusion. Usually due to high titre of anti-HPA-1a antibody in HPA-1a –ve patient.

Features

- Rare.
- Multiparous ♀ most commonly (previous pregnancies or transfusions).
- Caused by platelet-specific alloantibodies (usually anti-HPA-1a).
- Platelets ↓↓ with associated bleeding/bruising—may be severe and even life threatening.

Management

- IVIg if bleeding.
- Plasma exchange worth considering.
- If platelet transfusion needed, use random donor platelets (no evidence that HPA-1a superior).

Haematological emergencies

Hypercalcaemia

Clinical symptoms

- General—weakness, lassitude, weight loss.
- Mental changes—impaired concentration, drowsiness, personality change and coma.
- GIT—anorexia, nausea, vomiting, abdominal pain (peptic ulceration and pancreatitis are rare complications).
- Genitourinary—polyuria, polydipsia.

Clinical effects

- Cardiovascular—↓ QT interval on ECG, cardiac arrhythmias and hypertension.
- Renal—dehydration, renal failure and renal calculi.

Haematological causes

1. Myeloma.
2. High grade lymphoma.
3. Adult T-cell leukaemia/lymphoma (ATLL).
4. Acute lymphoblastic leukaemia.

Hypercalcaemia occurs in other clinical situations including metastatic carcinoma of breast, prostate and lung. Theories for occurrence in haematological malignancy include increased bone resorption mediated by osteoclasts under the influence of locally or systemically released cytokines such as PTH-related peptide, TGF, TNF-α, M-CSF, interleukins and prostaglandins. Increased intestinal absorption of calcium secondary to increased 1,25-hydroxycholecalciferol.

Normal range for plasma [Ca^{2+}] 2.12–2.65mmol/L. 40% of plasma Ca^{2+} is bound to albumin. Most laboratories measure the total plasma Ca^{2+} although only unbound Ca^{2+} is physiologically active. For accurate measurement of plasma or serum Ca^{2+} blood sampling should be taken from an uncuffed arm, i.e. without the use of a tourniquet.

Correct for albumin	
Albumin <40g/L	corrected calcium = (Ca^{2+}) + 0.02 [40–(Albumin)]
Albumin >45g/L	corrected calcium = (Ca^{2+}) – 0.02 [(Albumin)–45]

Management

▶ An emergency if Ca^{2+} >3.0mmol/L.

1. Rehydrate with normal saline 4–6L/24h.
2. Beware fluid overload—use loop diuretics and CVP monitoring if necessary.
3. Stop thiazide diuretics and consider regular loop diuretics.
4. Give bisphosphonates e.g. disodium pamidronate 60–90mg IV stat (*see table*).
5. Treat underlying malignancy.
6. Consider dialysis if complicating factors (CCF, advanced renal failure).
7. Other therapeutic options:
   - Calcitonin 200IU 8-hourly.

- Corticosteroids (e.g. prednisolone 60mg/d PO).
- Mithromycin 25μg/kg IV × 3 weekly.
- Plicamycin.

Treatment of hypercalcaemia with disodium pamidronate

Serum Ca^{2+} (mmol/L)	Pamidronate (mg)
Up to 3.0	15-30
3.0–3.5	30-60
3.5–4.0	60-90
>4.0	90

Infuse slowly (*see BNF*).
Response often takes 3–5d.

Hyperviscosity

Common haematological emergency. Defined as increase in whole blood viscosity as a result of an increase in either red cells, white cells or plasma components, usually Ig.

Commonest situations arise as a result of

- ↑ in red cell volume in polycythaemia rubra vera.
- High blast cell numbers in peripheral blood e.g. AML or ALL at presentation.
- Presence of monoclonal Ig e.g. Waldenström's macroglobulinaemia (IgM).

Clinical features—polycythaemia (e.g. PRV)

- Lethargy, itching, headaches, hypertension, plethora, arterial thromboses viz: MI, CVA and visual loss (central retinal artery occlusion).

▶ Emergency treatment

Isovolaemic venesection. Remove 500mL blood volume from large bore vein (antecubital usually) with simultaneous replacement into another vein of 500mL 0.9% saline. Repeat daily until PCV <0.45.

Clinical features—high WBC (e.g. AML)

- Dyspnoea and cough (pulmonary leucostasis); confusion, ↓ conscious level, isolated cranial nerve palsies (cerebral leucostasis), visual loss (retinal haemorrhage or CRVT).

▶ Emergency treatment

- Unless machine leucapheresis can be obtained immediately, venesect 500mL blood from large bore vein and replace isovolaemically with packed red cells if Hb <7.0g/dL—otherwise replace with 0.9% saline to avoid increasing whole blood viscosity.
- Arrange leucapheresis on cell separator machine. Use white cell interface programme to apherese with replacement fluids depending on Hb as above. 2h is usually maximum tolerated.
- Initiate tumour lysis prophylactic protocol (see *p560*) in preparation for chemotherapy.
- Start chemotherapy as soon as criteria allow (high urine volume of pH>8 and allopurinol commenced). This is crucial as leucapheresis in this situation is only a holding manoeuvre while the patient is prepared for chemotherapy.
- Continue leucapheresis daily until leucostasis symptoms resolved or until WBC <50 × 10^9/L.

Hypergammaglobulinaemia (e.g. Waldenström's)

Lethargy, headaches, memory loss, confusion, vertigo, visual disturbances from cerebral vessel sludging—rarely MI, CVA.

▶ Emergency treatment

- Unless immediate access to plasma exchange machine available, venesect 500mL blood from large bore vein with isovolaemic replacement with 0.9% saline unless Hb <7.0g/dL when use packed red cells.
- Arrange plasmapheresis on a cell separator machine using plasma exchange programme (see p584). Replacement fluids on criteria as above. Aim for 1–1.5 × blood volume exchange (usually 2.5–4.0L)

starting at lower end of range initially. Repeat daily until symptoms resolved.

- Maintenance plasma exchanges at 3–6 weekly intervals may be sufficient treatment for some forms of Waldenström's macroglobulinaemia. However, if hyperviscosity due to IgA myeloma or occasionally IgG myeloma, chemotherapy will need to be initiated.

Note

Diseases in which the abnormal Ig shows activity at lower temperature e.g. cold antibodies associated with CHAD (*see p118*) require maintenance of plasmapheresis inlet and outlet venous lines and all infusional fluids at 37°C. Polyclonal ↑ in Ig (e.g. some forms of cryoglobulinaemia) can also rarely cause hyperviscosity symptoms. Management is as above for monoclonal immunoglobulins.

Disseminated intravascular coagulation

Pathological process characterised by generalised intravascular activation of the haemostatic mechanism producing widespread fibrin formation, resultant activation of fibrinolysis, and consumption of platelets/coagulation factors (esp I, II, V). Usually the result of serious underlying disease but may itself become life threatening (through haemorrhage or thrombosis). Mortality in severe DIC may exceed >80%. Haemorrhage usually the dominant feature and is the result of excessive fibrinolysis, depletion of coagulation factors and platelets and inhibition of fibrin polymerisation by FDPs. Wide range of disorders may precipitate DIC.

Pathophysiology—DIC may be initiated by

- Exposure of blood to tissue factor (e.g. after trauma).
- Endothelial cell damage (e.g. by endotoxin or cytokines).
- Release of proteolytic enzymes into the blood (e.g. pancreas, snake venom).
- Infusion or release of activated clotting factors (factor IX concentrate).
- Massive thrombosis.
- Severe hypoxia and acidosis.

Causes of DIC

Tissue damage (release of tissue factor) e.g. trauma (esp brain or crush injury), thermal injury (burns, hyperthermia, hypothermia), surgery, shock, asphyxia/hypoxia, ischaemia/infarction, rhabdomyolysis, fat embolism.

Complications of pregnancy (release of tissue factor) e.g. amniotic fluid embolism, abruptio placentae, eclampsia and pre-eclampsia, retained dead fetus, uterine rupture, septic abortion, hydatidiform mole.

Neoplasia (release of tissue factor, TNF, proteases) e.g. solid tumours, leukaemias (esp. acute promyelocytic).

Infection (endotoxin release, endothelial cell damage) e.g. Gram –ve bacteria (e.g. meningococcus), Gram +ve bacteria (e.g. pneumococcus), anaerobes, *M tuberculosis*, toxic shock syndrome, viruses (e.g. Lassa fever), protozoa (e.g. malaria), fungi (e.g. candidiasis), Rocky Mountain spotted fever.

Vascular disorders (abnormal endothelium, platelet activation) e.g. giant haemangioma (Kasabach–Merritt syndrome), vascular tumours, aortic aneurysm, vascular surgery, cardiac bypass surgery, malignant hypertension, pulmonary embolism, acute MI, stroke, subarachnoid haemorrhage.

Immunological (complement activation, release of tissue factor) anaphylaxis, acute haemolytic transfusion reaction, heparin-associated thrombocytopenia, renal allograft rejection, acute vasculitis, drug reactions (quinine).

Proteolytic activation of coagulation factors e.g. pancreatitis, snake venom, insect bites.

Neonatal disorders e.g. infection, aspiration syndromes, small-for-dates infant, respiratory distress syndrome, purpura fulminans.

Other disorders e.g. fulminant hepatic failure, cirrhosis, Reye's syndrome, acute fatty liver of pregnancy, ARDS, therapy with fibrinolytic agents, therapy with factor IX concentrates, massive transfusion, acute intravascular haemolysis familial ATIII deficiency, homozygous protein C or S deficiency.

Clinical features	
Acute (uncompensated) DIC	Rapid and extensive activation of coagulation, fibrinolysis or both, with depletion of procoagulant factors and inhibitors and signifi cant haemorrhage.
Chronic (compensated) DIC	Slow consumption of factors with normal or increased levels; often asymptomatic or associated with thrombosis.

Clinical features may be masked by those of the disorder which precipitated it and rarely is the cause of DIC obscure. DIC should be considered in the management of any seriously ill patient. The specific features of DIC are:

- Ecchymoses, petechiae, oozing from venepuncture sites and post-op bleeding.
- Renal dysfunction, ARDS, cerebral dysfunction and skin necrosis due to microthrombi.
- MAHA.

Laboratory features

The following investigations are useful in establishing the diagnosis of DIC though the extent to which any single test may be abnormal reflects the underlying cause of DIC.

- D-dimers—more specific and convenient than FDP titre (performed on plasma sample). Significant ↑ of D-dimers plus depletion of coagulation factors ± platelets is necessary for diagnosis of DIC.
- PT—less sensitive, usually ↑ in moderately severe DIC but may be normal in chronic DIC.
- APTR—less useful. May be normal or even <normal, particularly in chronic DIC.
- Fibrinogen—↓ or falling fibrinogen levels are characteristic of many causes of DIC in the presence of D-dimers. Greatest falls are seen with tissue factor release.
- Platelet count—↓ or falling platelet counts are characteristic of acute DIC, most notably in association with infective causes.
- Blood film may show evidence of fragmentation (schistocytes) though the absence of this finding does not exclude the diagnosis of DIC.

- Antithrombin levels are frequently ↓ in DIC and degree of reduction in plasma antithrombin and plasminogen may reflect severity.
- Factor assays rarely necessary or helpful. In severe DIC levels of most factors are reduced with the exception of FVIIIc and von Willebrand factor which may be increased due to release from endothelial cell storage sites.

Management of DIC

1. Identify and, if possible, remove the precipitating cause.
2. Supportive therapy as required (e.g. volume replacement for shock).
3. Replacement therapy if bleeding: platelet transfusion if platelets $<50 \times 10^9$/L, cryoprecipitate to replace fibrinogen, and FFP to replace other factors (10 units cryoprecipitate for every 3 units FFP).
4. Prophylactic platelet transfusion may be helpful if platelets $<20 \times 10^9$/L.
5. Monitor response with platelet count, PT, fibrinogen and D-dimers.
6. Heparin (IVI 5–10iu/kg/h) for DIC associated with APML, carcinoma, skin necrosis, purpura fulminans, microthrombosis affecting skin, kidney, bowel and large vessel thrombosis.
7. ATIII concentrate in intractable shock or fulminant hepatic necrosis.
8. Protein C concentrate in acquired purpura fulminans or severe neonatal DIC.

Haematological emergencies

Overdosage of thrombolytic therapy

- Large doses of any thrombolytic agent (streptokinase, urokinase, TPA) will cause primary fibrinolysis by proteolytic destruction of circulating fibrinogen and consumption of plasminogen and its major inhibitor α2-antiplasmin.
- Overdosage is associated with high risk of severe haemorrhage particularly at recent venepuncture sites or surgical wounds; intracranial haemorrhage occurs in 0.5–1% of patients treated with thrombolytic therapy.
- Superficial bleeding at venepuncture site may be managed with local pressure and the infusion continued.
- Bleeding at other sites or where pressure cannot be applied necessitates cessation of thrombolytic therapy ($t_{1/2}$<30mins) and determination of the thrombin time (if used to monitor thrombolytic therapy) or fibrinogen level. If strongly indicated and bleeding minimal or stopped the infusion may be restarted at 50% the initial dose when the thrombin time has returned to the lower end of the therapeutic range (1.5 × baseline).

Treatment of serious bleeding after thrombolytic therapy

- Stop thrombolytic infusion immediately.
- Discontinue any simultaneous heparin infusion and any antiplatelet agents.
- Apply pressure to bleeding sites, ensure good venous access and commence volume expansion.
- Check fibrinogen and APTR.
- Transfuse 10 units cryoprecipitate.
- Monitor fibrinogen, repeat cryoprecipitate to maintain fibrinogen >1.0g/L.
- If still bleeding, transfuse 2–4 units FFP.
- If bleeding time >9 mins, transfuse 10 units platelets.
- If bleeding time <9 mins, commence tranexamic acid.

Haematological emergencies

Heparin overdosage

The most serious complication of heparin overdosage is haemorrhage. The therapeutic range using the APTT is 1.5–2.5× average normal control. The plasma $t^{1/2}$ following IV administration is 1–2h. The $t_{½}$ after SC administration is considerably longer.

Management guidelines—APTT > therapeutic range

Without haemorrhage	***Continuous IV infusion*** stop infusion, if markedly elevated, recheck after 0.5–1h; restart at lower dose when APTT in therapeutic range ***Intermittent SC heparin*** reduce dose recheck 6h after administration
With haemorrhage	***Continuous IV infusion*** stop infusion; if bleeding continues, administer protamine sulphate by slow IV injection (1mg neutralises 100iu heparin, max dose 40mg/injection) ***Intermittent SC heparin*** if protamine is required, administer 50% of calculated neutralisation dose 1h after heparin administration and 25% after 2h

Haematological emergencies

Heparin-induced thrombocytopenia (HIT)

Uncommon but sometimes life-threatening condition due to immune complex-mediated thrombocytopenia in patients treated with heparin. Early recognition reduces morbidity and mortality.

Incidence

Estimated incidence 1–3% of patients receiving heparin for ≥1week. Occurs both with full dose regimens and 'minidose' regimens (5000IU bd) or low doses used for 'flushing' IV lines. Less common with low molecular weight heparin.

Pathogenesis

IgG antibodies formed in response to heparin therapy form immune complexes with heparin and PF4, bind to platelet Fc receptors, trigger aggregation and cause thrombocytopenia. Thrombin activation causes vascular thrombosis and microthrombi cause microvascular occlusion.

Clinical features

- HIT causes a fall in the platelet count ~8d (4–14d) after a patient's first exposure to heparin but may occur within 1–3d in a patient who has recently had prior exposure to heparin.
- Platelet count generally falls to $\sim 60 \times 10^9$/L but may fall to $< 20 \times 10^9$/L.
- Venous and arterial thromboses occur in up to 15%.
- Bleeding is rare.
- Microvascular occlusion may cause progressive gangrene extending proximally from the extremities and necessitating amputation. In patients with HITT (thrombocytopenia and thrombosis) limb amputation is required in ~10% and mortality approaches 20%.

HIT should be suspected in any patient on heparin in whom the platelet count falls to $< 100 \times 10^9$/L or drops by ≥30–40% or develops a new thromboembolic event 5–10d after ongoing heparin therapy.

►► **Heparin should be discontinued immediately and confirmatory investigations undertaken.**

Diagnostic test

ELISA using PF4 to detect antibodies to heparin-low molecular weight protein complex; may miss 5–10% of cases with antibodies to other proteins and up to 50% false positives after CABG.

Management

- Discontinue heparin (platelet count normally recovers in 2–5d).
- Substitute alternative anticoagulation where necessary and to prevent further thromboembolic events:
- **Recombinant hirudin**
  - Thrombin inhibitor; anticoagulant effect lasts ~40min.
  - Slow IV bolus followed by IVI.
  - Dose determined by body weight and renal function (*see product literature*).
  - Monitor 4h after IV bolus dose using APTT or ecarin clotting time (ECT); target range 1.5–2.5 × mean normal APTT; reduce target to

1.5 if concomitant warfarin therapy and discontinue hirudin when INR ≥2.0.
  - Adverse effects bleeding (esp. with warfarin), anaemia, haematoma, fever and abnormal LFTs.
- **Argatroban**
  - Thrombin inhibitor; $t_{½}$ ~45min.
  - Initiate IV infusion at dose of 2μg/kg/min.
  - Check APTT at 2h and adjust dose for APTT 1.5–3 × baseline (max 100s).
  - ↓ dose by 75% if hepatic insufficiency.
  - Side effect—bleeding.
- **Danaparoid**
  - A heparinoid with low level cross-reactivity with HIT antibodies.
  - IV bolus dose by weight (*see product literature*) followed by decremental infusion schedule and maintenance infusion.
  - Monitor by factor Xa inhibition assay 4h after dose (target range 0.5–0.8U/ml).
  - Prolonged $t_{½}$ of 25h.
  - Side effect—bleeding.

►► Low molecular weight heparins frequently cross-react with HIT antibodies and are not recommended.

Warfarin overdosage

Haemorrhage is a potentially serious complication of anticoagulant therapy and may occur with an INR in the therapeutic range if there are local predisposing factors e.g. peptic ulceration or recent surgery, or if NSAIDs are given concurrently.

Management guidelines

INR	Action
>7.0	Without haemorrhage: stop warfarin & consider a single 5–10mg oral dose of vitamin K if high bleeding risk; review INR daily
4.5–7.0	Without haemorrhage: stop warfarin & review INR in 2d
>4.5	With severe life-threatening haemorrhage: give factor IX concentrate (50U/kg) or FFP (1L for an adult), consider a single 2–5mg IV dose of vitamin K
>4.5	With less severe haemorrhage: e.g. haematuria or epistaxis, withhold warfarin for ≥1d and consider a single 0.5–2mg IV dose of vitamin K
2.0–4.5	With haemorrhage: investigate the possibility of an underlying local cause; reduce warfarin dose if necessary; give FFP/factor IX concentrate only if haemorrhage is serious or life threatening

Vitamin K administration to patients on warfarin therapy

Effect of vitamin K is delayed several hours even with IV administration. Doses >2 mg cause unpredictable and prolonged resistance to oral anticoagulants and should be avoided in most circumstances where prolonged warfarin therapy is necessary. Particular care must be taken in patients with prosthetic cardiac valves who may require heparin therapy for several weeks to achieve adequate anticoagulation if a large dose of vitamin K has been administered.

Haematological emergencies

Massive blood transfusion

Massive transfusion defined as replacement of >1 blood volume (5L) in less than 24h. Haemostatic failure may result from dilution or consumption of coagulation factors and platelets, DIC, systemic fibrinolysis or acquired platelet dysfunction.

Pathophysiology

- ***Dilution/consumption*** e.g. replacement of intravascular volume with fluids lacking coagulation factors or platelets e.g. packed red cells and crystalloids.
- ***DIC*** may follow tissue damage, hypoxia, acidosis, sepsis or haemolytic transfusion reaction. Causes coagulopathy due to consumption of platelets and coagulation factors, fibrinolysis and circulating fibrin degradation products (*see p512*).
- ***Systemic fibrinolysis*** particularly associated with liver disease; causes rapid lysis of thrombi at surgical sites and plasmin-induced fibrinogenolysis; may be assessed by the euglobulin lysis time.
- ***Platelet dysfunction*** may be due to circulating FDPs, exhausted platelets activated by intravascular trauma or effects of transfusion of stored platelets.

Investigations

- Baseline tests
  - Haematocrit.
  - Platelet count.
  - Fibrinogen.
  - PT.
  - APTT ratio.
  - D-dimers.
- Frequent reassessment of tests to monitor effect of, and need for, further replacement therapy.

Management		
Haematocrit	<0.30	Transfuse red cells
Platelet count	$<75 \times 10^9$/L	Transfuse platelets
Fibrinogen	<1.0g/L	Transfuse cryoprecipitate
PT ± APTT ratio	>1.5 × control	Transfuse FFP

Red cell transfusion

- Full crossmatch takes 30–40 minutes.
- Uncrossmatched group-specific blood can be available in 10 minutes.
- Uncrossmatched group O Rh (D) –ve blood may be transfused in the emergency situation until group-specific blood can be made available; group O Rh (D) +ve red cells may be given to males and older women if necessary.

Platelet transfusion

- Usually available within 10–15 minutes.
- Standard adult dose (6 units equivalent) will raise platelet count by $\sim 60 \times 10^9$/L in absence of dilution or consumption.

- As platelets do not carry Rh antigens, type incompatible platelets may be administered when necessary; Rh immune globulin should be administered when a Rh –ve patient has received Rh +ve platelets.
- 6 units of platelets contain ~300mL plasma.

Fresh frozen plasma

- Takes up to 30 minutes to thaw; dose required ~10mL/kg.
- Use immediately for optimum replacement of coagulation factors.
- Each unit contains ~200–280mL plasma and 0.7–1.0iu/mL activity of each coagulation factor
- ABO group compatible FFP should be administered—no crossmatch is required.
- If large volumes infused, serum [Ca^{2+}] should be monitored to exclude hypocalcaemia due to citrate toxicity.

Cryoprecipitate

- Precipitate formed when FFP is thawed at 4°C; resuspended in 10–15mL plasma and refrozen at –18°C; takes up to 15 minutes to thaw and pool.
- No grouping required.
- Contains 80–100IU FVIIIC, 100–250mg fibrinogen, 50–60mg fibronectin and 40–70% of the original von Willebrand factor.
- Should be used immediately for optimum replacement of fibrinogen and factor VIIIC.
- Infusion of 8–10 bags raises fibrinogen concentration by 0.6–1.0g/L in a 70kg patient.

Paraparesis/spinal collapse

May be due to tumour in the cord, spinal dura or meninges or by extension of a vertebral tumour into the spinal canal with compression of the cord or as a result of vertebral collapse.

Spinal cord compression from vertebral collapse in a haematological patient is most commonly due to myeloma (in up to 20% of patients) but may occur in a patient with Hodgkin's disease (3–8%) or occasionally non-Hodgkin's lymphoma. Spinal cord involvement by leukaemia is most common in AML, less so in ALL and CGL and least common in CLL.

Onset of paraplegia may be preceded for days or weeks by paraesthesia but in some patients the onset of paraplegia may follow initial symptoms by only a few hours.

Symptoms suggestive of spinal cord compression require urgent assessment by CT or MRI and referral to a neurosurgical unit for assessment for surgical decompression. Where this is not possible early radiotherapy may provide symptomatic improvement. However, if treatment is delayed until paraparesis has developed, this often proves to be irreversible despite surgery and/or radiotherapy.

Haematological emergencies

Leucostasis

Term is applied both to organ damage due to 'sludging' of leucocytes in the capillaries of a patient with high circulating blast count and to the lodging and growth of leukaemic blasts, usually in AML, in the vascular tree eroding the vessel wall and producing tumours and haemorrhage.

Features

- More common in AML and blast crisis of CML.
- Leucostatic tumours are associated with an exponential increase in blasts in the peripheral blood and, prior to the development of effective chemotherapy, haemorrhage from intracerebral tumours was not an uncommon cause of death.
- Pulmonary or cerebral leucostasis are serious complications which may occur in patients who present with a blast count $>50 \times 10^9$/L.
- Leucocyte thrombi may cause plugging of pulmonary or cerebral capillaries. Vascular rupture and tissue infiltration may occur.
- Less common manifestations are priapism and vascular insufficiency.
- Pulmonary leucostasis causes progressive dyspnoea of sudden onset associated with fever, tachypnoea, hypoxaemia, diffuse crepitations and a diffuse interstitial infiltrate on CXR.
- Pulmonary haemorrhage and haemoptysis may occur. More common with monocytic leukaemias and the microgranular variant of acute promyelocytic leukaemia. Differentiation from bacterial or fungal pneumonia may be difficult.
- Cerebral leucostasis may cause a variety of neurological abnormalities.
- Anaemia may protect a patient with marked leucocytosis from the effects of increased whole blood viscosity. Transfusion of RBCs to correct anaemia prior to chemotherapy may initiate leucostasis.

Management

Urgent leucapheresis is required for a patient with marked leucostasis ($>200\times 10^9$/L) or in any patient in whom leucostasis is suspected. Chemotherapy may be commenced concomitantly to further reduce the leucocyte count but may be associated with a high incidence of pulmonary and CNS haemorrhage.

Haematological emergencies

Thrombotic thrombocytopenic purpura

Definition

Fulminant disease of unknown aetiology characterised by increased platelet aggregation and occlusion of arterioles and capillaries of the microcirculation. Considerable overlap in pathophysiology and clinical features with HUS—fundamental abnormality may be identical.

Incidence:

Rare, ~1 in 500,000 per year. ♀:♂ = 2:1. HUS much commoner in children, TTP commoner in adults—peak age incidence is 40 years, and 90% of cases <60 years old. There is some case clustering.

Clinical features

- Classical description is of a *pentad* of features:
  1. **Microangiopathic haemolytic anaemia**.
  2. **Severe thrombocytopenia**.
  3. **Neurological involvement**.
  4. **Renal impairment**.
  5. **Fever**.

  In practice, few patients have the full monty. 50–70% have renal abnormalities (*cf.* nearly all with HUS) and they are less severe. Neurological involvement is more prevalent in TTP than HUS. 40% of TTP patients have fever.
- *Haemolysis*—severe and intravascular causing jaundice.
- *Thrombocytopenia*—severe, mucosal haemorrhage likely and intracranial haemorrhage may be fatal.
- *Neurological*—from mild depression and confusion→visual defects, coma and status epilepticus.
- *Renal*—haematuria, proteinuria, oliguria and ↑ urea and creatinine. HUS >TTP.
- *Fever*—very variable, weakness and nausea common.
- *Other disease features*: serious venous thromboses at unusual sites (e.g. sagittal sinus—microthrombi in the brain seen on MRI scan). Abdominal pain severe enough to mimic an acute abdomen is sometimes seen due to mesenteric ischaemia. Diarrhoea is common, particularly bloody in HUS.

Diagnosis and investigations

- Made on the clinical features above—exclude other diseases e.g. cerebral lupus, sepsis with DIC.
- FBC shows severe anaemia and thrombocytopenia.
- Blood film shows gross fragmentation of red cells, spherocytes and nucleated red cells with polychromasia.
- Reticulocytes ↑↑ (>15%).
- LDH ↑↑ (>1000iu/L).
- Clotting screen including fibrinogen and FDPs usually normal (*cf.* DIC).
- Serum haptoglobin low or absent.
- Urinary haemosiderin +ve.
- Unconjugated bilirubin ↑.
- DAT –ve.
- BM hypercellular.

- U&E show increases (HUS > TTP).
- Proteinuria and haematuria.
- Renal biopsy shows microthrombi.
- Stool culture for *E. coli* 0157 +ve in most cases of HUS in children, less often in adult TTP.
- MRI brain scan shows microthrombi and occasional intracranial haemorrhage.
- **Lumbar puncture – do not proceed with LP unless scans clear and there is suspicion of infective meningitis.**
- Look for evidence of viral infection. Association of syndrome with HIV, SLE, cyclosporin usage and the 3rd trimester of pregnancy.

Treatment is a haematological emergency—seek expert help immediately

1. Unless antecubital venous access is excellent, insert a large bore central apheresis catheter (may need blood product support).
2. May need ITU level of care and ventilation.
3. ***Initiate plasmapheresis as soon as possible.***
   Exchange 1–1.5 × plasma volume daily until clinical improvement.
   May need 3–4L exchanges. Replacement fluid should be solely FFP.
   In the event of delayed access to cell separator facilities, start IV infusions of FFP making intravascular space with diuretics if necessary.
   Once response achieved, ↓ frequency of exchanges gradually.
   If no response obtained within one week, change FFP replacement to *cryosupernatant* (rationale: it lacks high molecular weight multimers of von Willebrand factor postulated in endothelial damage disease triggers).
4. Give RBC as necessary but reserve platelet transfusions for severe mucosal or intracranial bleeding as reports suggest they may worsen the disease.
5. Cover for infection with IV broad spectrum antibiotics including teicoplanin if necessary to preserve the apheresis catheter.
6. Start anticonvulsants if fitting.
7. Most would start high dose steroids (prednisolone 2mg/kg/d PO) with gastric protection although evidence is equivocal.
8. Aspirin/dipyridamole/heparin may be considered for non-responders.
9. Refractory patients (~10%) should be considered for IV vincristine.
10. Still refractory patients may achieve remission with splenectomy.
11. Response to treatment may be dramatic e.g. ventilated, comatose patient watching TV in the afternoon after plasma exchange in the morning!

Prognosis

- 90% respond to plasma exchange with FFP replacement.
- ~30% will relapse. Most respond again to further plasma exchange but leaves 15% who become chronic relapsers.
- Role of prophylaxis for chronic relapsers unclear. Intermittent FFP infusions or continuous low dose aspirin may help individual cases.

Sickle crisis

Management

- ▶ Early and effective treatment of crises essential (hospital).
- ▶ Rest patient and start IV fluids and O_2 (patients often dehydrated through poor oral intake of fluid + excessive loss if fever).
- ▶ Start empirical antibiotic therapy (e.g. cephalosporin) if infection is suspected whilst culture results (blood, urine or sputum) are awaited.
- ▶ Analgesia usually required—e.g. intravenous opiates (diamorphine/morphine) especially when patients are first admitted to hospital. Switch later to oral medication after the initial crisis abates.
- ▶ Consider exchange blood transfusion (if neurological symptoms, stroke or visceral damage). Aim to ↓ HbS to <30%.
- ▶ Exchange transfusion if PaO_2 <60mm on air (▶chest syndrome).
- ▶ α-adrenergic stimulators for priapism.
- ▶ Seek advice of senior haematology staff.
- ▶ Consider regular blood transfusion if *crises frequent* or *anaemia is severe* or patient has had *CVA/abnormal brain scan.*
- ▶ Top-up transfusion if Hb <4.5g/dL (hunt for cause).

Transfusion and splenectomy may be lifesaving in children with splenic sequestration.

www.bcshguidelines.com/pdf/SICKLE.V4_0802.pdf

Haematological emergencies

Supportive care

14

Quality of life

In managing any disease problem a key objective is to improve the quality of a patient's survival as well as its duration. Part of the clinical decision-making process takes into account quality of life (QoL) in judging the most appropriate treatment.

Defining quality of life precisely is not easy; it has been described as a measure of the difference at a particular time point between the hopes and expectations of the individual and that individual's present experiences. QoL is multifaceted and can only be assessed by the individual since it takes into account many aspects of that individual's life and their current perception of what, for them, is good QoL in their specific circumstances.

A clear distinction exists between performance scores (e.g. Karnofsky or WHO) which record functional status and assess independence; these are assessed by the physician according to pre-set criteria. They have erroneously been considered to be surrogate markers of QoL.

Patient QoL as assessed by the treating physician has been shown to be unreliable in an oncological setting.

There is no single determinant of good QoL. A number of qualities which go to make up QoL are capable of assessment; these include *ability to carry on normal physical activities, ability to work, to engage in normal social activities, a sense of general well-being* and a *perception of health.*

Several validated instruments now exist to measure QoL; these mainly involve questionnaires completed by the patient. They are simple to complete and involve 'yes' or 'no' answers to specific questions, answers on a linear analogue scale or the use of 4- or 7- point Likert scales.

Available QoL instruments include

- Functional Living Index – Cancer (FLIC)[1]
- Functional Assessment of Cancer Therapy (FACT)[2]
- European Organisation for Research and Treatment in Cancer (EORTC) Quality of Life Questionnaire C-30 (QLQ C30)[3]

Data from validated QoL questionnaires are now accepted as a requirement and a clinical end point in many major clinical trials, especially in malignancies, particularly those where survival differences are minimal between contrasting therapy approaches. Where survivals are minimally affected it is then essential to focus on treatments which will offer the best QoL.

Schipper, H. *et al.* (1984) Measuring the quality of life of cancer patients: the Functional Living Index–Cancer: development and validation. *J Clin Oncol*, **2**, 472–483; Cella, D.F. *et al.* (1993) The Functional Assessment of Cancer Therapy scale: development and validation of the general measure. *J Clin Oncol*, **11**, 570–579; Aaronson, N.K. *et al.* (1993) The European Organization for Research and Treatment of Cancer QLQ-C30: a quality-of-life instrument for use in international clinical trials in oncology. *J Natl Cancer Inst*, **85**, 365–376.

Supportive care

Pain management

Pain is a clinical problem in diverse haematological disorders, notably in sickle cell disease, haemophilia and myeloma. Acknowledgement of the need to manage pain effectively is an essential part of successful patient care and management in clinical haematology.

Pain may be local or generalised. More than one type of pain may be present and causes may be multifactorial. It is most important to listen to the patient and give him/her the chance to talk about their pain(s). Not only will this help determine an appropriate therapeutic strategy, the act of listening and allowing the patient to talk about their pains and associated anxieties is part of the pain management process.

Engaging the patient in 'measuring' their pain is often helpful; it enables specific goals to be set and provides a means to assess the effectiveness of the analgesic strategy.

Basic to the control of pain is to manage and remove the pathological process causing pain, wherever this is possible. Analgesia must be part of an integrated care plan which takes this into account.

Analgesic requirements should be recorded regularly as these form a valuable 'semi-quantitative' end point of pain measurement. Reduction in requirements, for example, is an indicator that attempts to remove or control the underlying cause are succeeding.

Managing pain successfully involves patient and family/carer participation, a collaborative multidisciplinary approach in most categories of haematological disorder related pain; medication should aim to provide continuous pain relief wherever possible with a minimum of drug related side effects

Analgesics

Simple non-opioid analgesics	Paracetamol: 1g 4–6 hourly, oral as tablets or liquid; suppositories available. No contraindication in liver disease; useful in mild to moderate pain.
Anti-inflammatory drugs	Ibuprofen 800mg or diclofenac 75–100mg bd as slow release formulations can be synergistic with other analgesics; combined formulations of diclofenac with misoprostol may reduce risks of gastric irritation bleeding; useful in combination with paracetamol or weak opioids
Weak opioids	Dextropropoxyphene 100mg usually combined with paracetamol 1g as coproxamol tablets; usual dosage is 2 tablets 6 hourly or codeine 30–60mg or dihydrocodeine 30–60mg up to 4 hourly provide effective analgesia for moderate pain. Confusion, drowsiness may be associated with initial usage in some. Weak (and strong) opioids cause constipation; usually requires simple laxatives
Strong opioids	Morphine available as liquid or tablets commencing at 5–10mg and given 4 hourly is treatment of choice

in severe pain. Once daily requirements are established patients can be 'converted' to 12 hourly slow release morphine preparations. Breakthrough pain can be treated with additional doses of 5–10mg morphine. Diamorphine preferred for parenteral usage. Highly soluble and suitable for use in a syringe driver for continuous administration or as a 4 hourly injection.

Alternatives to opioids Tramadol may be given orally. Fentanyl given as slow release transdermal patches may be a valuable alternative to slow release morphine for moderate to severe chronic pain.

For chronic pain give analgesia PO regularly, wherever possible.

- Pain control is very specific to the individual patient, there is no 'correct' formula other than the combination of measures which alleviate the pain.
- The clinician should work 'upwards' or 'downwards' through the levels of available analgesics to achieve control.
- Constipation due to analgesics should be managed with aperients.
- Nausea or vomiting may occur in up to 50% patients with strong opiates; cyclizine 50mg 8 hourly, metoclopramide 10mg 6 hourly or haloperidol 1.5mg 12 hourly are available options to limit nausea or vomiting.
- Additional general measures include
  - Radiotherapy for localised cancer pain.
  - Physical methods e.g. TENS or consideration of nerve root block.
  - Surgery, especially in myeloma where stabilising fractures and pinning will relieve pain and allow mobility.
  - Encouraging/allowing patients to utilise 'alternative' approaches. including relaxation techniques, aromatherapy, hypnosis, etc.
- Additional drug therapy
  - Antidepressants e.g. amitriptyline may help in neuropathic pain.
  - Anticonvulsants e.g. carbamazepine may be helpful in neuropathic pains especially in post-herpetic neuralgia.
  - Corticosteroids, particularly dexamethasone, to relieve leukaemic bone pain in late stage disease.

Many hospitals also run specific pain clinics. The support and expertise available should be enlisted particularly for difficult problems with persistent localised pain e.g. post-herpetic neuralgia. For long term painful conditions it is essential to work with medical and nursing colleagues in Primary Care and in Palliative Care so that the patient receives appropriate support in the community setting.

Psychological support

Many haematological disorders are long term conditions; the specific diagnosis can be seen to 'label' the patient as different or ill and therefore will exert a profound influence on their life and that of their immediate family or carers. Patients (and their families) experience and demonstrate a number of reactions to their diagnosis, the clinical haematologist needs to have an awareness of this and respond accordingly.

Reactions to serious diagnosis include
- Numbness.
- Denial.
- Anger.
- Guilt.
- Depression.
- Loneliness.

Ultimately most patients come to acceptance of their condition; carers/partners will also go through a similar range of reactions. The clinician needs to be aware of the way in which news of a diagnosis is likely to affect a patient and his/her family/carers and respond appropriately. In the first instance this will often involve the need to impart the diagnosis, what it means and what needs to be done clinically. There is no 'right way' to impart bad or difficult news. It is very important to make and take time to tell the patient of the diagnosis. Wherever possible this should be done in a quiet, private setting. Numbness at learning of a serious diagnosis often means that very little is taken in initially other than the diagnostic label. The various reactions listed above may subsequently emerge during the time the patient comes to accept the diagnosis, what it means and what is to be done clinically.

Within the haematological team there should be support available to the patient and family/carers which can provide them with practical information about the disease and its management. Simply knowing there is a sympathetic ear may be all that is required in the way of support; however, for some patients and families/carers more specialised support may be needed e.g. availability of formal counselling or access to psychological or psychiatric support.

Use can be made of local or national patient support groups; knowledge of others in similar predicaments can help diffuse anger and loneliness. Support groups can also be a valuable resource in providing information and experience which patients and families/carers find helpful.

The most effective psychological support for haematological patients is to see them as individuals and not 'diseases'.

Supportive care

Protocols and procedures

Note

Please check local protocols since these may differ to those outlined in this handbook.

Acute leukaemia – investigation

Haematology
- FBC, blood film, reticulocytes, ESR.
- Serum B_{12}, red cell folate, and ferritin.
- Blood group, antibody screen and DAT.
- Coagulation screen, INR, APTT, fibrinogen (and XDPs if bleeding).
- BM aspirate for morphology, cytogenetics, immunophenotype (and peripheral blood if relevant) plus samples required by the MRC trials.
- BM trephine biopsy.

Biochemistry
- U&E, LFTs.
- Ca^{2+}, phosphate, random glucose.
- LDH.
- Serum and urine lysozyme (if M4 or M5 AML suspected).

Virology
- Hepatitis BsAg.
- Hepatitis A antibody.
- Hepatitis C antibody.
- HIV I and II antibody (counselling and consent required).
- CMV IgG and IgM.

Immunology
- Serum immunoglobulins.
- Autoantibody screen profile.
- HLA type—Class 1 always in case HLA matched platelets are required, Class 1 and 2 if allogeneic transplant indicated.

Bacteriology
- Baseline blood cultures.
- Throat swab.
- MSU.
- Stool for fungal culture.
- Nose swab for MRSA if transferred from another hospital/unit.

Cardiology
- ECG.
- Echocardiogram, only if in cardiac failure or infective endocarditis suspected or significant cardiac history.

Radiology
- CXR.
- Sinus radiographs.

Other
- If any evidence of severe dental caries or gum disease refer patient for dental assessment *before* chemotherapy.
- Consider semen storage.

Protocols and procedures

Platelet storage and administration

Storage

Platelets should be stored at room temperature (20–22°C) in a platelet agitator until infused. Helps to retain function. Use before expiry date on pack.

- Platelet packs should be inspected before infusion—platelet packs that look visibly pink due to RBC contamination should not be used.
  - Occasionally fine fibrinoid strands may be seen in concentrates (give a slightly stringy or cloudy appearance). Such strands disperse with gentle massage and are safe to use.
  - Occasionally larger aggregates of platelets and/or white cell clumps are seen in the bags which do not disperse with gentle massage. Such bags are dangerous and should never be infused.

Dosage and timing

- A single dose of platelets is generally supplied as a single bag.
- Represents a standard transfusion dose although twice this amount may be required to cover insertions of central lines or minor surgery.
- Occasionally double doses may be required for patients becoming refractory.
- The frequency of platelet transfusion will be determined by clinical circumstances. In general, a patient who is well, afebrile and with no evidence of new bruising or bleeding need only have a platelet count maintained above 10×10^9/L. May be achieved with platelets given as infrequently as every 2–4 days with this estimate being guided on daily platelet counts.
- Patients who are infected or bleeding have much greater platelet requirements—aim to keep the platelet count $>20 \times 10^9$/L. This will usually mean daily platelet infusions for the duration of this clinical episode.
- Platelet counts of $<10 \times 10^9$/L should always be avoided but within these constraints the fewer platelets transfused the better since this reduces the risk of alloimmunisation to HLA and platelet antigens.
- Anyone with a *persistent* platelet count $<10 \times 10^9$/L should be started on tranexamic acid 1g qds PO or IV unless specific contraindications exist such as genitourinary tract bleeding.

Choice of blood group for platelet support

At diagnosis, all patients should have a blood group and CMV antibody status determined. Patients should receive platelets of their own blood group as far as possible. Due to fluctuations in supply, this is not always possible and the choice is less critical than for red cell transfusions as platelet ABO blood group antigen expression is weak and the recipient is exposed only to donor plasma.

Patient's blood group	first choice	second choice
O	O	A
A	A	O
B	B (if available)	A preferably or O
AB	A	O

- Rh (D) +ve patients may receive Rh (D) +ve or Rh (D) –ve products.
- Rh (D) –ve patients should receive Rh (D) –ve platelets.

- Occasionally necessary to give Rh (D) +ve platelets to Rh (D) –ve patients. The Blood Bank should be informed as all future red cell transfusions must be Rh (D) –ve. Anti-D administration may be given to such patients routinely or may be reserved for women of child-bearing age (dose: 250iu (50μg). Anti-D SC immediately after the transfusion.

Platelet transfusion support

See p546 and p650.

Platelet reactions and refractoriness

Reactions to platelet transfusion are common and range from mild temperatures to rigors. The development of an urticarial rash is also frequently seen. When a transfusion reaction develops, the following steps should be taken:

- ▶ Stop the transfusion.
- ▶ Give 10mg chlorphenamine (chlorpheniramine) IV and 1g of paracetamol PO.
- ▶ Cover future transfusions with chlorpheniramine and paracetamol 30 mins pre-transfusion.

- Hydrocortisone 100mg IV stat may be (sparingly) used for refractory reactions
- Pethidine is a suitable alternative for severe reactions and is almost invariably effective. Give 25mg IV stat with repeat dose if necessary or set up an IVI of 25–50mg IV over 8h.
- The possibility of generation of HLA and platelet-specific antibodies should also be considered (*see below*).

Platelet refractoriness

Occasionally patients show little/no increment in the platelet count after platelet transfusions. This is called platelet refractoriness. May be due to physical or immunological mechanisms in the patient. The commonest physical mechanism is of platelet circulatory half-life reduction caused by concurrent sepsis or coagulopathy e.g. DIC. Immunological causes include induction of anti-HLA antibodies due to allosensitisation from previous transfusions or generation of anti-platelet antibodies such as in ITP. Investigation should be considered if platelet transfusions fail to maintain a platelet count $>10 \times 10^9$/L at all times.

Proceed as follows

1. Check FBC pre-platelet infusion, 1 and 12h post-infusion to assess the rate of platelet count decay. Failure to show a rise of platelet count by at least 10×10^9/L at 1h or any rise after 12h post-infusion merits further testing.
2. Samples should be sent to a blood transfusion centre for HLA and platelet antibody screening (10mL EDTA samples and 20mL serum).
3. The patient's own HLA type should be checked.
4. If HLA or platelet antibodies are identified, the provision of HLA or platelet antigen matched platelet products may improve the platelet transfusion responsiveness.

Platelet refractoriness—More than two-thirds of patients receiving multiple transfusion with random platelets develop anti-HLA antibodies. Refractoriness defined as failure of 2 consecutive transfusions to give corrected increment of $>7.5\times 10^9$/L 1h after platelet transfusion in absence of fever, infection, severe bleeding, splenomegaly, or DIC.

GvHD—Rare complication where there is engraftment of donor lymphocytes in platelet concentrate in severely immunocompromised patients.

Calculating platelet increment $[(P_1–P_0) \times SA]/n$

P_0 = platelet count pre-transfusion ($\times 10^9$/L)
P_1 = platelet count post-transfusion ($\times 10^9$/L)
SA = surface area
n = number of units of platelets transfused

Corrected increment 60 min after transfusion $>7.5 \times 10^9$/L indicates successful platelet transfusion ($P_1–P_0$).

Hows, J.M. & Brozovic, R. (1992) in *ABC of Transfusion* 2nd edn BMJ Publications.

Prophylactic regimen for neutropenic patients

Infective risk is related to the severity and duration of neutropenia. Higher risk is associated with concurrent immunological defects e.g. hypogammaglobulinaemia in myeloma, T-cell defects e.g. HIV disease, additional immunosuppressive agents e.g. cyclosporin post-transplant, and older patients. Principal risk is from bacterial organisms but fungi and viruses, especially herpes (HSV, HZV) and CMV are also seen in prolonged neutropenia.

Typical protocols include

- ***Isolation procedures***—strict handwashing by all patient contacts is the only isolation measure of universally proven benefit. Others include visitor restriction, gloves, aprons, gowns, masks and full reverse barrier nursing. Isolation rooms with positive pressure filtered air will prevent fungal infection.
- ***Drinks***—avoid mains tap water/still mineral water (use boiled water or sparkling mineral water). Avoid unpasteurised milk and freshly squeezed fruit juice.
- ***Food***—avoid cream, ice-cream, soft, blue or ripened cheeses, live yoghurt, raw eggs or derived foods e.g. mayonnaise and soufflés, cold chicken, meat paté, raw fish/shellfish, unpeeled fresh vegetables/salads, unpeeled fruit, uncooked herbs and spices, ground pepper (contains *Aspergillus* spores).
- ***General mouthcare***—antiseptic mouthwash e.g. Corsadyl 10mL 4 hourly swish and spit. If soreness develops, substitute Difflam mouthwash. For discrete oral ulcers, use topical Adcortyl in Orobase; for generalised ulceration use 0.9% saline mouthwash hourly, swish and spit. Corsodyl toothpaste should replace standard preparations. Oral antifungal prophylaxis should be nystatin susp. 1mL 4 hourly swish and spit or swallow, or amphotericin lozenges one to suck slowly 4 hourly.
- ***Antibacterial prophylaxis***—aim to alter flora and prevent exogenous colonisation. Principal agents: ciprofloxacin 250mg bd or cotrimoxazole 480mg bd or colistin 1.5MU tds and neomycin 500mg qds. All given PO starting 48h after antifungal prophylaxis.
- ***Antifungal prophylaxis***—a systemic imidazole compound is most routinely used e.g. fluconazole 100mg PO od. Itraconazole liquid 2.5mg/kg bd PO may offer additional protection against *Aspergillus*.
- ***Antiviral prophylaxis***—Acyclovir is the most useful drug at preventing herpes reactivation. Dose is dependent on degree of immunosuppression and thus the likely organism to be encountered. 400mg bd will prevent HSV reactivation e.g. post-standard chemotherapy; 400mg qds may prevent HZV reactivation e.g. post-SCT; 800mg tds or more may prevent CMV reactivation post-allogeneic SCT.
- ***Additional prophylaxis for specials situations***—history of, or radiological evidence of, tuberculosis (TB). Consideration should be given to standard anti-TB prophylaxis e.g. rimactazid/pyridoxine particularly if prolonged neutropenia expected. Splenectomised patient—at extra risk from encapsulated organisms particularly *Streptococcus pneumoniae*, *Haemophilus influenzae* and *Neisseria meningitidis*. Use penicillin V 500mg

od PO or erythromycin 250 mg od PO if penicillin allergic as prophylaxis switching to high dose amoxicillin/cefotaxime if febrile. Post-SCT (see *p*294).

Guidelines for use of IV antibiotics in neutropenic patients

Urgent action required if neutropenic patient develops

- Single fever spike >38°C.
- 2 fever spikes >37.5°C 1h apart.
- Symptoms or signs of sepsis even without fever.

Assessment

- Search for localising symptoms or signs of infection.
- Full clinical examination noting BP, pulse, mouth, chest, perineum, line sites, skin and fundi.
- O_2 saturation (pulse oximetry).
- FBC, U&E, creatinine, LFTs, CRP, INR, APTT, fibrinogen.
- Perform a septic screen:
  - 3 sets of blood cultures (10mL per bottle optimises organism recovery) if central line present, take paired peripheral and central samples.
  - Single further blood culture set if non-response at 48–72h or condition changes.
- Swab relevant sites: wounds, central line exit site, throat.
- Sputum culture.
- MSSU.
- Faeces if symptomatic incl. *C difficile* toxin.
- Viral serology if clinically relevant.
- CXR.
- Other imaging as relevant, consider sinus x-ray.
- Consider bronchoalveolar lavage if chest infiltrates present.
- Consider risk of invasive fungal infection: CT chest if high risk.

Empirical treatment

Start IV antibiotics to provide broad spectrum cover. Stop prophylactic ciprofloxacin. Follow local protocol if available.

First line: Tazocin 4.5g tds plus gentamicin 6mg/kg/day.

If patient has history of penicillin allergy use ceftazidime 2g tds instead of tazocin; if anaphylaxis with penicillin discuss with microbiologist.

If suspected line infection (exit site inflammation) add vancomycin 1g bd and consider line removal. Vancomycin dose should be split and administered through each lumen. May be locked in the line for 1h then flushed.

If there are signs of perianal sepsis, mucositis or intra-abdominal infection or if *C difficile* is suspected add metronidazole 500mg tds IV.

1. Patients on od gentamicin should have pre-dose level checked 24h after first dose then twice weekly if satisfactory.
2. Patients on vancomycin should have pre-dose levels checked immediately before 3rd or 4th dose (2nd if renal impairment) then twice weekly if satisfactory.

Reassess at 48–72h:

If no response to antibiotics and negative blood cultures:
Add vancomycin 1g bd.
If already on vancomycin, consider line removal.
Consider risk of invasive fungal infection. CT chest if high risk.

Reassess after further 48–72h:
If no response to antibiotics and negative blood cultures:

If high risk for invasive fungal infection:
Stop above antibiotics. Commence amphotericin 1mg/kg/day plus ciprofloxacin 500mg bd PO/IV. Stop prophylactic fluconazole/itraconazole.

If low risk for invasive fungal infection:
Switch antibiotics to meropenem 1g tds plus gentamicin 6mg/kg/day.

Reassess after further 48h:
If no response to amphotericin, change ciprofloxacin to meropenem 1g tds plus gentamicin 6mg/kg/day.

If not on amphotericin, consider switching to amphotericin 1mg/kg/day plus ciprofloxacin 500mg bd PO/IV. Stop prophylactic fluconazole/itraconazole.

Duration of therapy

If temperature responds but cultures are negative, continue anti-infective treatment until apyrexial for 72h or minimum 5d course. If still neutropenic restart prophylactic anti-infectives. Amphotericin should be continued until neutrophil regeneration or total dose of 1g administered.

Positive cultures

Antibiotic therapy may be changed on the basis of positive cultures.

Treatment of neutropenic sepsis when source unknown

▶▶ One of the commonest haemato-oncological emergencies.

- May be defined as the presence of symptoms or signs of infection in a patient with an absolute neutrophil count of $<1.0 \times 10^9/L$. In practice, the neutrophil count is often $<0.1 \times 10^9/L$.
- Similar clinical picture also seen in neutrophil function disorders such as MDS despite normal neutrophil numbers.
- ***Beware***—can occur without pyrexia, especially patients on steroids.

Immediate action

▶▶ Urgent clinical assessment.

- Follow ALS guidelines if cardiorespiratory arrest (rare).
- More commonly, clinical picture is more like cardiovascular shock ± respiratory embarrassment viz: tachycardia, hypotension, peripheral vasodilatation and tachypnoea. Occurs with both Gram +ve (now more common with indwelling central catheters) and Gram –ve organisms (less common but more fulminant).
- Immediate rapid infusion of albumin 4.5% or gelofusin to restore BP.
- Insert central catheter if not *in situ* and monitor CVP.
- Start O_2 by face mask if pulse oximetry shows saturations <95% (common) and consider arterial blood gas measurement—care with platelet counts $<20 \times 10^9/L$—manual pressure over puncture site for 30 mins.
- Perform full septic screen (*see p552*).
- Give the first dose of first line antibiotics immediately e.g ureidopenicillin and loading dose aminoglycoside (ceftazidime or ciprofloxacin if pre-existing renal impairment). Follow established protocols.
- If the event occurs while patient on first line antibiotics, vancomycin/ciprofloxacin or vancomycin/meropenem are suitable alternatives.
- Commence full ITU-type monitoring chart.
- Monitor urine output with urinary catheter if necessary—if renal shutdown has already occurred, give single bolus of IV frusemide. If no response, start renal dose dopamine.
- If BP not restored with colloid despite elevated CVP, consider inotropes.
- If O_2 saturations remain low despite 60% O_2 delivered by rebreathing mask, consider ventilation.
- ***Alert ITU giving details of current status.***

Subsequent actions

- Discuss with senior colleague.
- Amend antibiotics according to culture results or to suit likely source if cultures negative.
- Check aminoglycoside trough levels after loading dose and before second dose as renal impairment may determine reducing or withholding next dose. Consider switch to non-nephrotoxic cover e.g. ceftazidime/ciprofloxacin.
- Continue antibiotics for 7–10d minimum and usually until neutrophil recovery.

- If cultures show central line to be source of sepsis, remove immediately if patient not responding.

Treatment of neutropenic sepsis when source known/suspected

Central indwelling catheters

Very common. Organisms usually *Staph. epidermidis* but can be other *Staph* spp. and even Gram –ve organisms. May be erythema/exudate around entry or exit sites of line, tenderness/erythema over subcutaneous tunnel or discomfort over line tract. Blood cultures must be taken from each lumen and peripherally and labelled individually. Add vancomycin 1g bd IV if not in standard protocol. Split dose between all lumens unless cultures known to be +ve in one lumen only. Lock and leave in line for 1h, then flush through. If no response or clinical deterioration, ***remove line immediately.***

Perianal or periodontal

Both are common sites of infection in neutropenic patients. Perianal lesions may become secondarily infected if skin abraded. Add metronidazole 500mg IV tds to standard therapy. Painful SC abscesses may form and may require surgical incision. Gum disease and localized tooth infections/abscesses are frequently seen. Add metronidazole to therapy as above, arrange OPG and dental review as surgical intervention may be required in non-responders. If possible, best delayed until neutrophil recovery in most cases—then do electively before next course of chemotherapy.

Lung

Atypical organisms

Risk group

HIV infection, HCL, post-SCT.

Mycoplasma and other atypicals are commonly found and usually community acquired (except *Legionella*)—typically occur shortly after return to hospital and in patients with chronic lung disease.

Treatment

Azithromycin (or clarithromycin if IV preparation needed) is now treatment of choice—well absorbed and fewer side effects than erythromycin. 5d rather than 3d course may be needed.

Pneumocystis carinii pneumonia

Risk group

Lymphoid malignancy long-term treatment esp. ALL, steroid usage, purine analogues e.g. fludarabine and 2-CDA.

Treatment

High dose cotrimoxazole IV initially—watch renal function and adjust dose to creatinine. Give short pulse of steroid 0.5mg/kg at start of treatment. At-risk patients should remain on long-term prophylaxis until chemo finished and absolute CD4 lymphocyte count $>500 \times 10^6$/L. Use cotrimoxazole 480mg bd on Monday, Wednesday and Friday only, provided neutrophil count maintained $>1.0 \times 10^9$/L. Otherwise use nebulised pentamidine 300mg every 3 weeks with preceding nebulised salbutamol 2.5mg.

Fungal

Risk group
Prolonged, severe neutropenia, chronic steroid and antibiotic usage, GvHD. *Aspergillus* and other moulds increasingly common with intensive chemotherapy protocols and post-stem cell transplant esp. MUDs.

Treatment
- Amphotericin IV (*see p330*).
- Once neutrophil recovery has occurred, maintenance may be with oral itraconazole liquid 2.5mg/kg bd—may also be used for prophylaxis.

Viral—CMV

Risk group
Allogeneic SCT esp. MUDs where donor or recipient is CMV +ve. Disease usually due to reactivation rather than *de novo* infection. Apart from pneumonitis, may cause graft suppression, gastritis, oesophagitis, weight loss, hepatitis, retinitis, haemorrhagic cystitis and vertigo.

Treatment
Ganciclovir or foscarnet (*see CMV, p334*) + IV immunoglobulin. Lack of response, switch to the other drug.

Viral—HSV/HZV

Risk group
Rare causes of lung disease. SCT recipients at greatest risk esp. MUDs and intensively treated lymphoid malignancy.

Treatment
High dose IV acyclovir 5–10mg/kg tds IV for minimum 10d.

Viral—RSV

Risk group
Post-SCT recipients esp. MUDs.

Treatment
Consider ribovarin therapy.

TB and atypical mycobacteria

Risk group
Prolonged T-cell immunosuppression e.g. chronic steroid or cyclosporin therapy, chronic GvHD, previous history and/or treatment for TB, HIV related disease.

Treatment
Often difficult to diagnose—empirical treatment required with standard triple therapy.

Prophylaxis for patients treated with purine analogues

The purine analogues fludarabine and 2-CDA used in standard lymphoproliferative protocols induce neutropenia in all cases. Nadir ~14d post-treatment initiation and neutrophil counts may fall to zero for several days or even weeks. They are therefore associated with the usual neutropenic infections. In addition, purine analogues have a particular property of inhibition of T4 helper lymphocyte subsets within weeks of initiation of therapy (nadir at 3 months) and may last for >1 year following cessation of therapy. This profound T4 function inhibition predisposes to fungal infection, as well as a higher incidence of Herpes zoster infection and PCP. ↓ lymphocyte function also predisposes to transfusion associated GvHD in passenger lymphocytes of donor blood transfusions.

The following preventive measures are recommended

Recommended

1. Irradiation of cellular blood products (2500cGy) from day 1 of initiation of therapy and continue until 2 years post-treatment.
2. PCP prophylaxis from start of therapy—usually cotrimoxazole 1 tablet bd Mondays, Wednesdays and Fridays. In patients who are already severely neutropenic, cotrimoxazole may be substituted by pentamidine nebulisers 300mg 3-weekly with 2.5mg of salbutamol nebuliser pre-treatment. PCP prophylaxis should continue until a year after the end of treatment.
3. HZV prophylaxis—acyclovir 400mg qds is the minimum continuous dose required to prevent HZV reactivation. Most physicians will not wish to have patients continuously on this dosage throughout the treatment cycle and for a year post-treatment so suggest: counsel patients about the risk of shingles and advised to contact the hospital immediately if shingles suspected. Patients who have already had a zoster reactivation should be maintained continuously on acyclovir 400mg qds and continuation of the purine analogue reviewed.

Optional

1. Anti-bacterial prophylaxis—consider use of ciprofloxacin 250mg bd PO from day 7⟶21 of each course.
2. Anti-fungal prophylaxis: Patients with no history of fungal reactivation should perform nystatin suspension 1mL qds mouthcare from day 7⟶21 of each course, taught symptoms of oral and genital thrush and supplied with fluconazole 200mg to be taken daily for 7d in the event of thrush.
3. Patients with previous history of suspected fungal infection with a mould-type organism e.g. *Aspergillus*—give itraconazole capsules 400mg daily or oral liquid 2.5mg/kg bd throughout treatment.

Protocols and procedures

Tumour lysis syndrome (TLS)

Potentially life threatening metabolic derangement resulting from treatment-induced or spontaneous tumour necrosis causing renal, cardiac or neurological complications. Usually occurs in rapidly proliferating, highly chemosensitive neoplasms with high tumour load: leukaemias with high WBC counts (ALL >50 × 10^9/L; AML >100 × 10^9/L; CML blast crisis >100 × 10^9/L; CLL >200 × 10^9/L; PLL or ATLL >100 × 10^9/L) and high grade NHL (particularly Burkitt lymphoma or high serum LDH). May occur before or up to 5 days (usually 48-72h) after initiation of chemotherapy.

Pathophysiology and clinical features

Rapid lysis of large numbers of tumour cells releases intracellular ions and metabolites into the circulation causing numerous metabolic abnormalities to develop rapidly:

- *Hyperuricaemia* due to metabolism of nucleic acid purines; (solubility decreased by high acidity); may cause arthralgia and renal colic.
- *Hyperkalaemia* due to rapid cell lysis; often earliest sign of TLS; aggravated by renal failure; may cause paraesthesiae, muscle weakness and arrhythmias.
- *Hyperphosphataemia* due to rapid cell lysis,; precipitates calcium phosphate in tissues (insolubility exacerbated by overzealous alkalinisation),
- *Hypocalcaemia* secondary to hyperphosphataemia; may cause paraesthesiae, tetany, carpo-pedal spasm, altered mental state, seizures and arrhythmias.
- *Acute renal failure* predisposed by volume depletion and pre-existing dysfunction; due to uric acid nephropathy, acute nephrocalcinosis and precipitation of xanthine; oliguria leads to volume overload and pulmonary oedema; uraemia causes malaise, lethargy, nausea, anorexia, pruritus and pericarditis; may require dialysis; usually reversible with prompt therapy.

Principles of management

1. Identify high risk patients, initiate preventative measures prior to chemotherapy and monitor for clinical and laboratory features of TLS.
2. Detect features of TLS promptly and initiate supportive therapy early.

Prevention and management

- Monitor daily weight bd, urine output, fluid balance, renal function, serum potassium, phosphate, calcium, uric acid and ECG for 72h after initiation of chemotherapy; monitor parameters at least three times daily in patients with TLS.
- Ensure aggresive intravenous hydration:
  - Aim for urine output >100mL/h (>3L/d) and total input >4Ld (3L/m^2/d) from 24–48h prior to chemotherapy and in high risk patients, until 48–72h after completion of chemotherapy.
  - Frusemide (20mg IV) may be given cautiously to maintain adequate diuresis in well hydrated patients; may be used to treat hyperkalaemia or fluid overload but may cause uric acid or calcium deposition in dehydrated patients; no proven benefit in initial treatment of TLS.
- Prevent hyperuricaemia:
  - Allopurinnol: xanthine oxidase inhibitor; 300–600mg/d PO for prophylaxis if renal function normal (100mg/d if creatine >100mmol/L) up to max 500mg/m^2/d for treatment of TLS; may be given IV if

necessary (max 600mg/d); side effects: rash, xanthine urolithiasis; reduce dose in renal impairment or mercaptopurine, 6-thioguanine or azathioprine therapy.
  - *Rasburicase*: recombinant urate oxidase; converts uric acid to water soluble metabolites without increasing excretion of xanthine and other purine metabolites; very rapidly ↓ uric acid levels and simplifies management of high risk patients; dose 200mg/kg/d IVI over 30 mins for 5–7 d; recommended in Burkitt lymphoma, high count leukaemia and as rescue treatment in hyperuricaemia plus rapidly rising creatinine, oliguria, phosphate ≥ 2mmol/L or K^+ ≥5.5mmol/L; side effects: fever, nausea, vomiting; less common: haemolysis, allergic reactions or anaphylaxis; contraindicated in G-6-PD deficiency and pregnancy.
- Alkalinisation of urine:
  - Not routine; administer $NaHCO_3$ PO (3g every 2h) or IV through central line (500mL 1.26% $NaHCO_3$ over 1h; 1L 5% dextrose over 4h; 500mL 0.9% NaCl over 1h, repeated 6 hourly) to increase urinary pH to 7.0 and maximise uric acid solubility.
  - Risk of more severe symptoms or hypocalcaemia and increased calcium phosphate precipitation in tubules.
  - Requires close monitoring of urinary pH (test all urine passed), serum bicarbonate and uric acid; withdraw IV sodium bicarbonate when serum bicarbonate >30 mmol/L, urinary pH>7.5 or serum uric acid normalised.
- Control of electrolytes
  - *Hyperkalaemia*: treat aggressively:
    1. Restrict dietary K^+ intake and eliminate K^+ from IV fluids.
    2. Use K^+-wasting diuretics with caution.
    3. Measure arterial blood gases (correction more difficult if acidosis).
    4. K^+ >5mmol/L, start calcium resonium 15g PO qds and increase hydration; recheck K^+ after 2h.
    5. K^+ >6mmol/L, check ECG; commence IVI of 50mL 50% dextrose with 20 U actrapid insulin over 1h.
    6. ECG changes or K^+ >6.5mmol/L, give 10mL calcium gluconate 10% or calcium chloride 10% IV cardioprotection.
  - *Hyperphosphataemia*:
    1. Commence oral phosphate binding agent, e.g. aluminium hydroxide 20–100mL or 4–20 capsules daily or Sevelamer 2.4–4.8g/d in divided doses; adjust dose according to serum phosphate.
    2. Infuse 50mL 50% dextrose with 20 U actrapid insulin IV over 1h.
- Dialysis
  - Seek renal and critical care consultations early if initial measures fail to control electrolyte abnormalities or renal failure.
  - Dialysis indicated if persistent hyperkalaemia (>6mmol/L) or hyperphosphataemia (>3.33mmol/L) despite treatment, fluid overload, rising urea or creatinine (>880mmol/L), hyperuricaemia (>0.6mmol/L) or symptomatic hypocalcaemia.
  - Haemodialysis achieves better phosphate and uric acid clearance than peritoneal dialysis.

Management of chronic bone marrow failure

Introduction

Common haematological problem. Occurs as result of marrow infiltrated with disease e.g. MDS, or following chemotherapy or other causes of marrow aplasia. Extent of RBC, WBC and platelet production failure varies greatly in individual clinical situations. Production failure may not affect all three cell lines equally.

Management

- Mainstay is supportive treatment with blood products and antibiotics.
- Underlying disease should be treated where possible.

Red cell production failure

- Where anaemia is due solely to absence of RBC production, transfusion requirement should be ~1 unit packed red cells/week. Suitable protocol is 3 unit transfusion every 3 weeks as day case.
- If requirement is greater, investigate for bleeding and haemolysis.
- If requirement is chronic e.g. a young patient with MDS, consider giving desferrioxamine as long-term iron chelation (*see p90*).
- Erythropoietin may be tried where some red cell production capacity remains and transfusion needs to be avoided or minimised e.g. Jehovah's Witnesses.

White cell production failure

- Mainstay of treatment is with antibiotics.
- Prompt treatment of fever in neutropenic patient with combination IV antibiotics is lifesaving.
- Simple mouthcare with Corsadyl or similar mouthwash, plus nystatin suspension orally reduces risk of bacterial and fungal colonisation in oropharynx. Dietary modifications may also be helpful.
- Role of prophylactic antibiotics remains controversial as resistance generation is an increasing problem.
- Ciprofloxacin 250mg bd PO is probably the best single agent.
- Patients with recurring foci of infection may have prophylaxis targeted to their usual or most likely organisms.
- Patients with neutropenia and low Igs who have developed bronchiectasis may benefit from regular infusions of IVIg 200mg/kg every 4 weeks ± rotating antibiotic courses.
- WBC infusions are not generally useful except in rare situations—they are toxic and cause HLA sensitisation.
- Haemopoietic growth factors should not be used routinely.
- Life-threatening infections despite IV antibiotics and anti-fungals can be considered for trial of G-CSF or GM-CSF at 5μg/kg/d SC.

Platelet production failure

Where low platelets are due solely to absence of platelet production, transfusion requirement should be ~1–2 adult dose packs/week. Tranexamic acid 1g qds PO may reduce clinical bleeding episodes and transfusion requirement. Thrombopoietin (TPO) is a potent *in vitro* platelet growth and maturation factor but its clinical role remains to be defined.

Venepuncture

Blood samples are best taken from an antecubital vein using a 21G needle and a Vacutainer™ system or syringe. If a large volume of blood is required a 21G butterfly may be inserted to facilitate changing the vacutainer sample bottle or the syringe.

A tourniquet should be gently applied to the upper arm and the antecubital fossa inspected and palpated for veins. In an obese individual antecubital veins may be more easily palpated than seen. The skin over the vein should be 'sterilised' (alcohol swab or Mediswab™) and allowed to dry. The needle should then be gently introduced along the line of the chosen vein at an angle of 45° to the skin surface. It may be helpful to attempt to penetrate the skin with the initial introduction of the needle and then slowly penetrate the vessel wall by continuing the forward movement of the needle. The tourniquet on the upper arm should be loosened once the needle has been inserted into the vein to reduce haemoconcentration. If a syringe is used the piston should be withdrawn slowly to prevent collapse of the vein. Once an adequate sample has been obtained, the tourniquet should be completely removed, a dry cotton wool ball applied gently above the site of venepuncture and gentle pressure increased as the needle is removed. Firm pressure should be directly applied to the venepuncture site for 3–5 minutes to ensure haemostasis and prevent extravasation and bruising. A small elastoplast or if allergic, suitable light dressing, should be applied to the venepuncture site.

In patients in whom it is difficult to obtain a sample, the arm should be kept warm, a sphygmomanometer cuff inflated on the upper arm to the diastolic pressure and the vein may be dilated by smacking the overlying skin. With patience it is rarely impossible to obtain a venous sample. In very obese individuals or those in whom iatrogenic thrombosis or sclerosis has occurred in the antecubital veins, the dorsal veins of the hand may be used for sampling, though a smaller gauge needle (23G) or butterfly is often necessary.

Protocols and procedures

Venesection

Aim of venesection or phlebotomy is the removal of blood for donation to the Blood Transfusion Service or as a therapeutic manoeuvre for a patient with haemochromatosis or polycythaemia rubra vera or for a patient who requires an exchange transfusion. In patients with haemochromatosis or PRV the therapeutic effect of the venesection programme to date should be assessed on a full blood count sample taken prior to venesection.

Procedure

- Patient or donor is best placed lying on a couch with the chosen arm placed comfortably on a supporting pillow.
- A large gauge needle attached to a collection pack containing anticoagulant is inserted in an antecubital vein or forearm vein after application of a sphygmomanometer cuff to the upper arm (inflated to diastolic pressure) and sterilisation of the skin. It is widespread practice to infiltrate the skin over the chosen vein with local anaesthetic (1% lidocaine (lignocaine)) prior to insertion of the large bore needle.
- Inflation of the sphygmomanometer cuff is maintained until the desired volume of blood is collected.
- The patient may assist the flow of blood by squeezing a soft ball or similar object in the hand of the arm from which the blood is drawn.
- Blood is allowed to drain into the collection pack until the desired volume has been obtained (usually 500mL).
- The volume collected may be monitored by suspension of the pack from a simple spring measuring device.
- The positioning of the collection pack below the patient's (or donor's) level facilitates blood flow into the bag.
- Once the desired volume has been collected the cuff is deflated, the line should be clamped and the needle removed and a dry cotton wool ball used to apply pressure to the venesection site.
- Direct firm pressure should be applied for 5 minutes and the site inspected for haemostasis prior to application of a firm bandage.
- The patient should slowly adopt the erect posture and should remain seated for several minutes if symptoms of lightheadedness occur.
- Patients should not be permitted to drive after venesection.
- The collected blood from a therapeutic venesection should be disposed of by incineration.

Note: for patients with PPP/PRV isovolaemic venesection is recommended to minimise volume depletion whilst still reducing Hct.

Protocols and procedures

Tunnelled central venous catheters

A tunnelled central venous catheter is required in all patients undergoing intensive cytotoxic chemotherapy and those undergoing bone marrow or peripheral blood stem cell transplantation. Also indicated for some patients on long-term regular transfusion programmes.

Catheter type

A double or triple lumen catheter preferred, and essential for patients undergoing transplantation procedures. Hickman catheters are available from Vygon UK and the Groshong lines (Bard) are available for use in all patients except those needing stem cell collections who will require apheresis catheters (Kimal).

Requirements

An x-ray screening room with facility for aseptic procedures or an operating theatre is required. A trained radiographer must be available for x-ray screening throughout the procedure. In addition a minimum of two staff are required for the safe execution of this procedure. One should be a member of medical staff (radiologist/surgeon/anaesthetist/haemato-oncologist) to insert the catheter and administer sedation and antibiotics and the other to generally assist. The second person can be an IV trained nurse.

Patient assessment

Assess for fitness for sedation and the ability to lie flat. Plan position of central venous catheter in advance. The first choice is the right subclavian vein, followed by the left subclavian vein. Check FBC and clotting screen. Platelets should be available if platelet count is less than 50×10^9/L.

Patient preparation

The patient should be well hydrated (↓ CVP makes procedure difficult), and fasting for 6h prior to the procedure as sedative drugs will be administered. Good peripheral venous access must be established (with Venflon™) before commencing central venous cannulation, for the administration of sedative drugs and prophylactic antibiotics as well as for emergency venous access.

Technique

Follow manufacturer's instructions. Sequence of stages during insertion is as follows:

1. Cannulation of the central vein, placement of guide wire and creation of the upper central wound.
2. Creation of lower peripheral wound, formation of subcutaneous tunnel and threading of the catheter through subcutaneous tunnel with cuff buried.
3. Placement of the vessel dilator/sheath in the central vein over the guide wire.
4. Placement of the catheter into the sheath.
5. Careful removal of the sheath whilst retaining position of catheter.
6. Suturing of the upper and lower wounds with suture around the body of the catheter close to the exit site to hold the catheter in position.
7. Manipulate catheter so tip lies in SVC above right atrium. Patency must be confirmed by easy aspiration of blood, and the catheter flushed with heparinised saline. Check position with standard PA chest radiograph.

Sedation and analgesia

IV sedation is used if the patient is particularly anxious before or during the procedure.

Prophylactic antibiotics

- Teicoplanin 400mg is administered by peripheral vein immediately prior to central venous cannulation.
- 400mg teicoplanin is also administered into the central venous catheter immediately after the insertion procedure (200mg is locked into each lumen for 1h and then the catheter is flushed with heparinised saline).

Catheter aftercare

- Catheter may be used immediately after above procedures. All patients should be educated in the care of their indwelling tunnelled intravenous catheter. This may include self-flushing of the catheter. Catheter should be flushed after each use with saline and locked with heparinised saline. Flush twice weekly when not in use.
- Urokinase may be used if line blockage occurs, insert urokinase and leave for 4–12h and remove.
- Clindamycin roll-on lotion may be applied to the exit site to minimise local infections.
- Upper wound suture is removed 7d post-insertion.
- Lower exit site suture can be removed at 2 weeks post-insertion for most lines and 3 weeks for apheresis lines to ensure SC embedding of the cuff.

Bone marrow examination

Bone marrow is the key investigation in haematology. It may prove ***diagostic*** in the follow-up of abnormal peripheral blood findings. It is an important ***staging*** procedure in defining the extent of disease, especially lymphoproliferative disorders. It is a helpful ***investigative*** procedure in unexplained anaemia, splenomegaly or selected cases of pyrexia of unknown origin (PUO). Preferred site for sampling→posterior iliac crest; aspirate and biopsy material can easily be obtained from this location. The anterior iliac crest is an alternative. The sternum is suitable only for marrow aspiration (*see below for contraindications*).

Marrow aspirate material provides information on

- Cytology of nucleated cells.
- Qualitative and semi-qualitative analysis of haematopoiesis.
- Assessment of iron stores.
- Smears for cytochemistry of atypical cells.

Suspensions of marrow cells in medium are suitable for

- Chromosome (cytogenetic) analysis.
- Immunophenotype studies using monoclonal antibodies directed against cell surface antigens.
- Aliquots of marrow can be cryopreserved for future molecular analysis.

Marrow trephine biopsy yields information on

- Marrow cellularity.
- Identification/classification of abnormal cellular infiltrates.
- Immunohistochemistry on infiltrates.

Note: Cytology of trephine imprints can be helpful, especially when aspirate yields a 'dry tap'. Trephine biopsy information complements that obtained at aspiration.

Contraindications

None, other than physical limitations e.g. pain or restricted mobility. Avoid sites of previous radiotherapy (inevitably grossly hypocellular and not representative).

Procedure

1. Bone marrow aspiration may be performed under local anaesthesia alone, but short acting intravenous benzodiazepines (e.g. midazolam) may be administered—with appropriate monitoring (pulse oximetry), oxygen administration and available resuscitation equipment—when trephine biopsy is performed. General anaesthesia rarely used (except in children).
2. Best position is with patient in L or R lateral position.
3. Skin and periosteum over the posterior iliac spine are infiltrated with local anaesthetic.
4. A small cutaneous incision is made, the aspirating needle is introduced through this and should penetrate the marrow cortex 3–10mm before removal of the trocar.
5. No more than 0.5–1mL marrow should be aspirated initially, and smears made promptly.

6. Further material can be aspirated and placed in EDTA or other anti-coagulant media for other studies.
7. An Islam or Jamshidi needle is preferred for trephine biopsy.
8. The needle is advanced through the same puncture site to penetrate the cortex.
9. The trocar is removed and using firm hand pressure the needle is rotated clockwise and should be advanced as far as possible.
10. The needle is removed by gentle anti-clockwise rotation. In this manner an experienced operator should regularly obtain biopsy samples of 25–35mm in length.
11. Simple pressure dressings are sufficient aftercare and minor discomfort at the location may be dealt with by simple analgesia such as paracetamol.

Administration of chemotherapy

Cytotoxic chemotherapeutic drugs may cause serious harm if not prescribed, dispensed and administered with great care. Drugs should be prescribed, dispensed and administered by an experienced multidisciplinary team with shared clear information on:

- The fitness of the patient to receive chemotherapy (e.g. recent FBC for myelosuppressive agents, renal function studies for cisplatinum).
- Appropriate protocol and chemotherapeutic regimen for the patient.
- Prescribed drugs and individualised dosage for the patient's surface area (*see p682*), taking note of cumulative maximum doses (e.g. anthracyclines).
- Appropriate supportive treatment required e.g. allopurinol, antiemetic prophylaxis, anti-infective prophylaxis, and hydration.

Chemotherapy for IV administration should be reformulated carefully in accordance with the manufacturer's instructions by an experienced pharmacist using a class B laminar airflow hood. Care should be taken to ensure that the drug is administered within the expiry time after it has been reformulated in the form chosen.

Many cytotoxic drugs are best administered as a slow IVI in dextrose or 0.9% saline over 30 minutes to 2h. *Vesicants* e.g. vincristine, daunorubicin, adriamycin and mitozantrone should be administered as a slow IV 'push'. However this should only be administered through the side access port of a freely flowing infusion of 0.9% saline or dextrose and should *never be injected directly into a peripheral vein.*

If the patient does not have an indwelling intravenous catheter (Hickman line), a Teflon or silicone intravenous cannula of adequate bore (≤21G) should be inserted into a vein of sufficient diameter to permit a freely flowing 0.9% saline infusion to be commenced. Site chosen should be one where cannula can be easily inserted and observed, can be fastened securely and will not be subject to movement during drug administration. The veins of the forearm are the most suitable for this purpose followed by those on the dorsum of the hand. Antecubital fossae and other sites close to joints are best avoided. The risk of extravasation (*see p578*) is increased by the use of a cannula which has not been inserted recently and by the use of steel (butterfly) cannulae.

A slow 'push' injection should be administered carefully into the side access port on the IV line with continuous observation of the drip chamber ensure that the infusion is continuing to run during injection of the cytotoxic drug. The patient should be asked whether any untoward sensations are being experienced at the site of the infusion and the site should be carefully observed to ensure that no extravasation is occurring. Patency of the IV site should be verified regularly throughout the procedure. The saline or dextrose infusion should be continued for 30 minutes after the chemotherapy administration has been completed before the cannula is removed.

The administration of potentially extravasable chemotherapy, site of cannulation, condition of the site and any symptoms associated with administration should be clearly documented in the patient's notes.

Antiemetics for chemotherapy

Classification of drugs

Dopamine antagonist—block D_2 receptors in the chemoreceptor trigger zone (CTZ). Examples are metoclopramide and domperidone—both have additional effect on enhancing gastric emptying. Side effects include extrapyramidal reactions and occasionally oculogyric crisis.

Phenothiazines—examples are prochlorperazine and cyclizine—particular benefit in opioid-induced nausea. Side effects include anticholinergic effects and drowsiness.

Benzodiazepine—lorazepam commonest used. Advantages are long $t^{1/2}$ and additional anxiolytic effect. Side effects include drowsiness.

$5HT_3$ antagonists—block $5HT_3$ receptors in the CTZ. Examples include ondansetron, granisetron and tropesitron. Side effects include headaches, bowel disturbance and rashes.

Cannabinoids—nabilone is the major drug. Side effects include depersonalisation experiences.

Steroids—examples are dexamethasone and predniso(lo)ne. Side effects include fungal infection predisposition, hypertension, irritability and sleeplessness, gastric erosions and, with chronic use, diabetes and osteoporosis.

Emesis with chemotherapy

Categorised as: anticipatory, early or late.

Anticipatory—occurs in advance of chemotherapy. Psychogenic in origin, it occurs in patients with previous bad experiences of nausea and vomiting and almost unknown prior to first dose. May be largely prevented by ensuring a positive experience with first dose by use of prophylactic antiemetics.

Early—occurs within minutes of IV chemotherapy administration or within hours of oral chemotherapy. The easiest to respond to antiemetics generally.

Late—occurs after the end of a chemotherapy course—up to 7d. The most difficult form to treat—requires continuation of antiemetics throughout post chemo period and even the newer agents such as the $5HT_3$ receptor antagonists are relatively ineffective.

Antiemetics may be used singly or in combination. Choices determined largely by patient preferences and degree of emetic potential of the chemo regimen to be used. These may be divided into high, medium and low.

Highly emetogenic regimens

Examples include cisplatinum, high dose cyclophosphamide and TBI. Suitable cocktail might be domperidone, $5HT_3$ antagonist and dexamethasone ± lorazepam.

Medium emetogenic regimens
Examples include anthracyclines, cytosine arabinoside. Suitable cocktail might be domperidone, cyclizine ± $5HT_3$ antagonist ± lorazepam.

Low emetogenic regimens
Examples include chlorambucil, vinca alkaloids, 6MP, fludarabine and most steroid-containing protocols. Suitable choice would be metoclopramide or domperidone as single agent.

Intrathecal chemotherapy

Usage

- Given for both prophylaxis and treatment of CNS disease.
- May be used in addition to other CNS disease strategies such as high dose IV methotrexate or cranial irradiation.
- CNS involvement is detected by presence of blasts on CSF cytospin.
- The **ONLY** cytotoxic drugs used intrathecally are:
  - Methotrexate.
  - Cytosine arabinoside (ara-C).
  - Hydrocortisone.
- All have strict upper dosage limits—***follow the protocol***.

▶▶ ***Never use any other cytotoxic drugs for intrathecal injection—fatal consequences may ensue.***

Common protocols

1. **CNS prophylaxis for ALL and high grade NHL:**
   – methotrexate $10mg/m^2$ (max 12.5mg) × 6 injections at weekly intervals.
2. **CNS prophylaxis for AML:**
   – ara-C $30mg/m^2$ (max 50mg), dosage schedule varies.
3. **CNS treatment for ALL:**
   Triple IT regimen viz:
   methotrexate $15mg/m^2$ (max 12.5–15mg).
   ara-C $30mg/m^2$ (max 50mg).
   hydrocortisone $15mg/m^2$.
   Usually given twice weekly until CSF clear of blasts then weekly to a maximum of 6 total courses. Consider using folinic acid rescue.

Technique

- Standard contraindications to lumbar puncture apply—alternatives will be needed in these situations. Cytotoxics should be made up freshly in smallest possible volume in a sterile pharmacy.
- Consider GA for children and IV sedation for adults.
- Use special LP 'blunt' needle or small gauge bevelled LP needle.
- Aim to remove the same volume of CSF as you are injecting intrathecally (may be several mL if giving triple chemotherapy).
- Take samples for CSF cytospin to determine blast cell concentration, microbiology for M/C/S, biochemistry for protein and glucose.
- Check syringe cytotoxic dose carefully with another person before connecting.
- Connect syringe and aspirate gently to confirm position in CSF. Inject slowly, drawing back at intervals to reconfirm position. Disconnect syringe and connect other syringes in turn if giving 'triple'.
- Follow standard post-LP precautions. Document procedure in notes.
- Repeated IT chemotherapy carries risk of CSF leakage and post-LP headache. Manometry pre-injection may help assess whether less CSF should be withdrawn pre-injection.
- A syndrome of methotrexate-induced neurotoxicity occurs in a few patients presenting with features of meningo-encephalitis. Aetiology is unknown. Treat with short pulse of high dose steroids.

  ▶ ***Do not give further IT methotrexate to these patients.***

Protocols and procedures

Management of extravasation

Inappropriate or accidental administration of chemotherapy into subcutaneous tissue rather than into the intravenous compartment causes pain, erythema and inflammation which may lead to sloughing of the skin and severe tissue necrosis. Appropriate early treatment can prevent the most serious consequences of extravasation. All chemotherapy units should have a protocol with which all staff administering chemotherapy are familiar and a regularly updated extravasation kit for the management of extravasation giving first aid instructions and further directions.

The risk of tissue damage relates to the drug's ability to bind to DNA, to kill replicating cells, to cause tissue or vascular dilatation and its pH, osmolarity, concentration, volume and formulation components e.g. alcohol, polyethylene glycol.

Drugs may be divided into three risk groups:

Group 1: Vesicants
Aclarubicin; amsacrine; carmustine; cisplatinum; dacarbazine; dactinomycin; daunorubicin; docetaxel; doxorubicin; epirubicin; idarubicin; mitomycin; mustine; paclitaxel; plicamycin; treosulfan; vinblastine; vincristine; vindesine.

Group 2: Irritants (may cause local inflammation, pain and necrosis)
Carboplatin; etoposide; liposomal daunorubicin; methotrexate; mitoxantrone (mitozantrone).

Group 3: Non-vesicants
Asparaginase; bleomycin; cladribine; cyclophosphamide; cytarabine; fludarabine; fluorouracil; gemcitabine; ifosfamide; melphalan; pentostatin; raltitrexed; thiotepa; aldesleukin (IL-2).

Symptoms and signs

- Burning, stinging or pain at the injection site.
- Induration, swelling, venous discolouration/erythema at injection site.
- No blood return.
- Reduced flow rate.
- Increased resistance to administration.

Pre-extravasation syndrome

- Severe phlebitis and/or local hypersensitivity.
- Local risk factors e.g. difficult cannulation and one patient symptom.
- Withdraw IV therapy immediately to prevent progression to extravasation.

Type I extravasation

- Bleb or blister with defined area of induration around site of extravasation.
- Often due to rapid IV bolus injection with excessive pressure.

Type II extravasation

- Diffuse boggy tissue injury with dispersal into the intracellular space.
- Associated with IV infusion or IV bolus into side arm port of infusion with dislodged cannula.

General treatment guidelines

- Stop the infusion, disconnect the IV line but do not remove the cannula.
- Mark the area of injury around the cannula tip.
- Seek the help of a more experienced individual if available.
- Aspirate the site of extravasation to remove as much of the offending drug as possible through cannula with a fresh 10mL syringe; this may be facilitated with SC injection of 0.9% saline.
- Remove the cannula.
- Administer 100mg hydrocortisone intravenously at another site.
- Administer a further 100mg hydrocortisone locally by 6–8 SC injections around the area of injury.
- Administer SC injections of specific antidote where available.
- Apply 1% hydrocortisone cream to the area and repeat bd whilst erythema persists.
- Cover with gauze and apply heat to disperse the drug or cool to localise the extravasation.
- Administer oral antihistamine (terfenadine 60mg/chlorpheniramine 4mg).
- Administer analgesia if required (indomethacin 25mg tds).
- Document site and extent of extravasation and treatment in case notes.
- Photograph site if possible.
- Complete a 'Green Card' to report the extravasation episode.
- Monitor injured site twice daily for erythema, induration, blistering or necrosis.
- Photograph injured site weekly until healed.

Specific procedures following extravasation

Group 1:	Vesicant drugs
All vesicants except vinca alkaloids & cisplatinum	Apply cold pack instantly. SC dexamethasone 4mg around margins. Elevate limb but encourage movement. Reapply cold pack for 24h.
Actinomycin D	Infiltrate area with 1–3mL 3% sodium thiosulphate.
Aclarubicin **Daunorubicin** **Doxorubicin** **Epirubicin** **Idarubicin** **Mitomycin**	Topical DMSO painted every 2h followed by hydrocortisone cream and 30 mins cold compression. Repeated for 24h thereafter DMSO and hydrocortisone should be alternated every 3h; if blistering occurs stop DMSO.
Cisplatinum	Infiltrate area with 1-3mL 3% sodium thiosulphate, aspirate off then administer 1500 units hyaluronidase and apply heat and compression.
Carmustine	Infiltrate area with 1–3mL sodium bicarbonate diluted to plicamycin 2.1%, avoid normal tissue at the margins, leave 2 mins then aspirate off.
Docetaxel **Paclitaxel**	Infiltrate area with 1–3mL of a mixture of 100mg hydrocortisone and 4mg chlorphenamine (chlorpheniramine) as 0.2mL pin-cushion injections, followed by 1500U of hyaluronidase then warm compression alternated with topical antihistamine cream; hydrocortisone and antihistamine creams should be applied alternately for 3d. In severe cases administer 1g sodium cromoglicate PO as soon as possible.
Chlormethine (mustine)	Infiltrate area with 1–3mL 3% sodium thiosulphate then infiltrate with 100mg hydrocortisone, apply cold compression intermittently for 12h.
Vincristine, vinblastine & vindesine	Infiltrate area with 1500 units of hyaluronidase as 0.2mL SC injections over and around the affected area; apply heat and compression for 24h then apply topical non-steroidal anti-inflammatory cream to the area qds.

Group 2: Irritant drugs

- Aspirate as much as possible.
- Administer 100mg hydrocortisone IV.
- Administer 100mg hydrocortisone SC at multiple sites around margins of extravasation.
- Apply topical hydrocortisone.
- Cover area with an ice pack.
- Manage symptoms.

Group 3: Non-vesicant drugs

- Aspirate as much as possible.
- Disperse extravasated drug with SC hyaluronidase injection around the area.
- Apply heat and compression to aid dispersal.
- Manage symptoms.

Protocols and procedures

Splenectomy

Splenectomy is an established procedure in management of selected haematological disorders. Removal of the spleen is usually required for one or more of the following reasons:

- Extreme enlargement.
- Hyperfunction.
- Autoimmune activity.
- Diagnostic and therapeutic purposes.

Indications include:

- ***Lymphoproliferative disorders***, e.g. CLL, mantle zone lymphoma, hairy cell leukaemia. Reasons include massive organomegaly, occurrence of autoimmune complications and for diagnostic and/or therapeutic purposes.
- ***Myeloproliferative disorders***—commonly used in myelofibrosis to reduce transfusion requirements, abdominal discomfort from massive splenic enlargement and may reduce constitutional symptoms e.g. weight loss and night sweats. Occasionally used in the management of chronic myeloid leukaemia.
- ***Autoimmune conditions***—an accepted treatment in autoimmune thrombocytopenic purpura and autoimmune haemolytic anaemia following the failure of immunosuppression with corticosteroids and immunoglobulin (in the case of thrombocytopenic purpura). The procedure is not curative but may result in prolonged remissions and certainly will have steroid-sparing effect.
- ***Hereditary disorders***—reduces red cell sequestration and transfusion requirements in homozygous β-thalassaemia. Recurrent, severe hereditary spherocytosis. Rare indications include pyruvate kinase deficiency and type 1 Gaucher's disease. Other circumstances where splenectomy may help include Felty's syndrome.
- ***Staging splenectomy*** is no longer a routine procedure for non-Hodgkin's lymphoma or Hodgkin's disease.

The clinician has to balance the risks and benefits of the procedure in an individual patient bearing in mind the *long-term risk of post-splenectomy sepsis* as well as immediate surgical factors. There are now established consensus guidelines for carrying out splenectomy.

Pre-operatively the need for the procedure is agreed with the patient and surgical team. At least 2 weeks pre-operatively immunisation with pneumococcal and *Haemophilus* vaccine should be given. Meningococcal vaccine may be offered but this covers sub-types A and C only and does not give long-lasting immunity. Peri-operative thromboembolic risks should be considered (e.g. standard surgical risks and those posed by the rebound thrombocytosis after splenectomy). Low dose heparin may be appropriate peri-operatively followed by low dose aspirin (may require modification in thrombocytopenia or if platelet dysfunction). Before discharge, patients must be given a leaflet/card which they carry. Life-long prophylaxis with penicillin V 250mg bd recommended or erythromycin 250mg bd if the patient is allergic to penicillin. The patient and his/her family must be advised to report urgently profound systemic symptoms, most promptly to their nearest local A&E department.

Re-vaccination with pneumococcal vaccine every 5 years recommended. Asplenic patients travelling to malarial areas must be meticulous in taking anti-malarial prophylaxis (greater risk of severe illness from *Plasmodium falciparum*).

Guidelines for the prevention and treatment of infections in patients with an absent or dysfunctional spleen. (2002) *Clinical Medicine*, **2**, 440–443

www.bcshguidelines.com/pdf/spleen12.pdf

Plasma exchange (plasmapheresis)

Plasmapheresis is the therapeutic removal of plasma from the peripheral blood usually carried out by a cell separator machine. The removed plasma is replaced isovolaemically usually by albumin/saline combinations depending on indication, plasma albumin level and frequency of exchange. Blood products may also be given as part of replacement which is useful in patients with fluid intolerance e.g. on renal dialysis. The exception to this is TTP where the replacement fluid is always FFP or cryosupernatant. ~1–1.5 × plasma volume is exchanged in each procedure, i.e. 2.5–4L for average adult. Procedure takes 2–4h depending on volume to be exchanged and the line flow rates. Procedure may need to be repeated daily until response e.g. TTP, or until a total volume exchange has been achieved e.g. 10–15L over 2 weeks (e.g. Guillain–Barré syndrome), or monthly to control hyperviscosity (e.g. Waldenström's macroglobulinaemia).

Indications—generally accepted in:

- Hyperviscosity syndromes.
- Guillain–Barré syndrome resistant to IVIg.
- Myasthenia gravis: peri-operatively for thymectomy, and refractory disease.
- Paraproteinaemic neuropathy.
- Goodpasture's syndrome.
- Thrombotic thrombocytopenia purpura.
- Post-transfusion purpura.
- Cold haemagglutinin disease.

Efficacy contentious but may be indicated in:

- Severe warm type AIHA.
- Lupus, Wegener's and other vasculitides.
- Rheumatoid arthritis.
- Peripheral neuropathies other than paraproteinaemic neuropathy.
- Multiple sclerosis.
- Chronic inflammatory demyelinating polyradiculopathy.
- Eaton–Lambert syndrome.
- Renal transplant rejection.

Venous access

If exchange is to be performed via peripheral veins, one large antecubital vein is required sufficient to tolerate cannulation by a 16G butterfly needle as the drawing line (return line need only be 18G). If not possible, make arrangements for insertion of a central line prior to the planned exchanges inserting a double lumen renal dialysis type catheter of 16G or larger. Regular medication due immediately prior to exchange may be best deferred until immediately post-exchange particularly for drugs which are predominantly protein bound (see *facing page*).

Problems with apheresis

General—patient anxiety, discomfort and boredom.

Citrate toxicity—parasthesiae, tremors, tetany.

Vascular and cardiac—poor venous access giving poor flow rates.

Extravasation, with haematoma at puncture sites, local vein thrombosis—during and after procedure, sepsis at puncture sites, hypo/hypervolaemia, vasovagal attacks, arrhythmias.

Metabolic and pharmacological—hypoalbuminaemia, hypoglycaemia, removal of drugs (plasma bound).

Allergic reactions—including anaphylaxis.

Drugs>75% bound: If drugs on the list below are due immediately prior to exchange, delay administration until after procedure.

Beta blockers
Propranolol
Timolol
Penbutolol

Ca^{2+} channel blockers
Diltiazem
Nifedipine
Verapamil

Anti-arrhythmics
Amiodarone
Propofenone
Quinidine
Digitoxin (Digoxin is OK)

Diuretics
Furosemide (frusemide)
Metolazone
Bendroflumethazide (bendrofluazide)
Diazoxide
Acetazolamide

Hypolipidaemics
Clofibrate

Gout drugs
Probenecid
Sulfinpyrazone

Analgesics
NSAIDs (all)
Aspirin
Coproxamol

Benzodiazepines
All

Antidepressants
All

Antiepileptics
Carbamazepine
Phenytoin
Sodium valproate

Antipsychotics
Chlorpromazine
Haloperidol
Thioridazine

Antifungal agents
Amphotericin B
Ketoconazole

Antihistamines
Chlorpheniramine

Antimalarials
Mepacrine
Pyrimethamine

Antibiotics
Cloxacillin
Flucloxacillin
Penicillin V
Sulphonamide
Doxycycline

Anti-TB
Rifampicin

Anticoagulants
Heparin
Warfarin

Thyroid Drugs
Thyroxine
Tri-iodothyronine
Propylthiouracil

Oestrogens and progestogens
All

Hypoglycaemics
Tolbutamide
Glipizide
Gliclazide
Glibenclamide
Chlorpropamide

Leucapheresis

Leucapheresis is the removal from the peripheral blood of white blood cells, usually leukaemic blasts, via a cell separation machine.

Procedure

Usually now a standard computer controlled programme on modern machines e.g. Cobe Spectra™ or Fenwall CS™. May be performed manually in an emergency (see *p510*).

Indications

In patients with high WBC e.g. AML, CML and with symptoms or signs of leucostasis, leucapheresis should be performed urgently. Leucostatic features are less common in lymphoid than in myeloid malignancies.

Leucostatic features

- Confusion.
- Decreased conscious level.
- Fits.
- Retinal haemorrhages.
- Papilloedema.
- Hypoxia and miliary shadowing on CXR.
- Bleeding and coronary ischaemia.

Should not be performed routinely just because of a high WBC. Leucostatic clinical features are the indication. Conversely, leucostasis may occur in some patients with AML without a very high blast count but these patients should be considered for leucapheresis.

Chemotherapy should be started as soon as possible after leucapheresis as WBC will 'rebound' quickly due to outpouring of cells from marrow. Leucapheresis may need to be repeated daily until chemotherapy has suppressed marrow.

Other indications

- Leucapheresis should be performed routinely at diagnosis of CML in patients <60 for stem cell cryopreservation which can be used in the future as a stem cell rescue procedure.
- Leucapheresis may be used as an alternative to chemotherapy in low grade haematological malignancies in pregnancy.

Protocols and procedures

Anticoagulation therapy – heparin

For acute thrombosis DVT/PE start with heparin and warfarin simultaneously. Essential to confirm diagnosis—but start treatment whilst awaiting results of investigations. When warfarin stable—stop heparin.

Heparin

Main advantage over oral anticoagulation is immediate anticoagulant effect and short $t_{1/2}$. Two main products: ***standard unfractionated heparin (UFH)***, a mixture of polysaccharide chains, mean MW 15,000, $t_{1/2}$ 1.0–1.5h, and ***low molecular weight heparin (LMWH)***, fragments of UFH (mean MW 5000) with longer $t_{1/2}$ (3–6h) and greater bioavailability. LMWH has significant advantages: one daily SC injection, no monitoring, no dose adjustment, low risk of HITT. Heparins act by potentiating coagulation inhibitor antithrombin (AT) resulting in antithrombin and anti-Xa activity. Both UFH and LMWH depend on renal clearance.

Therapeutic anticoagulation

LMWH—given SC once daily on basis of weight (*see individual products for dosage*). Usually continued for 4–7 days until warfarin effect, INR>2.0.

Standard IV UFH—initial IV bolus 5000iu in 0.9% saline given over 30 mins (lower loading dose for small adult/child). Follow with 15–25iu/kg/h using a solution of 25,000iu heparin in 50mL 0.9% saline (= 500iu/mL) and a motorised pump, e.g. for 80kg adult dose is 80 × 25 = 2000iu/h. Monitor IVI with APTT ratio, aim for ratio of 1.5–2.5, check 6h after starting treatment. Adjust dose as shown opposite.

Check APTT ratio 10h after dose change; daily thereafter. Use fresh venous sample—do not take from line. Continue heparin until INR in therapeutic range for warfarin—takes ~5 days; massive ileo-femoral thrombosis and severe PE may require 7–10 days' heparin.

Contraindications—caution if renal, hepatic impairment, recent surgery, known bleeding diathesis, severe hypertension.

Immediate complications of therapy

Bleeding occurs even when APTT ratio within the therapeutic range but risk ↑ with ↑APTT ratio. Treatment: Stop heparin until APTT ratio <2.5. In life-threatening bleeding use protamine sulphate: 1mg/100iu of heparin given in preceding hour. ***Thrombocytopenia***—Mild ↓ platelets common early in heparin therapy; not significant. Severe thrombocytopenia less common (HITT); occurs 6–10d after therapy begun; may be associated thrombosis. Stop heparin. Give alternative antithrombin drug such as lepirudin or danaparoid. Do not start warfarin until thrombocytopenia resolved.

Prophylactic anticoagulation

LMWH now used in preference to UFH. LMWH given at low dose SC once daily. Recommended dose usually greater for orthopaedic surgery than general surgery. Continue until patient discharged and mobile.

Moderate/high risk patients

LMWH given 2h pre-op and once daily (*see BNF for dosage*). UFH SC 5000iu 2h before surgery and bd until patient is mobile.

Medical patients are also at risk of VTE and should be assessed for risk and considered for LMWH prophylaxis.

Conclusions

The increased convenience and proven efficacy means that for most clinical situations LMWH will now be preferred to UFH.

Heparin infusion adjustment

APTR	>5.0	4.1–5.0	3.1–4.0	2.5–3.0	**TARGET (1.5–2.5)**	<1.2	1.5–2.5
DOSE	Stop* ↓500U/h	↓300U/h	↓100U/h	↓50U/h	**No change**	↑400U/h	↑200U/h

* Nil for 0.5–1.0h; check APTT ratio

Doses and dose adjustments (UFH) should follow local guidelines.

Weitz, J.I. (1997) Low-molecular-weight heparins. *N Engl J Med*, **337**, 688–698.

Oral anticoagulation

Warfarin is the drug of choice; few side effects, well tolerated. A vitamin K antagonist, it takes ~72h to be effective; stable state takes 5–7d. $t_{1/2}$~35h. Circulates mainly bound to albumin; free warfarin is active. Many drugs ↑ warfarin effect by displacing it from albumin. Monitored by PT using the international normalised ratio (INR).

Administration
Given daily. Usually given with heparin on day 1. If massive thrombosis, delay warfarin for 2–3d. Standard adult regimen = 10mg/d for 2d. Load with caution using reduced dose if liver disease, interacting drugs, patient >80 years. Check INR <1.4 before loading. Check INR daily for first 4 days (see Appendix II, Guidelines on oral anticoagulation: third edition, *Brit J Haematol* 1998, **101**, 374–378) on Day 3, ~16h after second dose, and adjust as follows.

Target INR usually 2.5 except for mechanical heart valves in mitral position when target is 3.0 or 3.5.

Complications
Haemorrhage. Easy bruising common within therapeutic range—is patient on aspirin? Rate of major bleeds ~2.7/100 treatment years, ↑ age ↑ INR. Rare side effects—alopecia, warfarin-induced skin necrosis, hypersensitivity, purple toe syndrome.

Management of over-anticoagulation: *See p522 for details*

Asymptomatic patient
INR >5.0—stop warfarin and reduce dose by at least 25%. Check INR within 1 week.

INR >8.0—consider oral vitamin K 1–5mg.

Symptomatic patient
Moderate bleeding, INR 5.0–8.0, give vitamin K 1mg slowly IV. INR >8.0: give vitamin K 1mg and FFP or factor concentrate. Severe bleeding: vitamin K 5mg IV, and concentrate containing factors II, VII, IX and X (e.g. beriplex). Observe in hospital. Vitamin K reverses over-anticoagulation in 24h. Look for causes of over-anticoagulation e.g. heart failure, alcohol, drugs.

Kearon, C. & Hirsh, J. (1997) Management of anticoagulation before and after elective surgery. *N Engl J Med*, **336**, 1506–1511.

Protocols and procedures

Management of needlestick injuries

Every doctor dealing with high risk patients is concerned to prevent exposure to blood and body fluids, particularly a needlestick injury. The UK DoH published guidance on post-exposure prophylaxis (PEP) for HIV in 1997 (tel 0203 9724385 for copy). Your hospital/GP surgery should have a policy for the prevention and management of contamination incidents—check this out.

Risk to health care workers

2 types of injury—***sharps injury*** where intact skin is breached by sharp object contaminated with blood/blood-stained body fluids or unfixed tissue, and ***contamination injury*** where blood/blood-stained body fluid comes into contact with mucous membranes or non-intact skin. HBV and HIV are the 2 major concerns. All health care workers should be vaccinated against HBV. Risk of contracting HIV from percutaneous exposure to HIV-infected blood is ~0.3%. The amount of blood injected and a high viral load in the patient's blood increase the risk.

General guidelines

Prevention

All health care workers must adopt universal precautions when handling blood/blood stained fluids—wear gloves, avoid blood spillage, use decontamination procedures if spillage occurs, label high risk specimens, care with needles (***do not resheath***), disposal in burn bins, etc.

Immediate action in event of exposure

- Encourage bleeding and/or wash under running water.
- Contact Occupational Health/A&E departments for help.
- Establish patient status *re* blood-borne viruses.
- Take blood from patient/test for viruses (*with consent*).
- Take blood from needlestick victim and store. Check HBV immunity/later tests if necessary.

Treatment

Decision to treat will be made by an experienced medical staff member. Treatment recommended for '*all health care workers exposed to high risk body fluids or tissues known to be, or strongly suspected to be, infected with HIV through percutaneous exposure, mucous membrane exposure or through exposure of broken skin.*' Zidovudine alone given as soon as possible ↓ risk of seroconversion by 80% but failures are well described. Prophylaxis with triple therapy now recommended. Treat for 4 wks as soon as possible with:

- Zidovudine 200mg tds/250mg bd + Lamivudine 150mg bd + Indinavir 800mg tds. A 'starter pack' should be available in an accessible place at all times.
- Known exposure to hepatitis B
  - No immunity—give HepB Ig 500mg IM; vaccinate immediately.
  - Known immunity with HepB Ab >100 IU/L in past 2 yr—no action.
  - Immunity—HepB Ab status not known—give booster dose.

Follow-up

Occupational Health Department appointment for advice *re* further management and tests. Counselling as required. 6 months after the incident a –ve test indicates infection has not occurred. Report incident to PHLS CDSC tel 0208 2006868. In Scotland to SCIEH tel 0141 9467120.

Cardo, D.M. *et al.* (1997) A case-control study of HIV seroconversion in health care workers after percutaneous exposure. Centers for Disease Control and Prevention Needlestick Surveillance Group. *N Engl J Med*, **337**, 1485–1490.

VAPEC-B

Vincristine, doxorubicin, prednisolone, etoposide, cyclophosphamide, bleomycin

Indication

Hodgkin's lymphoma stage IA or IIA only without B symptoms or bulky disease.

Schedule: 6-week chemotherapy and radiotherapy regimen given once only.

Days	Drug	Dose	Route	Comments
1–28	Prednisolone	50mg daily	PO	Take with food in morning; taper off after days 29–38; consider adding H_2 antagonist or PPI
1 & 15	Adriamycin (doxorubicin)	35mg/m^2	IV	Bolus injection via fast-running drip or IVI in 100mL 0.9% saline over 15 min
1	Cyclophosphamide	350mg/m^2	IV	IVI in 250mL 0.9% saline over 15min
15–19	Etoposide	100mg/m^2 for 5 consec. days	PT	Take 1h before food on empty stomach
8 & 22	Vincristine	1.4mg/m^2 (max 2mg)	IV	Bolus injection via fast-running drip; dilute in 20mL 0.9% saline as per national guideline
8 & 22	Bleomycin†	10,000iu/m^2	IV	IVI in 250mL 0.9% saline over 60 min
36	IF radiotherapy			

†Prescribe hydrocortisone 100mg IV before bleomycin.

Administration

- Involved field radiotherapy is given in week 6, 2 weeks after last dose of chemotherapy. The dose is 30–40Gy to the **initial** volume of the disease.
- Outpatient treatment.
- Consider sperm banking in males (low risk of infertility).

- Oral systemic PCP prophylaxis is recommended for the first 6 weeks.
- Oral systemic antifungal prophylaxis is optional.
- Antiemetic therapy for moderately emetogenic regimens on days 1 and 15.
- Delay doxorubicin, cyclophosphamide or etoposide by 1 week if platelets $<100 \times 10^9$/L or neutrophils $<1 \times 10^9$/L.
- Reduce cyclophosphamide to 75% dose if creatinine clearance 10–50mL/min, 50% dose if creatinine clearance <10mL/min.
- Reduce doxorubicin, vincristine and etoposide to 50% dose if serum bilirubin 1.7–2.5 × upper limit normal and 25% if 2.5–4 × upper limit normal. Caution with cyclophosphamide if hepatic impairment.
- **All cellular blood components should be irradiated indefinitely.**
- Total regimen 6 weeks' treatment.

ABVD

Adriamycin (doxorubicin), bleomycin, vinblastine, dacarbazine

Indication
Hodgkin's disease.

Schedule

28 day cycle		Day 1 (A)	Day 15 (B)
Doxorubicin	$25mg/m^2$ IV	X	X
Bleomycin	$10,000iu/m^2$ IV	X	X
Vinblastine	$6mg/m^2$ IV (max l0mg)	X	X
Dacarbazine	$375mg/m^2$ IVI in normal saline	X	X

Administration
- Out-patient regimen.
- Consider sperm banking in males.
- Add allopurinol 300mg/day throughout first treatment cycle.
- Antiemetic therapy for moderate emetogenic regimens.
- Consider doxorubicin dose reduction if significant liver impairment.
- Repeat treatment if WBC >3.5×10^9/L and platelet count >100×10^9/L.
- 25% dose reduction if WBC $2.5–3.5 \times 10^9$/L or platelets $75–100 \times 10^9$/L.
- Delay treatment 1 week if WBC <2.5×10^9/L or platelets <75×10^9/L.
- Treat to complete remission + 2 cycles.

Protocols and procedures

MOPP/ABVD

Chlormethine (mustine), vincristine, procarbazine, prednisolone, adriamycin (doxorubicin), bleomycin, vinblastine, dacarbazine.

Indication

Hodgkin's disease.

Schedule

8 week cycle

Chlormethine (mustine)	6mg/m^2 IV	days 1 & 8
Vincristine	1.4mg/m^2 IV (max. 2mg*)	days 1 & 8
Procarbazine	100mg/m^2 PO (max. 150mg)	days 1–14
Prednisolone	100mg/m^2 PO	days 1–14

		day 29	day 43
Doxorubicin	25mg/m^2 IV	X	X
Bleomycin	10,000 units/m^2 IV	X	X
Vinblastine	6mg/m^2 IV (max. 10mg)	X	X
Dacarbazine	375mg/m^2 IVI in N saline	X	X

•Original protocol put no maximum limit on vincristine dosage; higher doses are associated with severe neuropathy.

Administration

- Out-patient regimen.
- Consider sperm banking in males.
- Add allopurinol 300mg/d throughout first treatment cycle.
- Antiemetic therapy for highly emetogenic regimens.
- Alcohol prohibited with procarbazine; avoid monoamine oxidase inhibitors.
- Consider doxorubicin dose reduction if significant liver impairment.
- Repeat treatment if WBC >3.5 × 10^9/L and platelets >100 × 10^9/L.
- 25% dose reduction if WBC 2.5–3.5 × 10^9/L or platelets 75–100 × 10^9/L.
- Delay treatment 1 week if WBC <2.5 × 10^9/L or platelets <75 × 10^9/L.
- Treat for 12 months (6 cycles).

Protocols and procedures

CHOP

Cyclophosphamide, doxorubicin, vincristine, prednisolone.

Indications

- Intermediate and high grade non-Hodgkin's lymphoma.
- Low grade non-Hodgkin's lymphoma resistant to first-line therapy.

Schedule

21 day cycle		Day 1	2	3	4	5
Cyclophosphamide	750mg/m^2 IV	X				
Vincristine	1.4mg/m^2 IV (max. 2mg*)	X				
Doxorubicin	50mg/m^2 IV	X				
Prednisolone	50mg/m^2 (max 100mg) PO	X	X	X	X	X

*max 1mg for patients > 70 years

Administration

- Out-patient regimen.
- Consider sperm banking in males.
- Add allopurinol 300mg/d throughout first treatment cycle.
- Antiemetic therapy for moderately emetogenic regimens.
- Consider doxorubicin dose reduction if significant liver impairment.
- Repeat treatment when WBC $>3.0 \times 10^9$/L and platelets $>100 \times 10^9$/L.
- Treat to complete remission + 2 cycles (max 8 cycles).

R-CHOP

Rituximab, cyclophosphamide, doxorubicin, vincristine, prednisolone

Indication

- First line treatment of CD20+ diffuse large B cell lymphoma stage II, III or IV.

Schedule

21 day cycle	Day 1	2	3	4	5
Rituximab 375mg/m^2IV	X				
Cyclophosophamide 750mg/m^2IV	X				
Vincristine 1.4mg/m^2IV (max 2mg*)	X				
Doxorubicin 50mg/m^2IV	X				
Prednisolone 50mg/m^2 PO (max 100mg)	X	X	X	X	X

*max 1mg for patients>70 years.

Administration

- Outpatient regimen.
- Consider sperm banking in males.
- Add allopurinol 300mg/d throughout first treatment cycle.
- Antiemetic therapy for moderately emetogenic regimen.
- Administer rituximab *after* first dose of prednisolone on day 1 before administering chemotherapy.
- Premedication with paracetamol and chlorpheniramine should be administered before each rituximab infusion.
- Monitor closely for cytokine release syndrome: fever, chills, rigors within first 2 hours usually.
- Less common side effects include: flushing, angioedema, nausea, urticaria/rash, fatigue, headache, throat irritation, rhinitis, vomiting, tumour pain and features of tumour lysis syndrome, bronchospasm, hypotension.
- Interrupt rituximab infusion if severe dyspnoea, bronchospasm or hypoxia.
- Consider doxorubicin dose reduction if significant liver impairment.
- Repeat treatment when WBC>3.0 X 10^9 L and platelets >100 X 10^9/L.
- Treat to complete remission + 2 cycles, max 8 cycles.

DHAP

Dexamethasone, cytarabine, cisplatin

Indication
- Salvage chemotherapy for relapsed/refractory NHL and Hodgkin's lymphoma.
- Mobilisation of peripheral blood stem cells.

Schedule: 21–28 day cycle depending on count recovery

Days	Drug	Dose	Route	Comments
1–4	Dexamethasone	40mg	PO	Taken in the morning with food
1	Cisplatin	†100mg/m^2	IV	IVI in 500mL 0.9% saline over 1h
2	Cytarabine	†2g/m^2 X 2	IV	IVI in 1L 0.9% saline over 3h **twice** 12h apart

†cap surface area at 2m^2

Administration
- In-patient regimen.
- Ensure adequate venous access by inserting a dual lumen tunnelled central venous catheter.
- Severe myelosuppression (neutrophils <0.2 × 10^9/L and need for red cell and platelet transfusion support) should be expected.
- Allopurinol 300mg od PO (100mg if renal impairment) for first 2 cycles.
- Consider acyclovir prophylaxis if previous history of VZV or HSV reactivation.
- Antiemetic therapy for highly emetogenic regimens.
- Aggressive pre- and post-hydration including potassium/magnesium supplementation is required with cisplatin.
- Predsol 0.5% eye-drops qds until 5 days after completion of chemotherapy.
- Standard antimicrobial prophylaxis as dictated by local policy to cover duration of severe neutropenia.
- G-CSF 5–10mg/kg SC daily starting day +5 optional to shorten neutropenia and necessary to mobilise peripheral blood stem cells.
- Reduce cisplatin to 75% dose if creatinine clearance 45–60mL/min, 50% dose if creatinine clearance 30–45mL/min; do not give if creatinine clearance <30mL/min.
- Creatinine clearance should be assessed before each course of treatment.
- Cytarabine should be used with caution in severe renal impairment; consider reducing dose of cytarabine if hepatic impairment.
- Delay next cycle for 1 week if neutrophils <1.0 × 10^9/L or platelets <100 × 10^9/L.

- **Patients with Hodgkin's lymphoma and those in whom stem cell collection is planned within 2 weeks must receive irradiated cellular blood components to prevent transfusion associated graft versus host disease.**
- 2–6 cycles in total but usually consolidated with high dose therapy and autologous stem cell transplant in responding patients <65 years of age.

ESHAP

Etoposide, methylprednisolone, cytarabine, platinium

Indications

- Treatment of refractory/relapsed NHL and Hodgkin's lymphoma.
- Mobilisation of peripheral blood stem cells for NHL and Hodgkin's lymphoma.

Schedule: 21–28 day cycle as soon as neutrophils >1.0 × 10^9/L and platelets (unsupported) >100 × 10^9/L

Days	Drug	Dose	Route	Comments
1	Cytarabine	2g/m^2	IV	IVI in 500mL 0.9% saline over 2h
1–4	Etoposide	40–60mg/m^2	IV	IVI in 250mL 0.9% saline over 60 min
1–4	Cisplatin	25mg/m2	IV	IVI in 1L 0.9% saline over 24h
1–5	Methylpred.	500mg	IV	IVI in 100mL 0.9% saline over 30 min

Administration

- In-patient regimen.
- Ensure adequate venous access by inserting a dual lumen tunnelled central venous catheter.
- Severe myelosuppression (neutrophils <0.1 × 10^9/L and platelets <20 × 10^9/L) is expected.
- Add allopurinol 300mg (100mg if creatinine clearance <20mL/min) od for first 2 weeks.
- Antiemetic therapy for highly emetogenic regimens.
- Aggressive pre- and post-hydration including potassium/magnesium supplementation required with cisplatin.
- Predsol 0.5% eye-drops qds until 5 days after completion of chemotherapy.
- Give mouth care (nystatin and chlorhexidine M/W) and oral systemic antibacterial and antifungal prophylaxis until neutrophil recovery ≥ 1.0 × 10^9/L.
- Consider H_2 antagonist or PPI.
- Consider starting G-CSF 5mg/kg/day on day 7 either to shorten neutropenia or to facilitate peripheral blood stem cell collection around day 16.
- Reduce cisplatin to 50% dose if creatinine clearance 40–60mL/min; do not give if creatinine clearance <40mL/min.
- Reduce cytarabine to 50% dose and omit etoposide if serum bilirubin >50μmol/L.
- Creatinine clearance should be assessed before each course of treatment.

- **Patients with Hodgkin's lymphoma and those in whom stem cell collection is planned within 2 weeks must receive irradiated cellular blood components to prevent transfusion associated graft versus host disease.**
- 2-6 cycles in total but usually consolidated with high dose therapy and autologous stem cell transplant in responding patients <65 years of age.

Mini-BEAM

BCNU (carmustine), etoposide, cytarabine, melphalan

Indications

- Treatment of refractory/relapsed NHL and Hodgkin's lymphoma.
- To demonstrate persistent chemosensitivity of tumour.
- Mobilisation of peripheral blood stem cells.

Schedule

Days	Drug	Dose	Route	Comments
1	Carmustine	60mg/m^2	IV	IVI in 250mL 5% dextrose over 1h; avoid storage in PVC container for >24h
2–5	Cytarabine	100mg/m^2 **bd**	IV	IVI in 100mL 0.9% saline over 30 min
2–5	Etoposide	75mg/m^2	IV	IVI in 500mL 0.9% saline over 1h
6	Melphalan†‡	30mg/m2	IV	IVI in 100mL 0.9% saline within 30 min reconstitution

† Ensure adequate diuresis before administering melphalan.

‡ Ensure that melphalan is administered on a week day (Mondays or Tuesdays provide optimal timing for stem cell collection).

Administration

- In-patient regimen.
- Ensure adequate venous access by inserting a dual lumen tunnelled central venous catheter.
- Severe myelosuppression (neutrophils <0.1 × 10^9/L and platelets <20 × 10^9/L) is expected.
- Add allopurinol 300mg (100mg if creatinine clearance <20mL/min) od for first 2 weeks.
- Antiemetic therapy for moderately emetogenic regimens
- Give mouth care (nystatin and chlorhexidine M/W) and oral systemic antibacterial and antifungal prophylaxis until neutrophil recovery ≥1.0 × 10^9/L.
- Consider H_2 antagonist or PPI.
- Consider starting G-CSF 5mg/kg/d on day 9 either to shorten neutropenia or to facilitate peripheral blood stem cell collection around day 18.
- ***Note***: do not use mini-BEAM if creatinine clearance ≤40mL/min.
- **Patients with Hodgkin's lymphoma and those in whom stem cell collection is planned within 2 weeks must receive irradiated cellular blood components to prevent transfusion associated graft versus host disease.**

- A second course can be given when neutrophils >1.0 × 10^9/L and platelets (unsupported) >100 × 10^9/L; generally 4–6 weeks.
- Consolidate with high dose therapy and in responding patients autologous stem cell transplant.

BEAM (myeloablative conditioning regimen)

BCNU (carmustine), etoposide, cytarabine, melphalan

Indications

High dose chemotherapy consolidation for patients with:

- Aggressive NHL: chemosensitive relapse or poor prognostic disease.
- Hodgkin's lymphoma: refractory or second remission.
- Indolent NHL refractory to second-line therapy.

Schedule

Days	Drug	Dose	Route	Comments
–7	Carmustine	300mg/m^2	IV	IVI in 500mL 5% dextrose over 1h; avoid storage in PVC container for >24h
–6 to –3 (*inclusive*)	Cytarabine	200mg/m^2 **bd**	IV	IVI in 100mL 0.9% saline over 30 min
–6 to –3 (*inclusive*)	Etoposide	200mg/m^2	IV	IVI in 1L 0.9% saline over 2h
–2	Melphalan†	140mg/m^2	IV	IVI in 250mL 0.9% saline within 60min of reconstitution
0	**Thaw and reinfuse haematopoietic stem cells‡**			

†Ensure excretion of melphalan by aggressive hydration (± furosemide (frusemide)).

‡Ensure stem cell dose ≥ 2.0 × 10^6/L CD34+ cells; do not re-infuse stem cells within 24h of melphalan infusion.

Administration

- In-patient regimen.
- Ensure adequate venous access by inserting a dual lumen tunnelled central venous catheter.
- Severe myelosuppression (neutrophils <0.1 × 10^9/L and platelets <20 × 10^9/L) is expected.
- Add allopurinol 300mg (100mg if creatinine clearance <20mL/min) od for first week.
- Antiemetic therapy for highly emetogenic regimens.
- Give mouth care (nystatin and chlorhexidine M/W) and oral systemic antibacterial and antifungal prophylaxis until neutrophil recovery ≥ 1.0 × 10^9/L—refer to local protocol for patients with severe neutropenia.
- Consider H_2 antagonist or PPI
- Consider starting G-CSF 5mg/kg/day on day +5 to shorten the duration of neutropenia.
- Consider acyclovir antiviral prophylaxis if previous history of VZV or HSV reactivation.

- Consider oral systemic PCP prophylaxis for 6 months after count recovery—refer to local protocol.
- Do not use BEAM if creatinine clearance is <40mL/min
- **All patients must receive irradiated cellular blood components for *at least* 12 months post-SCT to prevent transfusion associated graft versus host disease.**

CVP

Cyclophosphamide, vincristine, prednisolone.

Indications
- Low grade non-Hodgkin's lymphoma.
- Advanced chronic lymphocytic leukaemia.

Schedule

21 day cycle		Day 1	2	3	4	5
Cyclophosphamide	750mg/m² IV	X				
Vincristine	1.4mg/m² IV (max. 2mg)*	X				
Prednisolone	60mg/m² (max 100mg) m² PO	X	X	X	X	X

*max 1mg in patients > 70.

Administration
- Out-patient regimen.
- Consider sperm banking in males.
- Add allopurinol 300mg/d throughout first treatment cycle.
- Antiemetic therapy for moderately emetogenic regimens.
- Consider doxorubicin dose reduction if significant liver impairment.
- Repeat treatment when WBC $>3.0 \times 10^9$/L and platelets $>100 \times 10^9$/L.
- Treat to complete remission + 2 cycles.

Protocols and procedures

Fludarabine and cyclophosphamide

Indications

- Third line therapy for CLL.
- Mantle cell lymphoma.

Schedule: 28 day cycle

Days	Drug	Dose	Route	Comments
1–3	Cyclophosphamide	250mg/m^2	IV	IV bolus in 50mL 0.9% saline immediately prior to fludarabine
1–3	Fludarabine	25mg/m^2	IV	IV bolus in 10mL 0.9% saline

Alternative oral schedule

Days	Drug	Dose	Route	Comments
1–5	Cyclophosphamide	150mg/m^{2†}	PO	
1–5	Fludarabine	24mg/m^{2†}	PO	

†Appropriate rounding to the next available tablet size.

Administration

- Out-patient regimen.
- Check direct antiglobulin test (DAGT) pre-treatment; **+ve DAGT is a relative contraindication to fludarabine therapy**.
- Allopurinol 300mg od PO (100mg if significant renal impairment) for first 2 cycles.
- Oral systemic PCP prophylaxis according to local protocol (generally 480mg bd tiw) throughout treatment and for 8 weeks after completion.
- Consider acyclovir prophylaxis if previous history of VZV or HSV reactivation.
- Antiemetic therapy for moderately emetogenic regimens.
- Reduce to 50% doses if renal impairment (creatinine clearance 30–60mL/min); do not give if creatinine clearance <30mL/min.
- Delay next cycle for 1 week if neutrophils $<1 \times 10^9$/L or platelets $<75 \times 10^9$/L.
- **All cellular blood components should be irradiated for 1 year after therapy to prevent transfusion associated graft versus host disease.**
- Administer 6 cycles.

Protocols and procedures

FMD

Fludarabine, mitoxantrone (mitozantrone), dexamethasone

Indications

- Follicular and other indolent NHL.(beyond second line)
- Waldenström's macroglobulinaemia. (beyond second line)
- Chronic lymphocytic leukaemia. (beyond second line)

Schedule: 28 day cycle

Days	Drug	Dose	Route	Comments
1–3	Fludarabine	$25mg/m^2$	IV	IV bolus in 10mL 0.9% NaCl
		or $40mg/m^2$	PO	
1	Mitoxantrone (mitozantrone)	$10mg/m^2$	IV	Bolus in fast-running drip or infusion in 100mL 0.9% saline over 15 min
1–5	Dexamethasone	20mg	PO/IV	

Administration

- Out-patient regimen.
- Check direct antiglobulin test (DAGT) pre-treatment and after each cycle; **positive DAGT is a relative contraindication to fludarabine therapy**.
- Allopurinol 300mg od PO (100mg if significant renal impairment) for first 2 cycles.
- Oral systemic PCP prophylaxis according to local protocol (generally 480mg bd tiw) throughout treatment and for 8 weeks after completion.
- Consider acyclovir prophylaxis if previous history of VZV or HSV reactivation.
- Antiemetic therapy for moderately emetogenic regimens.
- Consider H_2 antagonist or PPI.
- Reduce fludarabine to 50% dose if renal impairment (creatinine clearance 30–60mL/min); do not give if creatinine clearance <30mL/min.
- Reduce mitoxantrone (mitozantrone) to 50% dose if serum bilirubin >1.5 × upper limit normal and 25% if >3 × upper limit normal.
- Delay next cycle for 1 week if neutrophils $<1.5 \times 10^9$/L or platelets $<100 \times 10^9$/L.
- **All cellular blood components should be irradiated for 1 year after therapy to prevent transfusion associated graft versus host disease.**
- Repeat to maximum clinical response; usually 6 cycles.

Protocols and procedures

ABCM

Adriamycin (doxorubicin), BCNU (carmustine), cyclophosphamide, melphalan

Indication

Multiple myeloma.

Schedule

6 week cycle		**Day 1**	**22**
Doxorubicin	30mg/m^2 IV	X	
Carmustine	30mg/m^2 IV	X	
Cyclophosphamide	100mg/m^2 PO X 4 days		X
Melphalan	6mg/m^2 PO X 4 days		X

Administration

- Out-patient regimen.
- Consider sperm banking in males.
- Add allopurinol 300mg/day throughout first treatment cycle.
- Add infection prophylaxis with cotrimoxazole 2 tabs tiw and nystatin mouthwash/fluconazole 100mg/day.
- Antiemetic therapy for moderately emetogenic regimens.
- Repeat treatment when WBC >3.0 × 10^9/L and platelets >100 × 10^9/L.
- Treat to plateau phase (normally 4–8 courses).

Protocols and procedures

C-VAMP

Cyclophosphamide, vincristine, adriamycin (doxorubicin), methylprednisolone

Indications

- Multiple myeloma. Suitable for intensive therapy or resistant to alkylator therapy.

Schedule

21 day cycle		Day 1	2	3	4	5	8	15
Vincristine	0.4mg/day cont. IVI	X	X	X	X			
Doxorubicin	9mg/m^2/day cont. IVI	X	X	X	X			
Methylprednisolone	1.5g IV/PO	X	X	X	X	X		
Cyclophosphamide	500mg IV	X					X	X

Administration

- Out-patient regimen.
- Indwelling central venous catheter required with ambulatory infusion pump.
- Consider sperm banking in males.
- Add allopurinol 300mg/day throughout first treatment cycle.
- Add infection prophylaxis with cotrimoxazole 2 tabs tiw and nystatin mouthwash/fluconazole 100mg/day.
- Antiemetic therapy for mildly emetogenic regimens.
- Repeat treatment when WBC >2.0 × 10^9/L and platelets >100 × 10^9/L.
- Treat until maximum paraprotein and bone marrow response (normally 4–8 courses).

Protocols and procedures

VAD

Vincristine, adriamycin (doxorubicin), dexamethasone

Indication

- Multiple myeloma. Suitable for intensive therapy or resistant to alkylator therapy.

Schedule

21 day cycle		Day 1	2	3	4
Vincristine (continuous IVI)	0.4mg/day	X	X	X	X
Doxorubicin (continuous IVI)	9mg/m^2/day	X	X	X	X
Dexamethasone	40mg/day PO	X	X	X	X

(repeated days 9–12 and days 17–20 on first cycle only)

Administration

- Out-patient regimen.
- Indwelling central venous catheter required with ambulatory infusion pump.
- Consider sperm banking in males.
- Add allopurinol 300mg/day throughout first treatment cycle.
- Add infection prophylaxis with cotrimoxazole 2 tabs tiw and nystatin mouthwash/fluconazole 100mg/day.
- Antiemetic therapy for mildly emetogenic regimens.
- Repeat treatment when WBC >2.0 × 10^9/L and platelets >100× 10^9/L.
- Treat until maximum paraprotein and bone marrow response (normally 4–6 courses).

CVAD used in MRC/UKMF Study 'Myeloma IX' adds cyclophosphamide 500mg PO (or IV if preferred) on days 1, 8 and 15 of each cycle. Omit cyclophosphamide in patients with a serum creatinine >300μmol/L.

Protocols and procedures

Z-DEX

Idarubicin (zavedos), dexamethasone

Indications

Multiple myeloma suitable for intensive therapy or resistant to alkylator therapy.

Schedule: 21 day cycle

Days	Drug	Dose	Route	Comments
1–4	Idarubicin	Total dose 40mg/m^2 in divided doses over 4 days	PO	
1–4*	Dex.	40mg daily	PO	Take in the mornings; swallow whole with food

*Dexamethasone (Dex.) also on days 8–11 and days 15–18 for the first cycle only

Administration

- Out-patient regimen.
- Add allopurinol 300mg od PO (100mg if significant renal impairment) for first cycle.
- Antiemetic therapy for moderately emetogenic regimens.
- Commence H_2 antagonist or PPI.
- Nystatin and chlorhexidine mouthcare.
- Oral systemic PCP prophylaxis is recommended until 2 weeks after the end of treatment.
- Consider oral systemic antibacterial, antiviral and/or antifungal prophylaxis if patient is neutropenic.
- Reduce dose of idarubicin by 50% if bilirubin 20–50μmol/L; caution if bilirubin is >50μmol/L. Maximum cumulative dose = 400mg/m^2.
- Delay treatment for 1 week if neutrophils $<1.0 \times 10^9$/L or platelets $<50 \times 10^9$/L. Reintroduce at 300mg or 400mg per dose.
- Consider G-CSF if treatment delays are prolonged or frequent.
- Continue to maximal response, usually 4–6 cycles.

Protocols and procedures

C-Thal-Dex (CTD)

cyclophosphamide, thalidomide, dexamethasone

Indications

- Multiple myeloma: melphalan-resistant disease; myeloma-IX randomisation
- Waldenström's macroglobulinaemia.

Schedule: 21 day schedule

Days	Drug	Dose	Route	Comments
1,8,15	Cyclophos.	500mg	PO	
1–21	Thalidomide	100mg for 3 weeks then 200mg	PO	Pregnancy testing as below
1–4 & 12–15	Dexamethasone	40mg/day	PO	

Administration

- Out-patient regimen.
- **Women of childbearing potential must have negative pregnancy test within 24h before starting thalidomide, every 2–4 weeks while on thalidomide and 4 weeks after last dose**.
- Add allopurinol 300mg od PO (100mg if significant renal impairment) for first cycle.
- Antiemetic therapy for mildly emetogenic regimens.
- Commence H_2 antagonist or PPI.
- Consider regular laxative.
- Do not give cyclophosphamide if serum creatinine >300μmol/L after rehydration.
- Omit cyclophosphamide for 3 weeks if neutrophils $<1.0 \times 10^9$/L or platelets $<100 \times 10^9$/L. Reintroduce at 300mg or 400mg per dose.
- Consider G-CSF if treatment delays are prolonged or frequent
- Omit thalidomide for one cycle if grade 3/4 constipation, neuropathy, fatigue, sedation, rash, tremor or oedema; reintroduce at 50mg/day.
- Treat with full dose warfarin or LMW heparin if thromboembolic event. Stop thalidomide and restart at 50mg/day escalating on the subsequent cycle to 100mg/day.
- Repeat for 4–6 cycles

Protocols and procedures

Haematological investigations 16

Full blood count

Rapid analysis by the latest generation automated blood counters using either forward angle light scatter or impedance analysis provides enumeration of leucocytes, erythrocytes and platelets and quantification of haemoglobin, MCV plus derived values for haematocrit, MCH and MCHC, red cell distribution width (a measure of cell size scatter), mean platelet volume and platelet distribution width and a 5 parameter differential leucocyte count. The counter also flags samples which require direct morphological assessment by examination of a blood film.

Sample: peripheral blood EDTA; the sample should be analysed in the laboratory within 4h.

Blood film

Morphological assessment of red cells, leucocytes and platelets should be performed by an experienced individual of all samples in which the FBC has revealed any result significantly outside the normal range, samples in which a flag has been indicated by the automated counter and if clinically indicated. A manual differential leucocyte count may be performed and may differ from that produced by the automated counter most notably in patients with haematological disease affecting the leucocytes.

Sample: peripheral blood EDTA; the sample should be analysed in the laboratory within 4h. May be made directly from drop of blood or EDTA sample, air-dried and fixed.

Plasma viscosity

This test is a sensitive but non-specific index of plasma protein changes which result from inflammation or tissue damage. The plasma viscosity is unchanged by haematocrit variations and delay in analysis up to 24h and is therefore more reliable than the ESR. It is not affected by sex but is affected by age, exercise and pregnancy.

Sample: peripheral blood EDTA; the sample should be analysed in the laboratory within 24h.

ESR

This test is a sensitive but non-specific index of plasma protein changes which result from inflammation or tissue damage. The ESR is affected by haematocrit variations, red cell abnormalities (e.g. poikilocytosis, sickle cells) and delay in analysis and is therefore less reliable than measurement of the plasma viscosity. The ESR is affected by age, sex, menstrual cycle, pregnancy and drugs (e.g. OCP, steroids).

Sample: peripheral blood EDTA; the sample should be analysed in the laboratory within 4h.

Haematinic assays

Measurement of the serum B_{12} and red cell folate are necessary in the investigation of macrocytic anaemia, and serum ferritin in the investigation of microcytic anaemia in order to assess body stores of the relevant haematinic(s). *Serum* folate levels are an unreliable measurement of body stores of folate. The serum ferritin may be elevated as an acute phase protein in patients with underlying neoplasia or inflammatory disease (e.g. rheumatoid arthritis) and may give an erroneously normal level in an iron deficient patient.

Sample: clotted blood sample and peripheral blood EDTA.

Haemoglobin electrophoresis

This test is performed in the diagnosis of abnormal haemoglobin production (haemoglobinopathies or thalassaemia). It is usually performed on cellulose acetate at alkaline pH (8.9) but may be performed on citrate agar gel at acid pH (6.0) to detect certain haemoglobins more clearly. Haemoglobin electrophoresis has been largely replaced by HPLC analysis.

Sample: peripheral blood EDTA.

Haptoglobin

The serum haptoglobin should be measured in patients with suspected intravascular haemolysis and is frequently reduced in patients with extravascular haemolysis. It should generally be accompanied by estimation of the serum methaemalbumin, free plasma haemoglobin and urinary haemosiderin.

Sample: clotted blood.

Schumm's test

This spectrophotometric test for methaemalbumin (which has a distinctive absorption band at 558nm) should be measured in patients with suspected intravascular haemolysis and may be abnormal in patients with significant extravascular (generally splenic) haemolysis. It should generally be accompanied by estimation of the serum haptoglobin level, free plasma haemoglobin and urinary haemosiderin.

Sample: heparinised blood or clotted blood.

Kleihauer test

The Kleihauer test which exploits the resistance of fetal red cells to acid elution should be performed on all Rh(D) negative women who deliver a

Rh(D) positive infant. Fetal cells appear as darkly staining cells against a background of ghosts. An estimate of the required dose of anti-D can be made from the number of fetal cells in a low power field.

Sample: maternal peripheral blood EDTA.

Reticulocytes

Definition

- Immature RBCs formed in marrow and found in normal peripheral blood.
- Represent an intermediate maturation stage in marrow between the nucleated red cell and the mature red cell.
- No nucleus but retain some nucleic acid.

Detection and measurement

- Demonstrated by staining with supravital dye for the nucleic acid.
- Appear on blood film as larger than mature RBCs with fine lacy blue staining strands or dots.
- Some modern automated blood counters using laser technology can measure levels of reticulocytes directly.
- Usually expressed as a % of total red cells e.g. 5%, though absolute numbers can be derived from this and total red cell count.

Causes of ↑ reticulocyte counts

Marrow stimulation due to

- Bleeding.
- Haemolysis.
- Response to oral Fe therapy.
- Infection.
- Inflammation.
- Polycythaemia (any cause).
- Myeloproliferative disorders.
- Marrow recovery following chemotherapy or radiotherapy.
- Erythropoietin administration.

Causes of ↓ reticulocyte counts

Marrow infiltration due to

- Leukaemia.
- Myeloma.
- Lymphoma.
- Other malignancy.

Marrow underactivity (hypoplasia) due to

- Fe, folate or B_{12} deficiency. *Note:* return of reticulocytes is earliest sign of response to replacement therapy.
- Immediately post-chemotherapy or radiotherapy.
- Autoimmune disease especially rheumatoid arthritis.
- Malnutrition.
- Uraemia.
- Drugs.

- Aplastic anaemia (see p122).
- Red cell aplasia (see p126).

Urinary haemosiderin

Usage
The most widely used and reliable test for detection of chronic intravascular haemolysis.

Principle
Free Hb is released into the plasma during intravascular haemolysis. The haemoglobin binding proteins become saturated resulting in passage of haem-containing compounds into the urinary tract of which haemosiderin is the most readily detectable.

Method
1. A clean catch sample of urine is obtained from the patient.
2. Sample is spun down in a cytocentrifuge to obtain a cytospin preparation of urothelial cells.
3. Staining and rinsing with Perl's reagent (Prussian blue) is performed on the glass slides.
4. Examine under oil-immersion lens of microscope.
5. Haemosiderin stains as blue dots within urothelial cells.
6. Ignore all excess stain, staining outside cells or in debris all of which are common.
7. True positive is only when clear detection within urothelial squames is seen.

Cautions
An iron-staining +ve control sample should be run alongside test case to ensure stain has worked satisfactorily. Haemosiderinuria may not be detected for up to 72 hours after the initial onset of intravascular haemolysis so the test may miss haemolysis of very recent onset – repeat test in 3–7 days if –ve. Conversely, haemosiderinuria may persist for some time after a haemolytic process has stopped. Repeat in 7 days should confirm.

Causes of haemosiderinuria

Common causes	Red cell enzymopathies e.g. G6PD and PK deficiency but only during haemolytic episodes *Mycoplasma* pneumonia with anti-I cold haemagglutinin Sepsis Malaria Cold haemagglutinin disease TTP/HUS Severe extravascular haemolysis (may cause intravascular haemolysis)

Rarer causes	PNH Prosthetic heart valves Red cell incompatible transfusion reactions Unstable haemoglobins March haemoglobinuria

Ham's test

Usage

Diagnostic test for paroxysmal nocturnal haemoglobinuria (PNH). Now replaced by immunophenotyping methods.

Principle

- Abnormal sensitivity of RBCs from patients with PNH to the haemolytic action of complement.
- Complement is activated by acidification of patient's serum to pH of 6.2 which induces lysis of PNH red cells but not normal controls.

Specificity: high—similar reaction is produced only in the rare syndrome HEMPAS (a form of congenital dyserythropoietic anaemia type II) which should be easily distinguished morphologically.

Sensitivity: low—as the reaction is crucially dependent on the concentration of magnesium in the serum.

It appears to be a technically difficult test in most laboratories. Patients with only a low % of PNH cells may be missed at an early stage of the disease. Markedly abnormal PNH cells are usually picked up in ~75% of patients. Less abnormal cells are detected in only ~25% of patients.

Alternative tests

- Sucrose lysis—an alternative method of complement activation is by mixing serum with a low ionic strength solution such as sucrose. **Sensitivity** of this test is high but **specificity** is low—i.e. the opposite of the Ham's test.
- Immunophenotypic detection of the deficiency of the PIG transmembrane protein anchors in PNH cells is becoming a more widely used alternative *cf.* PNH section p124. Monoclonal antibodies to CD59 or CD55 (DAF) are used in flow cytometric analysis. Major advantage is that test can be performed on neutrophils and platelets in PB which are more numerous than the PNH red cells.

Immunophenotyping

Definition

Identification of cell surface proteins by reactivity with monoclonal antibodies of known specificity.

Uses

- Aids diagnosis and classification of haematological malignancy.

- Assess cellular clonality.
- Identify prognostic groups.
- Monitor minimal residual disease (MRD).

Terminology and methodology

Cell surface proteins are denoted according to their cluster differentiation (CD) number. These are allocated after international workshops define individual cell surface proteins by reactivity to monoclonal antibodies. Most cells will express many such proteins and pattern of expression allows cellular characterisation.

Monoclonal antibodies (MoAbs) are derived from single B-lymphocyte cell lines and have identical antigen binding domains known as ***idiotypes***. It is easy to generate large quantities of MoAbs for diagnostic use.

- Cell populations from e.g. PB or BM samples are incubated with a panel of MoAbs e.g. anti-CD4, anti-CD34 which are directly or indirectly bound to a fluorescent marker antibody e.g. FITC.
- Sample is passed through a fluorescence-activated cell sorter (FACS) machine.
- FACS instruments assign cells to a graphical plot by virtue of cell size and granularity detected as forward and side light scatter by the laser.
- Allows subpopulations of cells e.g. mononuclear cells in blood sample to be selected.
- The reactivity of this cell subpopulation to the MoAb panel can then be determined by fluorescence for each MoAb.
- A typical result for a CD4 T-lymphocyte population is shown: CD3, CD4 +ve; CD8, CD13, CD34, CD19 –ve.

Common diagnostic profiles

AML	CD13+, CD33+, ± CD 34, ± CD14 +ve.
cALL	CD10 and TdT +ve.
T-ALL	CD3, CD7, TdT +ve.
B-ALL	CD10, CD19, surface Ig +ve.
CLL	CD5, CD19, CD23, weak surface Ig +ve.

Clonality assessment

Particularly useful in determining whether there is a monoclonal B cell or plasma cell population.

▶ Monoclonal B cells from e.g. NHL will have surface expression of κ or λ light chains ***but not both***.

▶ Polyclonal B cells from e.g. patient with infectious mononucleosis will have both κ ***and*** λ expression.

Cytogenetics

Acquired somatic chromosomal abnormalities are common in haematological malignancies. Determination of patterns of cytogenetic abnormalities is known as ***karyotyping***.

Uses

- Aid diagnosis and classification of haematological malignancy.
- Assess clonality.
- Identify prognostic groups.
- Monitor minimal residual disease (MRD).
- Determine engraftment and chimerism post-allogeneic transplant.

Terminology

- Normal somatic cell has 46 chromosomes; 22 pairs and XX or XY.
- Numbered 1–22 in decreasing size order.
- 2 arms meet at centromere—short arm denoted **p**, long arm denoted **q**.
- Usually only visible during condensation at metaphase.
- Stimulants and cell culture used—colchicine to arrest cells in metaphase.
- Stained to identify regions and bands e.g. p1, q3.

Common abnormalities

- Whole chromosome gain e.g. trisomy 8 (+8).
- Whole chromosome loss e.g. monosomy 7 (–7).
- Partial gain e.g. 9q+ or partial loss e.g. 5q– .
- Translocation—material repositioned to another chromosome; usually reciprocal e.g. t(9;22)—the Philadelphia translocation.
- Inversion—part of chromosome runs in opposite direction e.g. inv(16) in M4Eo.
- Many translocations involve point mutations known as oncogenes, e.g. *BCR*, *ras*, *myc*, *bcl-2*.

Molecular cytogenetics

- Molecular revolution is further refining the specific abnormalities in the genesis of haematological malignancies.
- Techniques such as FISH (fluorescence *in situ* hybridisation) and PCR (polymerase chain reaction) can detect tiny amounts of abnormal genes.
- *BCR-ABL* probes are now used in diagnosis and monitoring of treatment response in CML.
- IgH and T-cell receptor (TCR) genes are useful in determining clonality of suspected B and T cell tumours respectively.
- Specific probes may be used in diagnosis and monitoring of subtypes of AML e.g. PML-RARA in AML M3.

Common karyotypic abnormalities

CML	
t(9;22)	Philadelphia chromosome translocation creates *BCR-ABL* chimeric gene.
AML	
t(8;21)	AML M2, involves *AML-ETO* genes—has better prognosis.
t(15;17)	AML M3 involves *PML-RARA* genes—has better prognosis.
inv(16)	AML M4Eo—has better prognosis.
–5, –7	Complex abnormalities have poor prognosis.
MDS	
–7, +8, +11	Poor prognosis.
5q– syndrome	Associated with refractory anaemia and better prognosis.
MPD	
20q– and +8	Common associations.
ALL	
t(9;22)	Philadelphia translocation, poor prognosis.
t(4;11)	Poor prognosis.
Hyperdiploidy	Increase in total chromosome number—good prognosis.
Hypodiploidy	Decrease in total chromosome number—bad prognosis.
T-ALL	
t(1;14)	Involves *tal-1* oncogene.
B-ALL and Burkitt's lymphoma	
t(8;14)	Involves *myc* and IgH genes, poor prognosis.
CLL	
+12, t(11;14)	
ATLL	
14q11	
NHL	
t(14;18)	Follicular lymphoma, involves *bcl-2* oncogene.
t(11;14)	Small cell lymphocytic lymphoma, involves *bcl-1* oncogene.
t(8;14)	Burkitt's lymphoma, involves *myc* and IgH genes.

HLA typing

HLA (human leucocyte antigen) system or MHC (major histocompatibility complex) is the name given to the highly polymorphic gene cluster region on chromosome 6 which codes for cell surface proteins involved in immune recognition.

The gene complex is subdivided into 2 regions

Class 1 The A, B and C loci.
These proteins are found on most nucleated cells and interact with CD8+ T lymphocytes.

Class 2 Comprising of DR, DP, DQ loci present only on B lymphocytes, monocytes, macrophages and activated T lymphocytes. Interact with CD4+ T lymphocytes.

- Class 1 and 2 genes are closely linked so one set of gene loci is usually inherited from each parent though there is a small amount of cross-over.
- There is ~1:4 chance of 2 siblings being HLA identical.
- There are other histocompatibility loci apart from the HLA system but these appear less important generally except during HLA matched stem cell transplantation when even differences in these minor systems may cause GvHD.

Typing methods

Class 1 and 2 antigens were originally defined by serological reactivity with maternal antisera containing pregnancy-induced HLA antibodies. Many problems with technique and too insensitive to detect many polymorphisms. Molecular techniques are increasingly employed such as SSP. Molecular characterisation is detecting vast Class 2 polymorphism.

Importance of HLA typing

- Matching donor/recipient pairs for renal, cardiac and marrow stem cell transplantation.
- Degree of matching more critical for stem cell than solid organ transplants.
- Sibling HLA matched stem cell transplantation is now treatment of choice for many malignancies.

- Unrelated donor stem cell transplants are increasingly performed but outcome is poorer due to HLA disparity. As molecular matching advances, improved accuracy will enable closer matches to be found and results should improve.

Functional tests of donor/recipient compatibility

- MLC (mixed lymphocyte culture)—now rarely used.
- CTLp (cytotoxic T lymphocyte precursor assays)—determine the frequency of cytotoxic T lymphocytes in the donor directed against the recipient—provides an assessment of GvHD occurring.

HLA related transfusion issues

- HLA on WBC and platelets may cause immunisation in recipients of blood and platelet transfusions.
- May cause refractoriness and/or febrile reactions to platelet transfusions.

- WBC depletion of products by filtration prevents this.
- Diagnosis of refractoriness confirmed by detection of HLA or platelet specific antibodies in patient's serum.
- Platelet transfusions matched to recipient HLA type may improve increments.

Blood transfusion

17

Using the blood transfusion laboratory

Requests for compatibility testing or blood grouping

Transfusion samples and forms must be clearly identified and clerical details match exactly. The form and sample should be signed by the person taking the sample as vouching for the identity of the potential recipient.

- 3 points of identification are required: patient's full name, date of birth, hospital number.
- Requests must be legible and clearly labelled with the name of the responsible clinician.
- Indication for transfusion should be specified.
- Indicate time for planned surgery.
- For major elective surgery where transfusion is usual with the procedure the laboratory should receive a G&S sample in advance (7 days)—allows identification of alloantibodies – the lab will arrange for appropriate blood units to be available.
- In genuine haemorrhagic emergencies ABO ± Rh (D) group compatible blood can be given *without* matching as the slight risk of this action far outweighs the immediate risk of death from exsanguination.
- Unmatched O Rh (D) –ve blood should *only* be used in extreme emergency when the patient's blood group is unknown or, if known, blood of the same ABO and Rh type is unavailable. Emergency grouping can be conducted in ~15 min; full laboratory compatibility testing can be completed in ≤1h. Can be ~20 min in emergencies (sending G&S sample to laboratory may save valuable time).

Hazards

- Most serious is ABO mismatch—almost invariably arises through clerical errors (at time of sampling) or when blood given to patient.
- The blood transfusion laboratory groups the blood sample received and assumes the sample has been correctly identified at the time of collection.

Issue and administration of blood and blood products

1. Units of blood are labelled as being matched for an individual patient.
2. Before administering the patient/recipient identity must be checked (see 3 point identity above).
3. Label details are rechecked by trained nursing staff at the bedside immediately prior to the transfusion *any discrepancies identified must be referred urgently to the blood bank and the clinician responsible for the patient – transfusion of that unit cannot proceed until any ambiguity about identity has been resolved.*
4. Unit of blood must be given within its expiry date.
5. Check for damage to the pack, discolouration of the contained red cells, or evidence of haemolysis.
6. Administration of the unit must commence <30 min after leaving the blood bank and be completed within 4h of commencing infusion.
7. Administration of blood products must be recorded in the case notes.
8. The unique number of given RBCs or blood products should be entered in the notes.
9. If given warm, ensure a safe approved warming procedure is used.

Blood transfusion

Maximum surgical blood ordering schedule (MSBOS)

A system of tailoring blood requirements to particular elective surgical procedures, including—importantly—procedures which do not usually require blood cover.

- The ABO group and Rh (D) type of the patient is determined on duplicate samples, and the serum screened for significant RBC ('atypical') antibodies. If there are no antibodies, the serum is kept available ('saved') for a determined period (usually a week)—this is the 'Group, Screen and Save' (G&S) procedure.
- If there are no atypical antibodies, and the planned surgery is likely to need peri-operative transfusion, the required number of red cell units are matched by routine tests, labelled and set aside in an accessible refrigerator. Storage conditions must meet certain standards (continuous recording of appropriate temperature, alarms, etc).
- If more blood is required than anticipated, extra units must be readily available. If the need is urgent, suitable arrangements—such as rapid matching (using the 'saved' serum) and despatch procedures—must enable the timely supply of blood.
- If there *are* atypical antibodies, which may occur in up to 10% patients, their specificity must be determined and, if clinically significant, sufficient (extra) red cell units *lacking* the relevant antigen provided and matched by detailed techniques. (These are often referred to as 'phenotyped red cells'.)
- If there is no 'MSBOS' more units must be matched than are usually required for transfusion, in order to give rapid access if extra blood is needed. Matched 'bespoke' blood is therefore unavailable for other patients for the 2–3 days set aside.
- A good MSBOS gives better access to blood stocks and enables more efficient use, in particular of O Rh(D) –ve blood. There is no good reason for regarding O Rh(D) –ve blood as a 'universal' donation type. It can be antigenic; and it is a precious resource, being available from <8% of the population.
- The surgical team must be confident in the system, and the blood bank staff committed to 'minimal barriers'. The cross-match : transfusion ratio of a blood bank may well become lower than 2 (i.e. overall <2 units matched for every unit transfused) which is an indication of efficient practices. It could even be nearer to 1 than to 2.
- MSBOS schedules will vary between hospitals—depending on demographic factors, general layout, access to the blood bank refrigerators, types of surgery etc.

Blood transfusion

Transfusion of red blood cells

Used acutely in the management of 'significant' blood loss following trauma or surgery or electively to manage anaemia *which is not correctable by other means*, e.g. correction of iron deficiency is by giving iron supplements, not by blood transfusion.

Indications for red cell transfusion	
Blood loss	Massive/acute
Bone marrow failure	Post-chemotherapy, leukaemias, etc. Supportive therapy with concentrated cells
Inherited RBC disorders	Homozygous β-thalassaemia Red cell aplasia, etc. Hb SS (some circumstances)
Acquired RBC disorders	Myelofibrosis Myelodysplasia Some chronic disorder anaemias Selected use in renal failure
Neonatal & exchange transfusions	Haemolytic disease of the newborn Meningococcal septicaemia Falciparum malaria

RBC transfusion is contraindicated in chronic iron deficiency anaemia; iron supplements will raise the haemoglobin in a safer and less costly manner. If patients are suffering marked anaemic symptoms then use of 2 units of concentrated cells will deal with this problem pending a response to iron. In severe megaloblastic anaemias RBCs should not be used; a rapid response to haematinics is expected. Transfusion can precipitate severe cardiac failure.

- Red cells have a shelf life of 35 days at 4°C and are supplied as concentrated red cells with PCV between 0.55 and 0.75. Most units in the UK are supplied in 'optimal additive solution', SAG-M*, which allows removal of all the plasma for preparation of other blood components and results in a less viscous product. The volume of a unit of concentrated cells is 280 ± 20mL. With adequate venous access it will flow easily through a standard blood giving set.
- In acute blood loss concentrated RBCs are adequate (whole blood not currently available in practice). Concentrated RBCs allow maintenance of oxygen delivery, and are often infused at the same time as other colloids.
- All blood in UK is leucodepleted at source.
- Irradiated RBCs are indicated to stop transfusion transmitted graft versus host disease e.g. following total body irradiation, bone marrow allografting or therapy with purine analogues (fludarabine, 2-CDA).
- Frozen RBCs similarly have plasma and some other constituents removed. They are expensive to process, store and handle; they must

be used within 24h after thawing. Clinical usage is restricted to patients with extremely rare blood groups or with highly problematic blood group alloantibodies.

In autoimmune haemolytic disorders transfusion can be lifesaving as a short term support pending a response to immunosuppression. As a general rule, most otherwise fit adult patients with chronic anaemia will tolerate Hb levels around 9.0–10.0g/dL without major problems. Transfusion therapy is more likely to be needed below this level

Transfusion procedure

Although fussy, strictly laid down hospital protocols must be followed for administration of blood and blood products. ***Errors carry the potential for major morbidity or fatality.***

1. Identity of label on each matched unit must match EXACTLY with the patient's identity.
2. The ABO and Rh groups on the blood pack and the compatibility report must correspond as must the donor number on the pack and compatibility form.
3. Units must show no sign of leakage or damage and be used within their expiry period.
4. The prescription of blood must be made by a registered medical practitioner and details of the product's administration must be recorded in the case record.
5. An IV line should be established and flushed with 0.9% saline solution ***before the pack is opened.***
6. No drug or other infusion solution should be added to any blood component.
7. Monitoring of the patient involves recording temperature, pulse and blood pressure before transfusion, every 15 min for the first hour and hourly until transfusion is finished.
8. Adverse events should be recorded meticulously.
9. Major reactions require immediate cessation of the transfusion and instigation of a full investigative protocol (see ***Emergencies: Transfusion reactions, p 502–504***).
10. Minor febrile reactions are not uncommon, their occurrence should be recorded, simple measures such as slowing the rate of infusion or administration of an antihistamine may deal with the problem; if not transfusion of the specific unit should be stopped.
11. An RBC pack should be given within 30 min of removal from the blood bank; the target infusion time for an individual unit should be ≤4h.

Platelet transfusion

May be given as prophylaxis against bleeding e.g. in patients undergoing intensive chemotherapy or to arrest overt haemorrhage e.g. in DIC. Platelets may be required to cover surgery and dentistry.

Indications for platelet transfusion	
↓ production due to BM failure/infiltration	Acute and chronic leukaemias Myelodysplasia Myeloproliferative disorders and myelofibrosis Marrow infiltration with other malignant tumours Post-chemotherapy or TBI Aplastic anaemia
↑ platelet destruction in peripheral circulation	Hypersplenism 2° splenic infiltration or portal hypertension Consumptive coagulopathies e.g. DIC Avoid in TTP (p530) Acute and chronic ITP (in emergencies only) Alloimmune thrombocytopenias e.g. PTP and perinatal thrombocytopenia (need to be HPA typed) Sepsis Drug induced
Platelet function abnormalities	Aspirin and NSAIDs Myelodysplasia Rare congenital disorders e.g. Bernard–Soulier
Dilutional	Massive blood transfusion—in practice not usually required unless some other haemostatic abnormality (e.g. consumption)
Cardiac bypass	Dilution and damage to platelets in extracorporeal circulation.

Indications for irradiated platelets

Recommended in immunosuppressed patients and haemopoietic stem cell transplant recipients to prevent transfusion-associated GvHD.

Indications for CMV negative platelets

1. Where CMV transmission may cause disease.
2. BM and PBSCT recipients who are CMV –ve.
3. Solid organ transplant recipients who are CMV –ve.
4. *In utero* and neonatal transfusion.
5. Aplastic anaemia.
6. GvHD.
7. Primary immunodeficiency syndromes.

Blood transfusion

Fresh frozen plasma (FFP)

FFP is prepared by removing plasma from a single donor unit by centrifugation within 8h of donation, snap frozen at –80°C and maintained deep frozen until use. Serological testing excludes HBV, HCV, HIV and the product is ABO and Rh (D) grouped. Group AB Rh (D) –ve FFP is suitable for all groups since it lacks anti-A and B, and will not sensitise Rh(D) –ve patients to Rh(D).

Factor	II	VII	IX	X
Range (u/dL)	53–121	41–140	32–102	61–150
Median	82.5	92.0	61.0	90.5

Indications for use

- Warfarin overdose—*see p522*.
- DIC (common causes include obstetric haemorrhage, postoperative complications, following trauma, severe infection, septicaemic shock, acute blood loss—*see p512*).
- Liver disease and biopsy.
- Massive blood transfusion—use of prophylactic FFP (1–2 units FFP/10 units of blood) and platelets is ***not supported by documented clinical benefit***. Give as dictated by coagulation tests.
- Isolated coagulation deficiencies where no specific concentrate is readily available.
- Treatment of thrombotic thrombocytopenia purpura/haemolytic uraemic syndrome (*see p468, 530*).
- Non-specific haemostatic failure in a bleeding patient e.g. following surgery, in intensive care with disturbed coagulation tests where no definite diagnosis is made.

Instructions for use

The average volume of 1 unit is 220–250mL.

Half-life of infused coagulation factors in FFP	
<12h	Factors V, VII, VIII, and protein C
>12 <24h	Factor IX and protein S
>24 <48h	Factor X
>48h	Fibrinogen, factors XI, XII, XIII, ATIII

- Defrost the bag in a waterbath (5 min) or at room temperature (20 min).
- Give as soon as possible and at least within the hour through a filter needle.
- Must be group compatible; if blood group not known, give 'all groups'.
- If recipient Rh (D) –ve ♀ of child bearing age given Rh (D) +ve plasma give anti-D (250u).
- Dose 10–15mL/kg body wt (usual starting dose in an adult = 2–4 units depending on the PT).

- Check PT and APTT before and 5 min after infusion to assess response.
- Note clinical response in bleeding patients; repeat as necessary, ***remember short half-life***.

Makris, M. *et al.* (1997) Emergency oral anticoagulant reversal: the relative efficacy of infusions of fresh frozen plasma and clotting factor concentrates on correction of coagulopathy. *Thrombosis Haemostasis*, **77** 477–80.

Cryoprecipitate

- Prepared by slow thawing of FFP at 4–6°C. Fresh plasma taken from a single donor is snap frozen then thawed at 4°C and a cryoprecipitate forms.
- Precipitate formed is cryoprecipitate which is then stored at –30°C.
- Rich in factors VIII, XIII, fibrinogen and von Willebrand factor.
  Per unit (bag):
  - Factor VIII and vWF ~80–100iu.
  - Fibrinogen ~250mg.
  - Factor XIII and fibronectin.
  - Does not contain other coagulation factors.
  - May contain anti-A and anti-B blood group antibodies.
- Formerly (but no longer) used for management of bleeding in factor VIII deficiency and von Willebrand's disease.
- Main clinical use for cryoprecipitate is as additional support for the clotting defects induced by massive transfusion and DIC.
- All donations are screened for HIV, HBV and HCV.

Indications for use

- Haemophilia A and vWD not treatment of choice where virally inactivated concentrates are available. May still have a role in acquired vWD when purified factor VIII products are ineffective.
- Hypo/dysfibrinogenaemia e.g. in DIC and liver disease/liver transplantation is used to treat and prevent bleeding.
- Of no proven value as empirical treatment in post-op or uraemic bleeding.

Instructions for use

- Keep frozen until required.
- Thaw at room temperature/37°C (takes 5–10 min); ***use immediately.***
- ABO compatibility not required.
- Give through filter needle.
- Dose depends on the indications for use and desired increment
  - Hypofibrinogenaemia: severe 2–4 bags/10kg body wt
    less severe 1–2 bags.
- Aim to keep fibrinogen >1g/L.
- Factor VIII minimum adult dose 5 bags.

Complications

Viral transmission—rare but reported. Reactions, fever, chills, allergic reactions.

Blood transfusion

Intravenous immunoglobulin

Used as antibody replacement in 1° and 2° antibody deficiency states, and as immune modulator.

Preparations of intravenous IgG (IVIg)

- Contain predominantly IgG (with small amounts of IgA and IgM).
- Prepared from large pool of normal donors e.g. >1000.
- Contain all subclasses of IgG encountered in normal population.

Uses	
Antibody replacement	
1° immune deficiency	2° immune deficiency
Transient hypogammaglobulinaemia of infancy	CLL
	Non-Hodgkin's lymphoma
Common variable immune deficiency	Multiple myeloma
Sex-linked hypogammaglobulinaemia	Post-BMT
Late-onset hypogammaglobulinaemia	
Hypogammaglobulinaemia + thymoma	
Immune modulation	
Autoimmune diseases	Antiviral activity
ITP	Prophylaxis/treatment of CMV in BMT patients
Autoimmune haemolytic anaemia	
Autoimmune neutropenia	B19-induced red cell aplasia
Red cell aplasia	Haemophagocytic syndromes (viral)
Coagulation factor inhibitors	
Post-transfusion purpura (PTP)	
Neonatal platelet alloimmunisation	
Thrombocytopenia in pregnancy	

Mechanisms of action

Not fully understood: natural anti-idiotypic antibodies suppress antibody production in patient; F_c receptor blockade on macrophages (thereby blocking RE function) and T/B lymphocytes (inhibits autoantibody production); suppression of production of inflammatory mediators (e.g. TNF-α, IL-1) produced by macrophages.

Administration

Usual dose 0.4g/kg/d × 5d (e.g. ITP, etc) or 0.2–0.4g/d × 1 day monthly (CLL, myeloma, etc). Check TPR and BP pre-infusion. With first infusion check TPR and BP ½ hourly for the first hour only. ***Side effects are more likely at the start of an infusion and in the first hour.*** (*See pack insert and BNF for details.*)

Complications

- Fevers, chills.
- Backache.
- Myalgic symptoms.
- Flushing.

- Nausea ± vomiting.
- Severe allergic reactions in IgA deficient patients (due to small amount of IgA in IVIg preparation).

Autologous blood transfusion

Allows patient to be transfused with his/her own red cells, avoiding (some) problems associated with transfusion of allogeneic (i.e. donor) blood, e.g. immunological incompatibility, risks of transmission of infection, and transfusion reactions. Useful for patients who wish not to receive allogeneic blood or who have irregular antibodies that make cross-matching difficult. Can be ***pre-deposit*** or ***intraoperative red cell salvage***.

Pre-deposit system

Involves collection of 2–4 units of blood: the first unit is collected ~2 weeks before the operation and the second is taken 7–10d prior to surgery. Iron replacement usually given. Some pre-deposit programmes use Epo (enables a larger number of units to be collected but *expensive*).

Advantages

- Can store RBCs up to 5 weeks at 4°C.
- May donate 2–4 units pre-op.
- Avoids many problems associated with allogeneic blood transfusion.

Disadvantages

- Generally requires Hb ≥11.0g/dL.
- Patients must be 'fit' for pre-donation programme (e.g. to donate 450mL 2–4 × pre-op) and live near transfusion centre.
- Requires close coordination between surgeon, patient and transfusion lab and fixed date for surgery.
- Little/no reduction in workload—blood must be treated in same way as regular donor units (including microbiological screening, grouping, compatibility testing, etc).
- Cost is high.
- Transfusion should be to donor *only*.
- Bacterial contamination of blood units may still occur.
- Patient may still require additional allogeneic units.
- Blood may be wasted if operation cancelled.
- Patients with epilepsy excluded (risk of seizures).

Intraoperative blood salvage

Allows blood lost during surgery to be reinfused into patients using suction catheters and filtration systems. Expensive and not widely used in the UK at present. Intraoperative blood salvage useful in cardiovascular surgery but may be used for almost any surgical procedure (provided no faecal contamination or risk of tumour dissemination).

1. Single use disposable canisters (e.g. Solcotrans™) where the patient is heparinised and anticoagulated blood is collected into ACD anticoagulant in the canister. Red cells reinfused after filtration through a microaggregate filter.
2. Automated or semi-automated salvage (e.g. Hemonetics Cell Saver™). Blood is collected, washed centrifugally, filtered and red cells held for reinfusion.

Other physical methods—pre-operative haemodilution

Involves reducing the Hb concentration prior to surgery. Reduces blood viscosity and red cell loss (through reduced haematocrit). Provides a bank of freshly collected autologous whole blood for return later.

- 2–3 units of blood are collected with replacement using crystalloids or colloid solutions.
- Hb is reduced to ~10 g/dL and haematocrit to 30% (0.3).
- O_2 transport improves (increased cardiac output).
- Used mainly in younger patients and in those with no pre-existing cardiopulmonary disease.

Pharmacological methods of blood saving

- Various drugs used to modify the coagulation and fibrinolytic systems, e.g. DDAVP.
- Platelet inhibitory drugs e.g. prostacyclin.
- Aprotinin widely used in cardiovascular surgery, liver transplantation and other surgical procedures.

Jehovah's Witnesses

- Religious sect numbering 120,000 in the UK.
- Pose ethical and management difficulties due to their refusal of blood transfusion, derived from a literal interpretation of a number of biblical passages (*Acts* 15:28–29).
- Jehovah's Witnesses still die during both elective and emergency surgery due to their beliefs.

Elective surgery—discuss

1. Risks of surgery and the specific risk of refusing blood.
2. Extent of religious belief (preferably alone to prevent any external pressure).
3. What blood derived products they personally are willing to accept e.g. albumin, FFP, platelets, etc?

If the surgeon agrees to an operation, communication then becomes paramount and the Jehovah's Witness should be referred to both an anaesthetist and haematologist—preferably when the patient is placed on the waiting list to allow time for any optimisation and for further counselling with their family.

Pre-operative considerations

- Timing (e.g. liver transplantation before clotting function deteriorates).
- Autologous blood transfusion—not permitted but may be acceptable to some.
- Morning list—to allow post-op observations during 'office hours'.
- Admission to ITU for invasive monitoring if required.
- Stop anticoagulants and NSAIDs.
- Optimise Hb—nutrition, B_{12}, folate, Fe, Epo.

Operative considerations

- ***Surgeon***
  Consultant
  Positioning of patient—to prevent venous congestion
  Tourniquets if possible
  Speed
  Meticulous haemostasis
- ***Anaesthetist***
  Consultant
  Regional blocks
  Hypotensive anaesthesia
  Hypothermia
  Isovolaemic haemodilution – permitted as long as blood remains linked to circulation
  Hypervolaemic haemodilution
  Intraoperative blood scavenging e.g. cellsavers
  Blood substitutes (fluorocarbons)
  Pharmacological methods to improve clotting e.g. DDAVP, tranexamic acid, aprotinin
- ***Post-operative considerations***
  Observation for re-bleed—HDU, senior surgeon review
  Optimise Hb—nutrition enteral or parenteral feeding, B_{12}, folate, Fe, erythropoietin
  Severe anaemia – IPPV to reduce oxygen demand
  Reduce phlebotomy and use paediatric vials
  Acid suppression to reduce GIT bleeding.

Emergency surgery

- Advanced directives.
- Early investigations CT, USS abdomen, pelvis.
- Low threshold to theatre.

Children

- Communication with parent.
- Judicial intervention if required.

Marsh, J.C. & Bevan, D.H. (2002) Haematological care of the Jehovah's Witness patient. *Br J Haematol*, **119**, 25–37.

Phone numbers and addresses 18

CancerBACUP

A major British cancer information and support charity; aims to provide clear, accurate, up-to-date information as well as sensitive and confidential support for patients and their families. Also provides assistance to health care professionals with specific enquiries relating to patients in their care.

CancerBACUP services for patient's and their families

- A national freephone cancer information service (tel 0808 800 1234), staffed by specialist oncology nurses.
- Cancer counselling service offering people the chance to talk through their concerns face to face (tel 0207 696 9003; fax 0207 696 9002)
- CancerBACUP produces excellent written information e.g. booklets on specific cancers, treatments and aspects of living with cancer and fact sheets on specific chemotherapy drugs, hormonal therapies, brain tumours and rare tumours. Available from CancerBACUP's administration (tel 0207 696 9003).

CancerBACUP services for health professionals

Medical Advisory Committee Statements produced by an expert panel on controversial or complex oncology issues including

- Clinical trials.
- Cancer screening—cervical, breast, prostate, colorectal and ovarian cancer.
- Breast cancer, the pill and hormone replacement therapy.
- Information on
  Support groups
  Sources of help
- Lists of booklets and factsheets.

Internet

CancerBACUP web site: www.cancerbacup.org.uk

Phone numbers and addresses

Leukaemia Research Fund (LRF)

The LRF is one of the major UK based research charities in the field of leukaemia and related conditions. It supports leukaemia research in major academic institutions; work supported ranges from basic science relating to the molecular genetics of leukaemogenesis to extensive case controlled studies into epidemiology of leukaemia and related disorders.

In addition to funding major research it provides information booklets on a range of (mainly) malignant blood disorders which are suitable for patients, their relatives and carers and also appropriate for non-specialist professional staff who become involved in specific aspects of the clinical care of the patient with leukaemia or a related disorder.

The stated aim of the fund is to improve treatments, find cures and prevent all forms of leukaemia and related cancers through a programme of nationally funded, high calibre research activities.

Booklets are available on the acute and chronic leukaemias, lymphomas including Hodgkin's disease, myeloma and related disorders, myelodysplasia myeloproliferative disorders and aplastic anaemia. A revised series of booklets was produced in 1997. Availability of such information on the wards or in the clinic is vary helpful to patients and their carers.

Address for the Leukaemia Research Fund
43 Great Ormond Street, London WC1N 3JJ
Telephone 0207 405 0101
e-mail: info@leukaemia.research.org.uk
www.leukres.demon.co.uk/lrfhome.htm

Phone numbers and addresses

NCRI Leukaemia Trials

Birmingham Clinical Trials Unit (BCTU)

For randomisation/entry of AML patients into MRC trials (AML14, AMLHR and AML15 trials).

Contacts:
BCTU
Park Grange
1 Somerset Road
Edgbaston
Birmingham B15 2RR

tel 0121 687 2310
fax 0121 687 2313
bctu@bham.ac.uk or H.Travers@bham.ac.uk
M.Nixon@bham.ac.uk or N.H.Hilken@bham.ac.uk
www.bctu.bham.ac.uk

CTSU

For randomisation into: CLL4, CLL5, PT1, UKALL XII and childhood ALL

CTSU
Harkness Building
Radcliffe Infirmary
Oxford OX2 6HE

tel 01865 240972
fax 01865 404849
Randomisation@ctsu.ox.ac.uk
www.ctsu.ox.ac.uk

Northern and Yorkshire Clinical Trials and Research Unit

For randomisation in: myeloma IX

NYCTRU
17 Springfield Mount
University of Leeds
Leeds
LS2 9NG

tel 0113 233 1476
fax 0113 343 1471
medseb@leeds.ac.uk
www.ukmf.org.uk

British Society for Haematology

BSH
100 White Lion Street
London N1 9PF

tel/fax 0207 713 0990
www.blackwellpublishing.com/uk/society/bsh/

Medical Research Council

20 Park Crescent
London W1N 4AL

tel 0207 636 5422

www.mrc.ac.uk

Haematology on-line

Haematology on-line

There are many Internet resources available for haematology, including organisations, journals, atlases, conference proceedings and newsgroups. The main difficulty with Internet resources is that they change so frequently and they are constantly being updated and outdated.

It would be impossible to list every known site, and we have provided only URLs for those we think are of most value.

General websites

Bloodline
www.bloodline.net

BloodMed
www.bloodmed.com

Hematologic Diseases (CliniWeb: Oregon Health Sciences University)
www.ohsu.edu/cliniweb/C15/C15.378.html

Hematology Case Studies (UC Davis School of Medicine)
medocs.ucdavis.edu/IMD/420A/course.htm

International Medical News
www.internationalmedicalnews.com

Medical Matrix
www.medmatrix.org/Index.asp

Meducation
www.meducation.com/

Medweb
www.medweb.emory.edu/medweb

MRC Molecular Haematology Unit
www.imm.ox.ac.uk/groups/mrc_molhaem

National Library of Medicine
www.nlm.nih.gov

Oncolink
www.oncolink.com

Oxford Haemophilia Centre
www.medicine.ox.ac.uk/ohc/

Oxford Regional Blood Club
www.btinternet.com/~phm/BloodClub.html

Sickle Hut
www.sicklehut.com

The Hematology Site
www.geocities.com/HotSprings/5340/

Atlases

Atlas of Hematology
www.medic.bgu.ac.il/mirrors/pathy/Pictures/atoras.html

Haematology on-line

Atlas of Hematology (Nagoya)
pathy.med.nagoya-u.ac.jp/atlas/doc/atlas.html

Cells of the blood (University of Leicester: Department of Microbiology and Immunology)
www-micro.msb.le.ac.uk/MBChB/bloodmap/Blood.html

Digital Image Study Sets (UC Davis School of Medicine)
medocs.ucdavis.edu/IMD/420A/dib

Hematology Image Atlas
www.hms.medweb.harvard.edu/HSHeme/AtlasTOC.htm

Introduction to Blood Morphology
www.hslib.washington.edu/courses/blood/intro.html

Journals and books

ASH Education Book
www.asheducationbook.org

Blood
www.bloodjournal.org/

Blood Cells, Molecules and Disease
www.scripps.edu/bcmd

British Journal of Haematology
www.blackwellpublishing.com/journals/bjh

British Medical Journal
bmj.bmjjournals.com

Cancer
caonline.amcancersoc.org

Haematologica
www.haematologica.it

Lancet
www.thelancet.com/

Nature
www.nature.com/

New England Journal of Medicine
content.nejm.org

Science
www.sciencemag.org

Societies and organisations

American Association of Blood Banks (AABB)
www.aabb.org

American Medical Association
www.ama-assn.org

American Society of Hematology
www.hematology.org/

Aplastic Anemia Foundation of America
www.medic.uth.tmc.edu/ptnt/00001045.htm

Bloodline
www.bloodline.net

British Blood Transfusion Society (BBTS)
www.bbts.org.uk

British Committee for Standards in Haematology
www.bcshguidelines.com

British Society for Haematology
www.b-s-h.org.uk

CancerBACUP
www.cancerbacup.org.uk/

European Bone Marrow Transplant Association
www.embt.org

Imperial Cancer Research Fund
www.cancerresearchuk.org

International Histiocytosis Organization (Histiocytosis Association of America)
www.histio.org

Leukemia Research Fund
dspace.dial.pipex.com/lrf-/

Leukemia Society of America
www.leukemia.org

Medical Research Council
www.mrc.ac.uk

National Blood Service
www.blood.co.uk

National Guidelines Clearinghouse
www.guidelines.gov

National Heart, Lung, and Blood Institute
www.nhlbi.nih.gov/

National Institutes of Health
www.nih.gov

NHS Centre for Reviews and Dissemination
www.york.ac.uk/inst/crd/

Royal College of Pathologists
www.rcpath.org

Royal College of Physicians
www.rcplondon.ac.uk

Royal Society of Medicine
www.roysocmed.ac.uk

Sickle Cell Information Centre Home
www.scinfo.org

Society for Hematopathology (Dartmouth College)
www.dartmouth.edu/~nlevy/wwwx.html

The Cochrane Library
www.update-software.com/cochrane/

UK NEQAS Schemes
www.ukneqas.org.uk

Wellcome Trust
www.wellcome.ac.uk/

World Federation of Hemophilia
www.wfh.org/

Guidelines and trials

cancerTrials (National Cancer Institute)
www.cancertrials.nci.nih.gov

Clinical practice guidelines: hematology (Canadian Medical Association)
www.cma.ca/cpgs/hema.htm

Clinical trials: hematology (CenterWatch)
www.centerwatch.com

Comprehensive Sickle Cell Center at Grady Health System
www.scinfo.org

National Guideline Clearinghouse (Agency for Health Care Policy and Research (AHCPR))
www.guidelines.gov

Charts and nomograms

20

Karnofsky performance status

Normal, no complaints; no evidence of disease	100%
Able to carry on normal activity; minor signs or symptoms of disease	90%
Normal activity with effort; some signs or symptoms of disease	80%
Cares for self; unable to carry on normal activity or to do active work	70%
Requires occasional assistance but is able to care for most of his/her needs	60%
Requires considerable assistance and frequent medical care	50%
Disabled; requires special care and assistance	40%
Severely disabled; hospitalisation is indicated although death not imminent	30%
Very sick; hospitalisation necessary	20%
Moribund; fatal processes progressing rapidly	10%
Dead	0%

WHO/ECOG performance status

0	Fully active; able to carry on all pre-disease performance without restriction.
1	Restricted in physically strenuous activity, but ambulatory and able to carry out work of a light or sedentary nature, e.g. light housework, office work.
2	Ambulatory and capable of all self-care but unable to carry out any work activities; up and about more than 50% of waking hours.
3	Capable of only limited self care, confined to bed or chair more than 50% of waking hours.
4	Completely disabled; cannot carry on any self care; totally confined to bed or chair.

Oken, M.M. *et al.* (1982) Toxicity and response criteria of the Eastern Cooperative Oncology Group *Am J Clin Oncol*, **5** 649.

Charts and nomograms

WHO haematological toxicity scale

Parameter	Grade 0	Grade 1	Grade 2	Grade 3	Grade 4
Haemoglobin (g/dL)	≥11.0	9.5–10.9	8.0–9.4	6.5–7.9	<6.5
Leucocytes ($\times 10^9$/L)	≥4.0	3.0–3.9	2.0–2.9	1.0–1.9	<1.0
Granulocytes ($\times 10^9$/L)	≥2.0	1.5–1.9	1.0–1.4	0.5–0.9	<0.5
Platelets ($\times 10^9$/L)	≥100	75–99	50–74	25–49	<25
Haemorrhage	none	petechiae	mild blood loss	gross blood loss	debilitating blood loss

Charts and nomograms

Body surface area nomogram

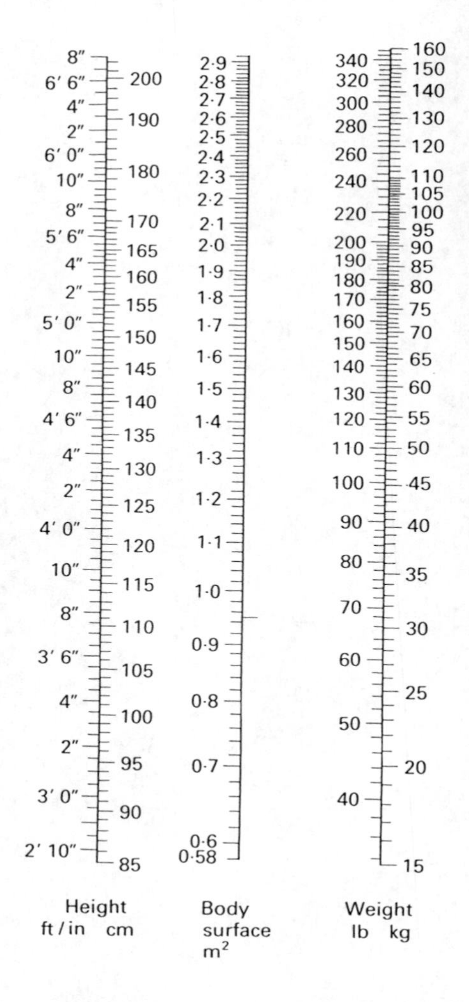

From Ramrakha, P. & Moore, K. (1997) *Oxford Handbook of Acute Medicine* (OUP), (with permission).

Charts and nomograms

Gentamicin dosage nomogram

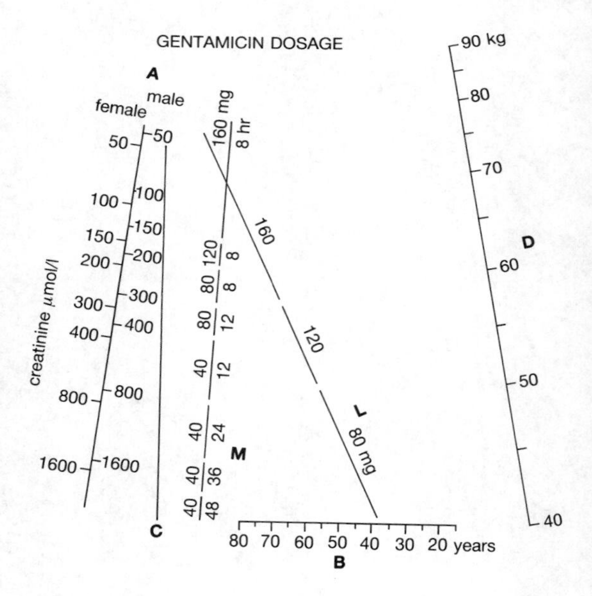

From Hope, R.A. *et al.* (1993) *Oxford Handbook of Clinical Medicine*, 3E (OUP) (with permission).

Charts and nomograms

The Sokal Score for CML prognostic groups	
Score	= Exp[0.0116 (age–43.4) + 0.0345 (spleen size–7.51) + 0.188 ([platelets/700]^2–0563) + 0.0887 (blasts–2.1)
Low risk	<0.8
Intermediate risk	= 0.8–1.2
High risk	>1.2

Normal ranges

Normal ranges (adults)

Haematology

Haemoglobin	13.0–18.0g/dL	(♂)
	11.5–16.5g/dL	(♀)
Haematocrit	0.40–0.52	(♂)
	0.36–0.47	(♀)
RCC	4.5–6.5 × 10^{12}/L	(♂)
	3.8–5.8 × 10^{12}/L	(♀)
MCV	77–95 fL	
MCH	27.0–32.0pg	
MCHC	32.0–36.0g/dL	
WBC	4.0–11.0 × 10^9/L	
Neutrophils	2.0–7.5 × 10^9/L	
Lymphocytes	1.5–4.5 × 10^9/L	
Eosinophils	0.04–0.4 × 10^9/L	
Basophils	0.0–0.1 × 10^9/L	
Monocytes	0.2–0.8 × 10^9/L	
Platelets	150–400 × 10^9/L	
Reticulocytes	0.5–2.5% (or 50–100 × 10^9/L)	
ESR	2–12 mm/1st hour (Westergren)	
Red cell mass	25–35mL/kg	(♂)
	20–30mL/kg	(♀)
Serum B_{12}	150–700ng/L	
Serum folate	2.0–11.0µg/L	
Red cell folate	150–700µg/L	
Serum ferritin	15–300µg/L (varies with sex and age)	
	14–200µg/L (premenopausal female)	
INR	0.8–1.2	
PT	12.0–14.0s	
APTT ratio	0.8–1.2	
APTT	26.0–33.5s	
Fibrinogen	2.0–4.0g/L	
Thrombin time	± 3s of control	
XDPs	<250µg/L	
D-dimer	<500ng/mL	
Factors II, V, VII, VIII, IX, X, XI, XII	50–150iu/dL	
RiCoF	45–150iu/dL	
vWF: Ag	50–150iu/dL	
Protein C	80–135u/dL	
Protein S	80–135u/dL	
Antithrombin III	80–120u/dL	
APCR	2.12–4.0	
Bleeding time	3–9min	

Normal ranges

Biochemistry and immunology

Serum urea	3.0–6.5mmol/L
	11.5–16.5g/dL
Serum creatinine	60–125μmol/L
Serum sodium	135–145mmol/L
Serum potassium	3.5–5.0mmol/v
Serum albumin	32–50g/L
Serum bilirubin	<17μmol/L
Serum alk phos	100–300iu/L
Serum calcium	2.15–2.55mmol/L
Serum LDH	200–450iu/L
Serum phosphate	0.7–1.5mmol/L
Serum total protein	63–80g/L
Serum urate	0.18–0.42mmol/L
Serum γ-GT	10–46iu/l
Serum iron	14–33μmol/L (♂)
	11–28μmol/L (♀)
Serum TIBC	45–75μmol/L
Serum ALT	5–42iu/L
Serum AST	5–42iu/L
Serum free T4	9–24pmol/L
Serum TSH	0.35–5.5mU/L
Immunology	
IgG	5.3–16.5g/L
IgA	0.8–4.0g/L
IgM	0.5–2.0g/L
Complement	
C3	0.89–2.09g/L
C4	0.12–0.53g/L
C1 esterase	0.11–0.36g/L
CH_{50}	80–120%
C-reactive protein	<6mg/L
Serum β_2-microglobulin	1.2–2.4mg/L
CSF proteins	
IgG	0.013–0.035g/l
Albumin	0.170–0.238g/L
Urine proteins	
Total protein	<150mg/24h
Albumin (24h)	<20mg/24h

Paediatric normal ranges

Full blood count

Age	Hb (g/dL)	MCV (fL)	Neuts	Lymph	Platelets
Birth	14.9–23.7	100–125	2.7–14.4	2–7.3	150–450
2 weeks	13.4–19.8	88–110	1.5–5.4	2.8–9.1	170–500
2 months	9.4–13.0	84–98	0.7–4.8	3.3–10.3	210–650
6 months	10.0–13.0	73–84	1–6	3.3–11.5	210–560
1 year	10.1–13.0	70–82	1–8	3.4–10.5	200–550
2–6 years	11.5–13.8	72–87	1.5–8.5	1.8–8.4	210–490
6–12 years	11.1–14.7	76–90	1.5–8	1.5–5	170–450
Adult ♂	12.1–16.6	77–92	1.5–6	1.5–4.5	180–430
Adult ♀	12.1–15.1	77–94	1.5–6	1.5–4.5	180–430

Neuts, neutrophils; lymph, lymphocytes and platelets (all × 10^9/L)

Haemostasis

Parameter	Neonate	Adult level
Platelet count	150–400 × 10^9/L	as adult
Prothrombin time	few sec longer than adult	up to 1 week
APTT	up to 25% increase	by 2–9 months
Thrombin time		as adult
Bleeding time	2–10 min	as adult
Fibrinogen	2.0–4.0g/L	as adult
Vit K factors		
Factor II	30–50% adult level	up to 6 months
Factor VII	30–50% adult level	by 1 month
Factor IX	20–50% adult level	up to 6 months
Factor X	30–50% adult level	up to 6 months
Factor V		as adult
Factor VIII	Variable: 50–200% adult level	
vW factor	usually raised (up to 3 × adult level)	
Factor XI	20–50% adult level	6–12 months
Factor XII	20–50% adult level	3–6 months
Factor XIII	50–100% adult level	1 month
FDP/XDP	up to twice adult level	by 7 days
AT	50–80% adult level	6–12 months
Protein C	30–50% adult level	up to 24 months
Protein S	30–50% adult level	3–6 months
Plasminogen	30–80% adult level	2 weeks

Normal ranges

Index